COLOR ATLAS
OF HISTOLOGY

COLOR ATLAS OF HISTOLOGY

STANLEY L. ERLANDSEN, PhD

Professor of Anatomy
Department of Cell Biology and Neuroanatomy
University of Minnesota School of Medicine
Minneapolis, Minnesota

JEAN E. MAGNEY, MS

Assistant Professor
Department of Cell Biology and Neuroanatomy
University of Minnesota School of Medicine
Minneapolis, Minnesota

With 561 *illustrations,* 328 *in color*

Mosby
Year Book

St. Louis Baltimore Boston Chicago London Philadelphia Sydney Toronto

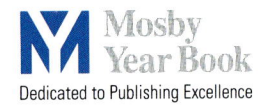

Mosby Year Book
Dedicated to Publishing Excellence

Editor: Kimberly Kist
Assistant Editor: Penny Rudolph
Project Manager: Peggy Fagen
Production Editor: Kathleen L. Teal
Design: Gail Morey Hudson

Copyright © 1992 by Mosby–Year Book, Inc.

A Mosby imprint of Mosby–Year Book, Inc.

All rights reserved. No part of this publication may be reproduced, stored in a retrieval system, or transmitted, in any form or by any means, electronic, mechanical, photocopying, recording, or otherwise, without prior written permission from the publisher.
Printed in the United States of America.

Permission to photocopy or reproduce solely for internal or personal use is permitted for libraries or other users registered with the Copyright Clearance Center, provided that the base fee of $4.00 per chapter plus $.10 per page is paid directly to the Copyright Clearance Center, 27 Congress Street, Salem, MA 01970. This consent does not extend to other kinds of copying, such as copying for general distribution, for advertising or promotional purposes, for creating new collected works, or for resale.

Printed in the United States of America

Mosby–Year Book, Inc.
11830 Westline Industrial Drive, St Louis, Mo 63146

ISBN 0-8016-1560-7

92 93 94 95 96 GW/CX/VH 9 8 7 6 5 4 3 2 1

This atlas is dedicated to the memory of

DR. DAVID G. CHASE

an indefatigable explorer of the microscopic world
who thrilled at the quest of the unknown,
and whose enthusiasm and wit
enriched the lives of all
who knew him.

PREFACE

IF A STUDENT is curious about the wondrous structure he or she inhabits, the study of histology can be fascinating. To make it exciting, we have included state of the art images from the work of scientists world-wide that elucidate not only structure but functions of cells and tissues. We have combined their pictures, which encompass a wide variety of imaging modalities and techniques (transmission and scanning electron micrographs, immunocytochemistry, histochemistry, confocal and dark field microscopy) with our own work and our teaching library of light micrographs to create an atlas that we think will help students integrate cellular structure with both the functions and biochemical properties of cells.

Current technologies used to create the images in this atlas are also used for laboratory investigation and clinical diagnosis. Introducing students, through this book, to the use of a multimedia approach to histology should help them develop better interpretive skills, inspire independent, original thinking about problem solving with microscopic material, and establish continuity between early class work and eventual professional practice.

The book is soft covered and spiral bound, making it suitable for use in the laboratory. The progression of information from cell to tissue to organ is arranged in chapters, each of which begins with a brief introduction or overview of the material contained therein. Within chapters, images are collected into "mini-lectures," groups of micrographs concerned with a single structure that examine it in different ways. Groupings are arranged on facing pages, which allows the student to compare and contrast structure and function. Legends are, for the most part, concise, and directly adjacent to the image being described for easy access. For pictures that are borrowed, the reader is referred to a list of contributors at the end of the text.

Stanley L. Erlandsen
Jean E. Magney

ACKNOWLEDGMENTS

THIS ATLAS WAS made possible by the generous contributions of numerous investigators who allowed us to incorporate their work. We are indebted to them for the extraordinary insight into structure and function provided by their images:

Adolph Ackerman; Jean Babel, A. Bischoff, and H. Spoendlin; Marianne Bachofen; P. Bagavandoss; Dorothy Bainton; Luciano Barajas; R.M. Bearman; Richard Blandau; Daniel Bodley; Daniel Branton; Ruth Bulger; Steven J. Burden; Kenneth Campbell; J.C. Cawley and F.G. Hayhoe; Marco Celio; David Chase; L.T. Chen; A. Kent Christensen; M. Costa J.B. Furness, A.C. Cuello, A.A.J. Verhofstad, H.W.J. Steinbusch, and R.P. Elde; Gwen Crabbe; Michael J. Cullen; Ernest Cutz; T. Daems and P. Brederoo; Ellen Roter Dirksen; Martin Dym; Tatsuo Ebe and S. Kobayashi; Richard Ellis; H.D. Fahimi; Marilyn Farquhar; Donald Fawcett; Frederic S. Fay; Alex Ferenczy; M.S. Forbes; Hisao Fujita; Tsunio Fujita; Giorgio Gabella; J.R. Garrett; Glenn Giesler; Norton B. Gilula; Gary Gorbsky; Peter Gould; A.D. Hally and Sybil M. Lloyd; Arthur R. Hand; Gretchen and Vincent Hascall; Orion Hegre and Robert Sorenson; Damon C. Herbert; John Heuser; Nobutaka Hirokawa; Tomas Hokfelt and Marianne Schultzberg; Karen Holbrook; A.F. Holstein; Ann L. Hubbard; E.B. Hunziker; Wei S. Hwang; Y. Ikeuchi; and T. Kanaseki; Susumu Ito; Ross Johnson; Albert Jones and E. Spring-Mills; Douglas Kelly; Shigeru Kobayashi; Charles Kuhn III; Lars-Inge Larsson; C.P. Leblond; I. Joel Leeb; Lee Leek; Paul Letourneau; G.D. Levine; John A. Long; Jeanette Lopez-Lewellyn; Mark Ludvigson; Adolfo Martinez-Palomo; Arvid B. Maunsbach; Jerry Maynard; Lawrence P. McCallister and Robert Hadek; Rosemary Mazanet and Clara Franzini-Armstrong; Masayuki Miyoshi; Pietro Motta; Marian Neutra; Lennart Nilsson; Phyllis Novikoff; Gary Olson; Lelio Orci; Lydia Osvaldo; Robert L. Owen; Sanford Palay and Victoria Chan-Palay; Janet Parkin; Laurie G. Paavola; David Phillips; Keith Porter; Giuliano Quintarelli; Elio Raviola; Robert S. Redman; J.-P. Revel, M. Rabinovitch, and M.J. DeStefano; Walter Rubin; Robert Schenk; Judith Schollmeyer; Melvin Schwartz; James O. Shaw; Judson Sheridan; Nicolae and Maia Simonescu; Christine and David Skerrow; David Smith; Sergei P. Sorokin; Franco Spinelli; Judith St. George; George and Charles Ploppet; Judy Strum; D. Szabo; Keiichi Tanaka; Bernard Tandler; Myron Tannenbaum; Jona C. Thaemert; Koji Uchizono; Jonathan Van Blerkom; J.H. Venable; S. Viragh; R. Vitale; Melvyn Weinstock; Leon Weiss; Carol Wells; Mark Willingham; Odile Grynszpan-Winograd; Richard Wood; Marie Yamada; D. Zucker-Franklin; and Barbara Zweber.

We also wish to thank Dr. Anna Mary Carpenter, who developed the histology slide collection at the University of Minnesota that was used as a source for most of the light micrographs in this atlas, and Dr. David W. Hamilton, Head of the Department of Cell Biology and Neuroanatomy, who so generously and enthusiastically supported the microfiche atlas upon which this volume is based. Others helped in the production of visual materials: Cathy Sulik organized and maintained the histology slide collection, Chris Frethem assisted in electron microscopy and photographic reproduction, Walter Gutzmer and Jerry Sedgewick provided photographic assistance, and Jackie Shipka, secretarial services.

At Mosby–Year Book, Kim Kist, Penny Rudolph, Peggy Fagen, and Kathy Teal were at all times patient and helpful to us, and we are very appreciative of their contributions.

Finally, we want to acknowledge many classes of medical students at Minnesota who enthusiastically used the Histology Microfiche Atlas and made many constructive comments during its development.

CONTENTS

1 Cell, 1
2 Epithelium, 12
3 Connective Tissue, 21
4 Cartilage, 29
5 Bone, 32
6 Peripheral Blood, 38
7 Bone Marrow, 42
8 Muscle, 50
9 Nerve, 59
10 Cardiovascular System, 67
11 Lymphoid System, 77
12 Exocrine Glands, 89
13 Endocrine Glands, 95
14 Skin, 104
15 Gastrointestinal Tract, 109
16 Liver, 124
17 Respiratory Tract, 130
18 Urinary Tract, 138
19 Male Reproductive Tract, 149
20 Female Reproductive Tract, 161

CHAPTER 1

CELL

CELLS COMPOSE THE four basic tissues of the body: **epithelium, connective tissue, muscle,** and **nerve.** Common to all mature cells, or cells at some time in their development, are **nuclei** and **cytoplasm** containing membranous compartments and cytoskeletal components. Cells vary considerably in size, shape, type, and distribution of organelles and, consequently, function. Despite these differences, by understanding the role of each organelle one can deduce general structural/functional correlates that lead to a clearer understanding of how cells work.

To obtain a better concept of the function of cells and their organelles, it is helpful to examine cells by a variety of methods. **Light microscopy** (LM) can be used with routine histologic stains **(hematoxylin and eosin; H&E)** to obtain information on the biochemical function and distribution of cellular components. The **basophilic** staining of nuclei by hematoxylin provides information on the distribution of inactive heterochromatin and the number of nucleoli, while cytoplasmic basophilia may reflect the presence of free or bound ribosomes (rough endoplasmic reticulum, RER) associated with protein synthesis or, in some other instances, the synthesis of sulfated mucosubstance destined for secretion. The intensity of cytoplasmic staining with eosin **(acidophilia)** generally reflects the relative abundance of cationic proteins. Mitochondria contain cationic proteins, such as cytochromes, which leads to intense cytoplasmic eosinophilia in cells involved in ion transport since they use abundant mitochondria to produce energy (ATP) to drive membrane pumps. **Transmission electron microscopy** (TEM) permits examination of the ultrastructure of organelles and cells, but interpretation of the fine structure, particularly in three dimensions, is hampered by the use of ultrathin sections needed for penetration of the sample by the electron beam. Visualization of the three-dimensional appearance of the surfaces of organelles, cells, and tissues can be better accomplished by using **scanning electron microscopy** (SEM); however, this method by itself does not necessarily provide information on the internal fine structure of cells. The **freeze-fracture** (FF) technique supplies information on the structure of membranes, particularly the distribution of intramembranous proteins related to the formation of cell junctions, but yields little information on the general structure of cells. Despite the limitations of each of the methods just described, when used collectively they enable us to obtain a comprehensive view of the structure and function of organelles and cells.

A typical cell will include the **nucleus, free ribosomes, polyribosomes,** and a variety of membranous organelles including **rough endoplasmic reticulum** (RER), **smooth endoplasmic reticulum** (SER), **Golgi apparatus, mitochondria, peroxisomes,** and components of the **lysosomal system. Cytoskeletal** organelles present within the cell include free **microtubules** and microtubular arrays including centrioles, basal bodies, flagella, and cilia; contractile proteins such as **actin** and **myosin;** and structural proteins comprising the **intermediate filaments** (desmin, glial fibrillary acidic protein, keratin, neurofilaments, nuclear lamins, and vimentin). Nonorganelle components that may be present within the cytoplasm of cells are **glycogen, lipid inclusions,** and **pigment.**

2   COLOR ATLAS OF HISTOLOGY

Composite Cell

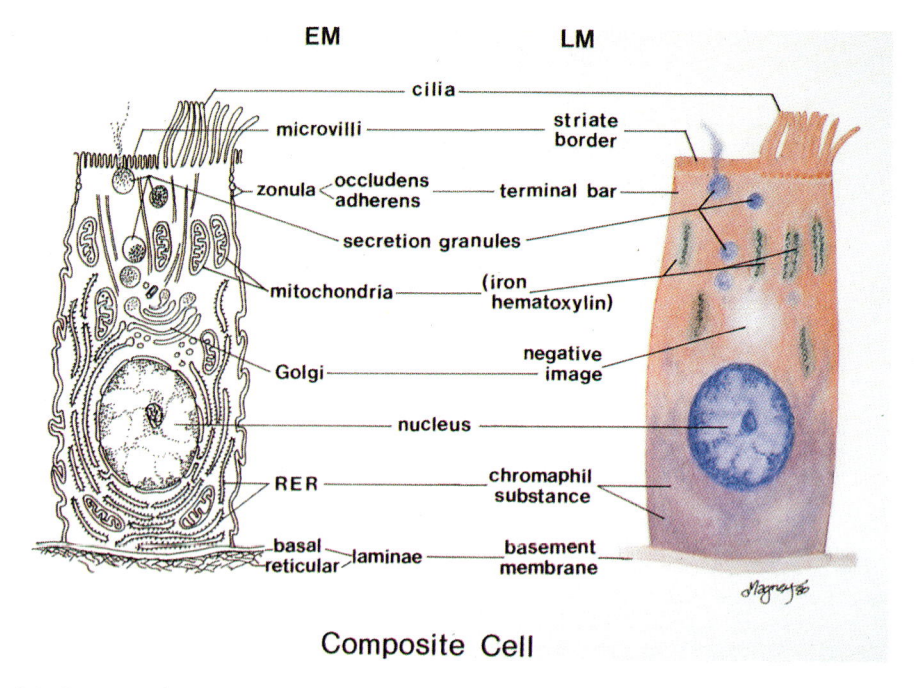

Fig. 1-1. Drawing of a composite, polarized epithelial cell comparing ultrastructural components as viewed by transmission electron microscopy (TEM) and light microscopy (LM). Mitochondria can be visualized at the LM level by the use of special stains, in this case, iron hematoxylin.

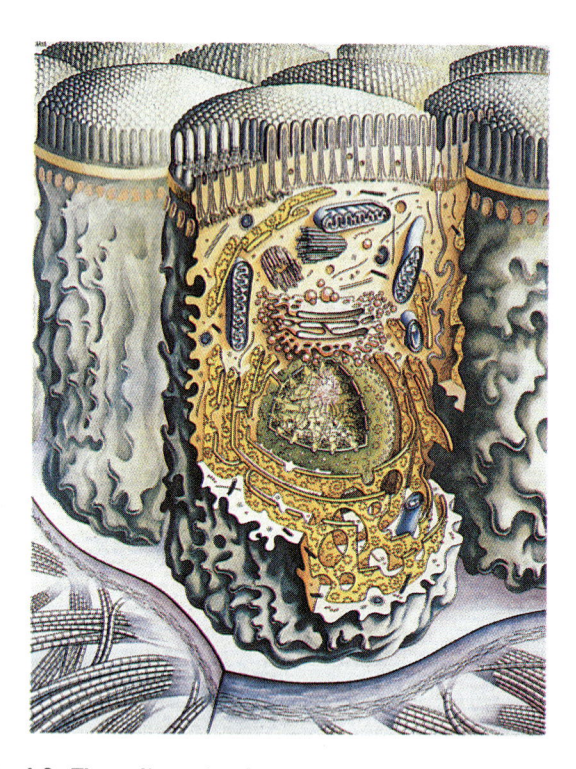

Fig. 1-2. Three-dimensional representation of simple columnar cells showing organelles, microvillous border (also known as brush or striate border), and basement membrane. The lateral borders of cells interdigitate, and junctional complexes at the apical borders connect them into a tissue called epithelium, which serves as a permeability barrier between body fluids and the external environment. Beneath the basement membrane is a connective tissue compartment containing collagen fibers and amorphous ground substance.

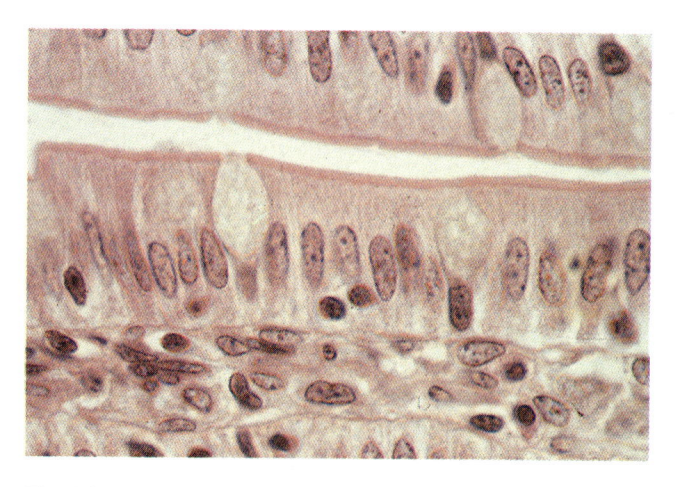

Fig. 1-3. Intestinal epithelium of simple columnar cells as seen by LM. Visible in the epithelium are mucus-secreting goblet cells, lymphocytes between the lateral borders of columnar cells, a microvillous border adjacent to the lumen, and the basement membrane subtended by connective tissue called the lamina propria. (H&E; ×1,600.)

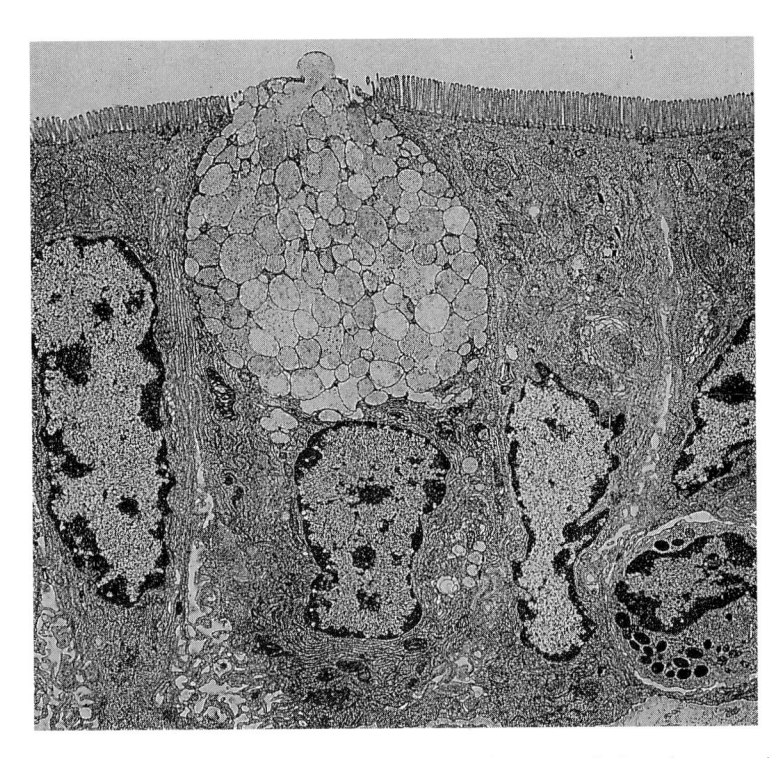

Fig. 1-4. Intestinal epithelium with a goblet cell seen by transmission electron micrograph (TEM). Compare with Figs. 1-2 and 1-3. Identify in the epithelium the mucus cell containing secretion granules, a microvillous border, nuclei, mitochondria, lateral cell borders, Golgi regions, and basement membrane. A wandering granulocyte (white blood cell) is seen between the epithelial cells at lower right. (×4,000.)

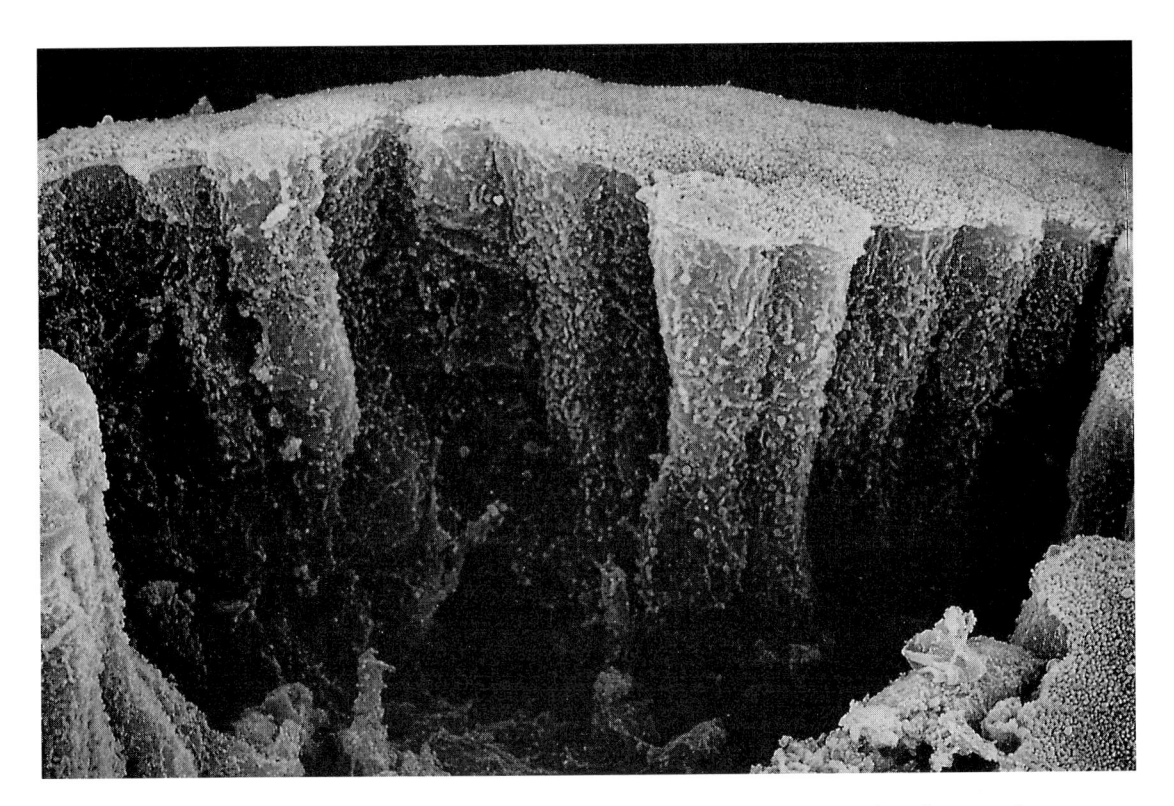

Fig. 1-5. Simple columnar epithelial cells of the gallbladder seen by scanning electron micrograph (SEM). Note that evaginations of lateral cell surfaces interdigitate with the membranes of adjacent cells. See Fig. 1-4 for the appearance of these membrane projections by TEM. (×2,400.)

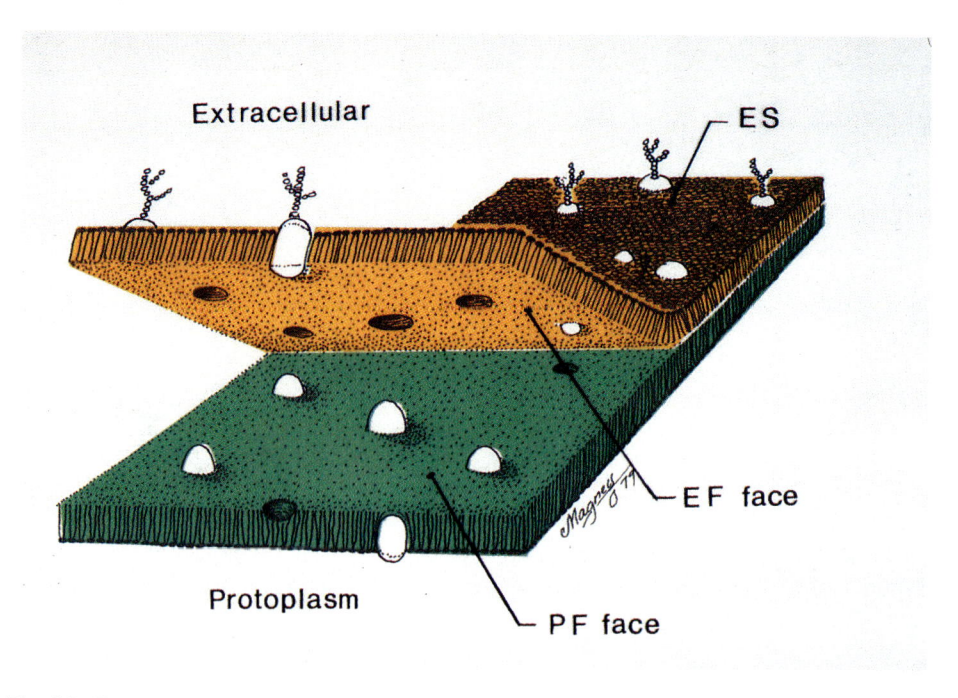

Fig. 1-6. Drawing of a cell membrane (plasmalemma) that has been freeze-fractured (FF). Note that the fracture plane passes through the lipid bilayer and that intramembranous particles tend to remain with the protoplasmic face (PF face). The extracellular face (EF face) is generally characterized by pits or depressions that remain when intramembranous particles pull free as a result of the fracture. *ES*, Extracellular surface.

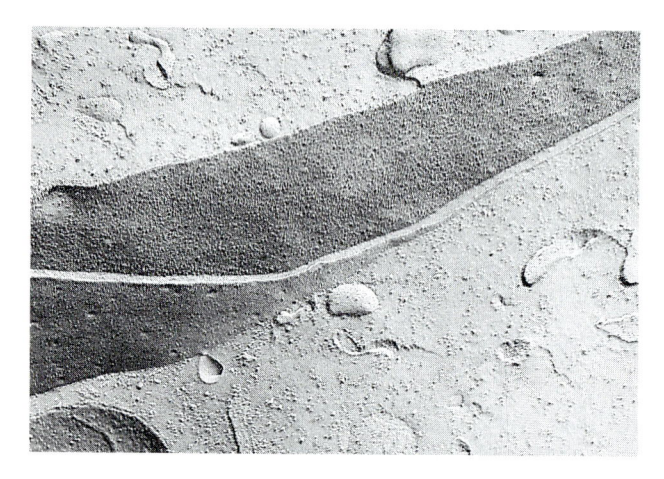

Fig. 1-7. Freeze fracture of two adjacent cells. The extracellular space passes diagonally from middle left to upper right, separating the particle-rich PF face of the top cell from the particle-poor EF face of the bottom cell at lower left. At mid-right, note the approximation of both leaflets (EF and PF) of the lower cell plasmalemma, as seen in cross-fracture. (×70,000.)

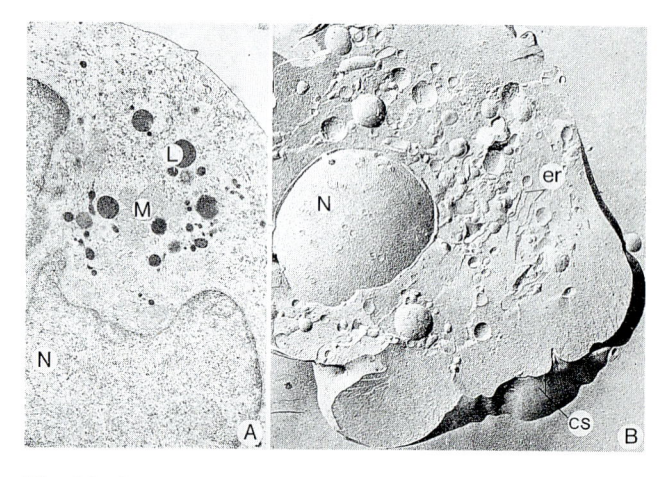

Fig. 1-8. Comparison of TEM and FF on the same cell type. **A,** TEM of a cell shows nucleus *(N)*, mitochondria *(M)*, lysosomes *(L)*, and cell surface (plasmalemma). (×17,000.) **B,** FF of a cell with nucleus *(N)* and nuclear pores, lysosomes, endoplasmic reticulum *(er)*, and the protoplasmic face of the cell plasmalemma *(CC)*. (×3,000.)

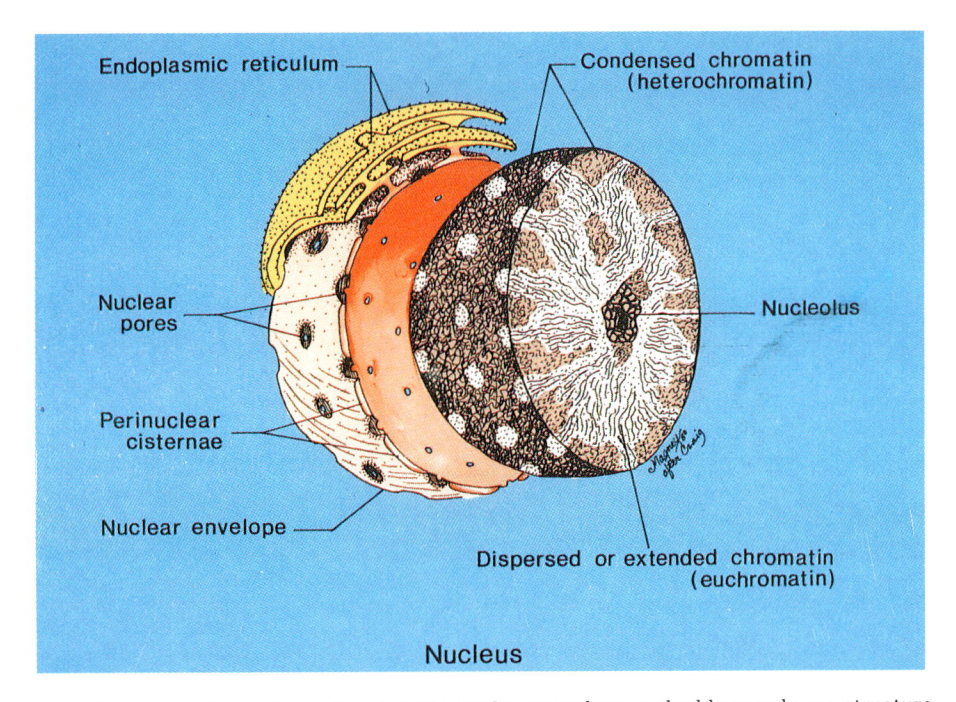

Fig. 1-9. Diagram of a nucleus showing the nuclear envelope, a double membrane structure with pores through which small molecules may pass between the cytoplasm and the nucleus. Cisternae of the endoplasmic reticulum may be directly connected to the nuclear envelope. Heterochromatin (inactive) is associated with the nuclear membrane, while euchromatin is actively involved with formation of RNA.

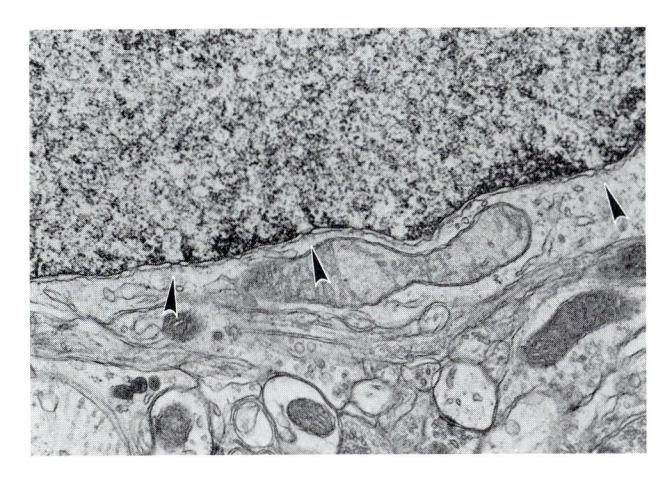

Fig. 1-10. TEM of a cell revealing diaphragm-covered pores *(arrowheads)* in the nuclear envelope. Note the difference between euchromatin and heterochromatin. (×29,000.)

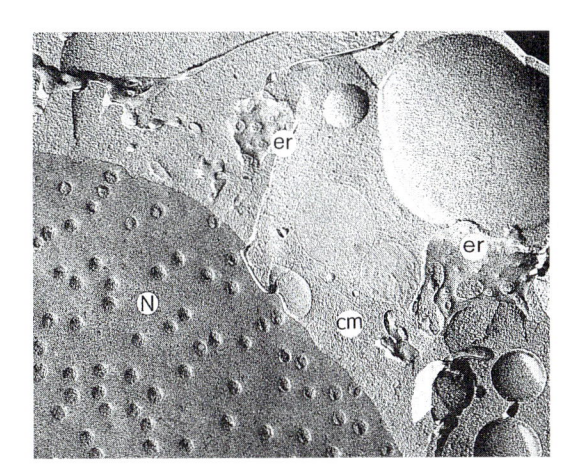

Fig. 1-11. Freeze fracture revealing pores in an otherwise smooth nuclear envelope. Surrounding the nucleus are the cytoplasmic matrix *(cm)* and elements of endoplasmic reticulum *(er)*. Direction of the platinum shadowing is from upper right in this FF. (×32,900.)

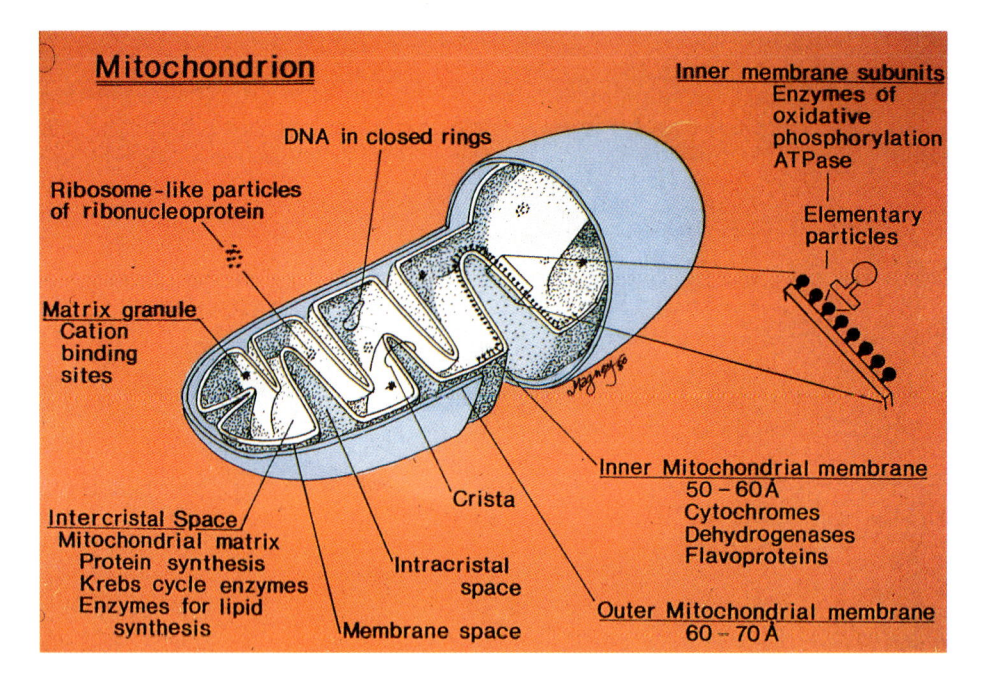

Fig. 1-12. Diagram of a mitochondrion illustrating the ultrastructural relationships of the two membranous compartments, the presence of cristae extending into the matrix, cation binding granules in the matrix, and the distribution of biochemical components such as DNA, ribosomes, and various respiratory enzymes.

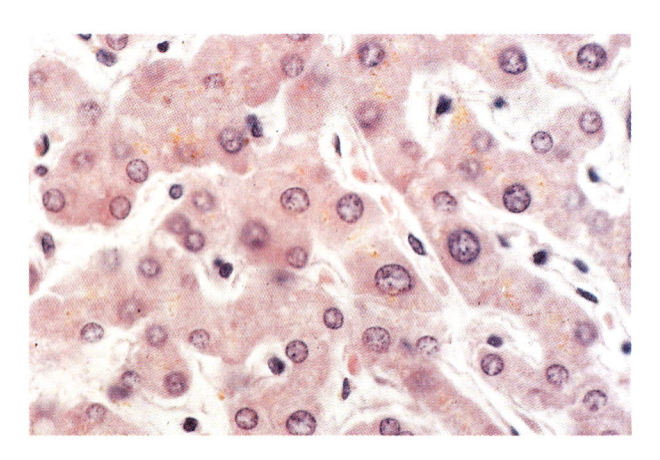

Fig. 1-13. LM of the liver. Note the large, vesicular nuclei of the liver cells, as well as the dark, more condensed nuclei of cells lining (or within) the vascular channels that separate rows of liver cells. This stain does not reveal the numerous mitochondria present within these cells. Compare this image with that in Fig. 1-16. (H&E; ×450.)

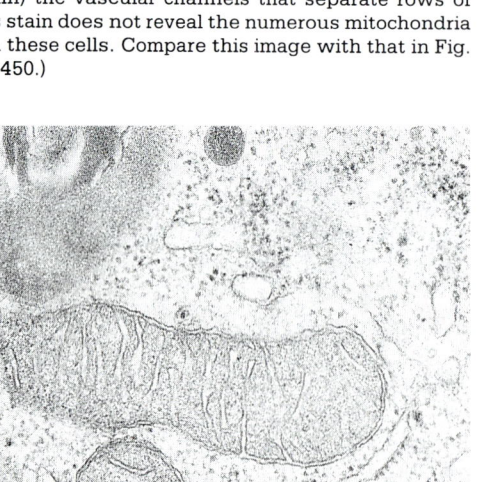

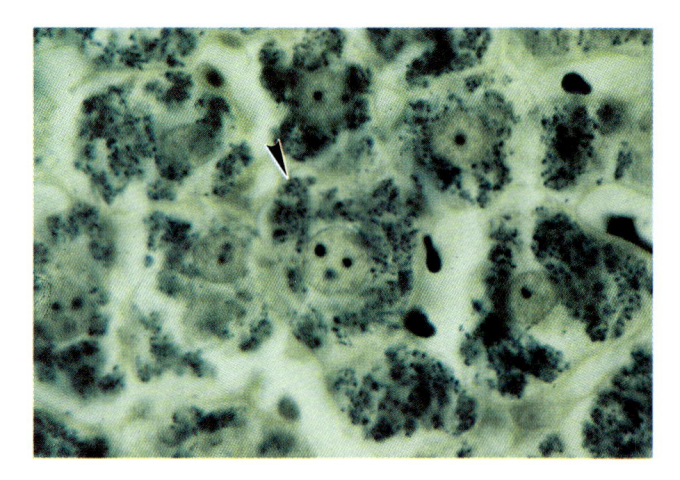

Fig. 1-14. LM of liver that has been stained with iron hematoxylin to demonstrate mitochondria *(arrowhead)* within the cytoplasm. The amorphous shapes in the vascular channels between liver cells are heavily stained red blood cells. (Iron hematoxylin; ×750.)

Fig. 1-15. TEM of intestinal epithelial cell cytoplasm showing several mitochondria adjacent to cisternae of RER and a lysosome. Compare the morphology of the tubular cristae and the matrix in the mitochondrion to the diagram shown in Fig. 1-12. (×34,000.)

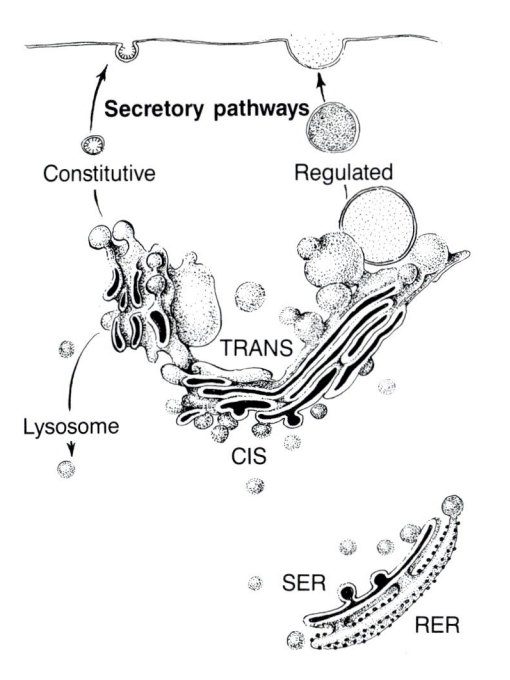

Post-Golgi
condensation
proteolysis

Golgi
glycosylation
CHO hydrolysis
phosphorylation
sulfation
proteolysis
sorting of proteins

Endoplasmic Reticulum
translation
signal proteolysis
protein segregation
primary glycosylation

Fig. 1-16. Schematic drawing of the Golgi apparatus depicting the relationships between the synthesis of proteins in the rough endoplasmic reticulum (RER) and the functional compartments traversed until these secretory proteins are released by exocytosis. The constitutive pathway is nonregulated and consists of dilute packing of proteins that are continuously discharged from the cell. The regulated pathway utilizes storage of product in secretion granules that are released on stimulation by secretogogues.

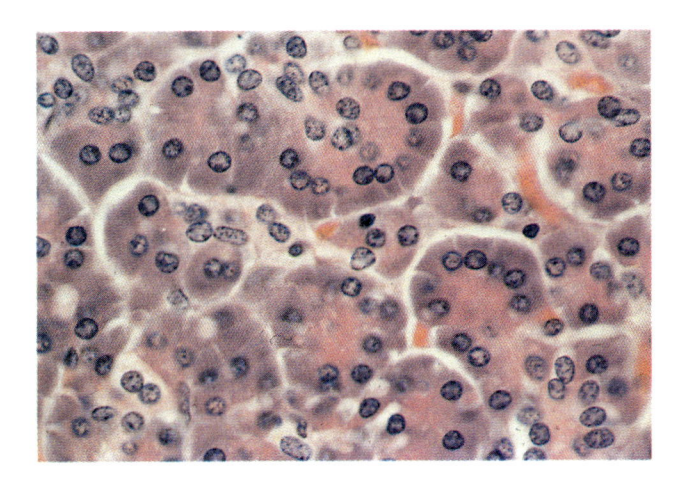

Fig. 1-17. High-magnification LM revealing the structure of the pancreatic acinus. Nuclei are located near the base of the cells; the Golgi apparatus lies in a supranuclear position but is not visible with this stain. Compare this image with Fig. 1-18, which is also pancreas. (H&E; ×350.)

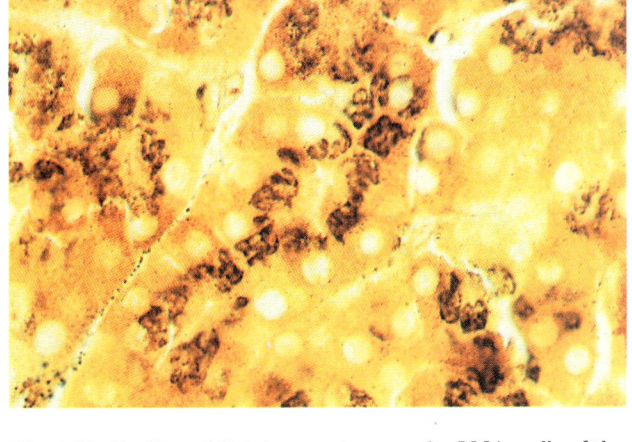

Fig. 1-18. Profiles of Golgi apparatus seen by LM in cells of the pancreatic acini, lying between unstained nuclei and cell apices. Secretions of these cells are released through the apical membranes into the lumen of the acinus. (Silver impregnation and gold toning; ×500.)

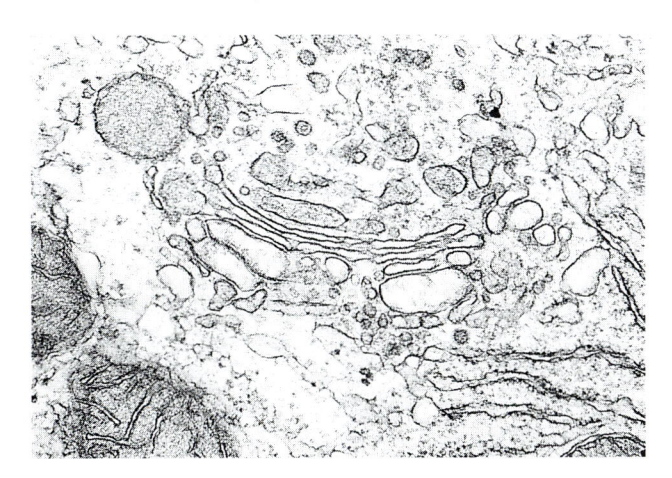

Fig. 1-19. TEM of a liver cell showing a Golgi apparatus with three to five cisternae. The *cis* face of the cisternae is oriented toward the RER, while the dilated rims of the opposite *trans* face gives rise to vesicles/vacuoles that form secretion granules. (×33,100.)

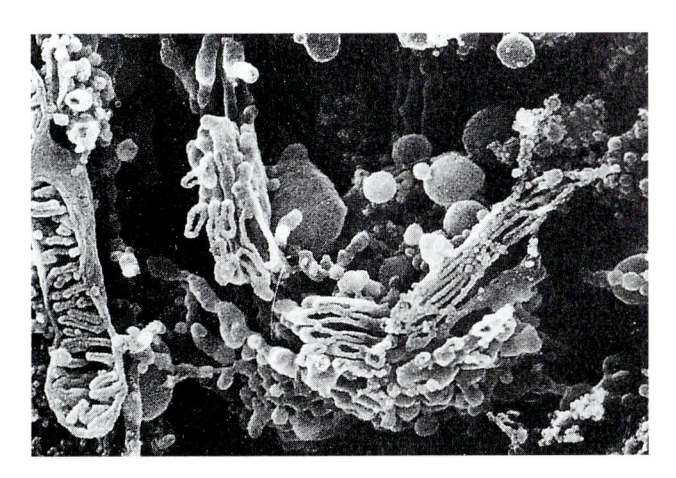

Fig. 1-20. SEM of the Golgi apparatus in an extracted cell, which reveals the spatial relationships between adjacent cisternae of the Golgi apparatus and forming vesicles. In the adjacent fractured mitochondrion, note the organization of cristae within the matrix (compare to Figs. 1-12 and 1-15). (×6,300.)

8 COLOR ATLAS OF HISTOLOGY

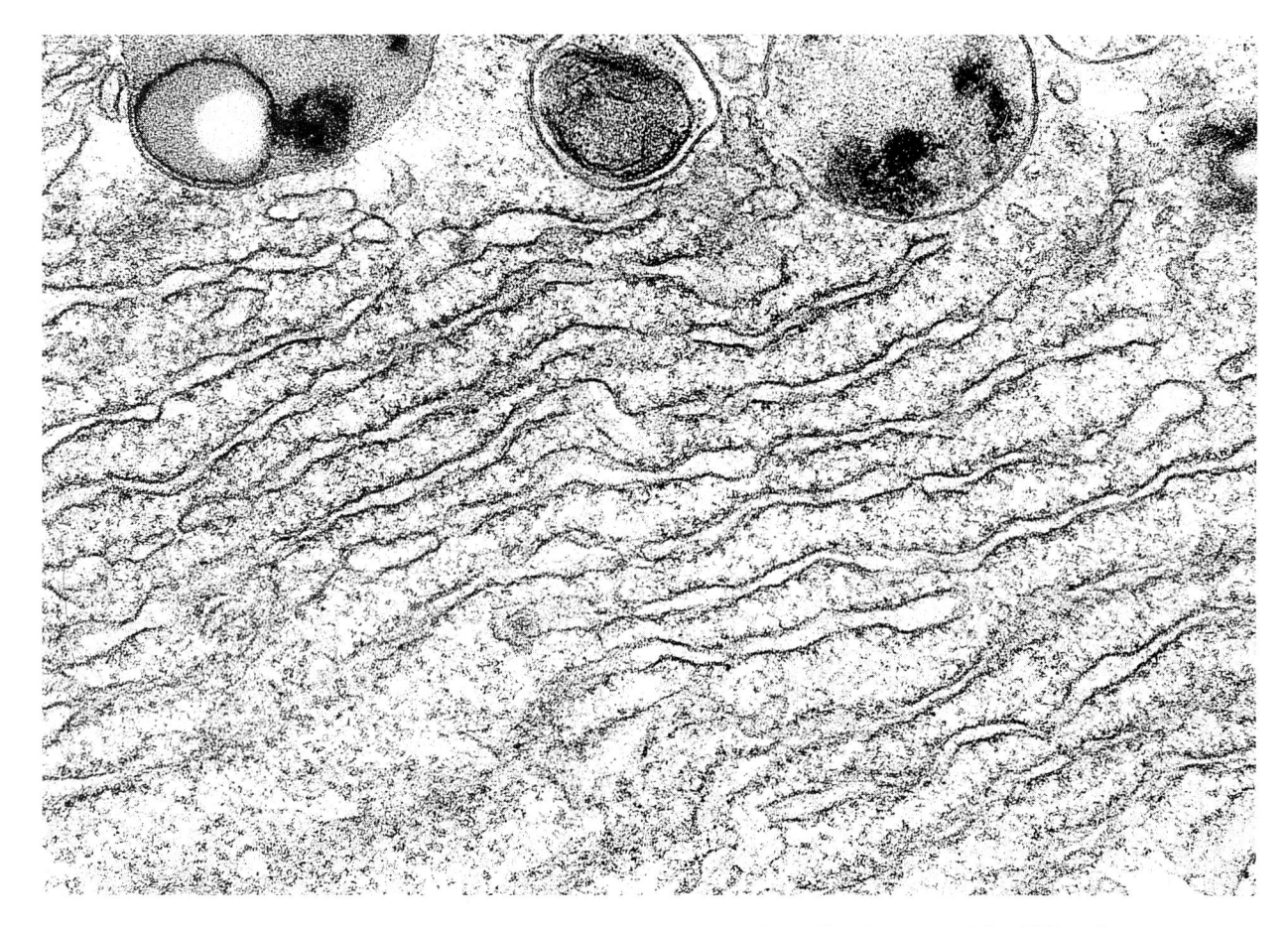

Fig. 1-21. TEM of liver cell cytoplasm showing an array of parallel cisternae of the RER and several adjacent lysosomes containing dense whorls of membranous elements called myelin figures. (×83,300.)

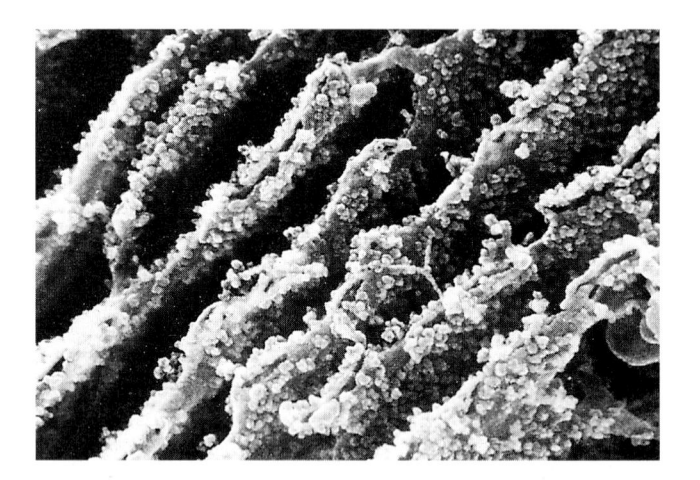

Fig. 1-22. SEM of cisternae of the RER. Ribosomes, seen attached to the cytosolic surface of the endoplasmic reticulum, transcribe mRNA as they synthesize proteins which are then sequestered within the cisternae of the RER before transfer to the Golgi apparatus for packaging. (×20,500.)

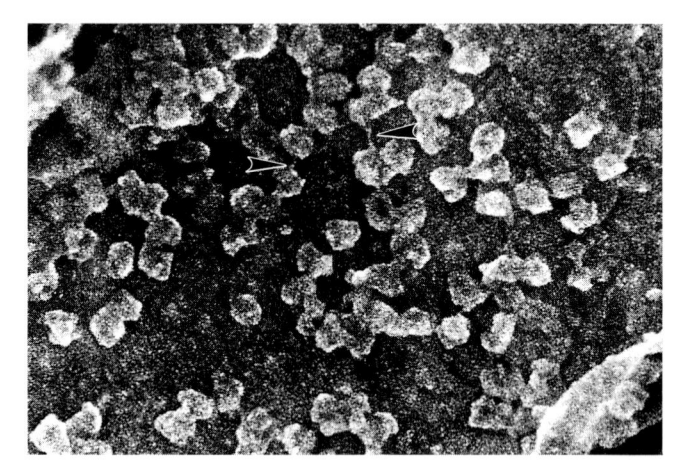

Fig. 1-23. High-resolution SEM of the cytosolic surface of the RER. Ribosomes and polyribosomes (linked by messenger RNA, *arrowheads*) can be seen on the surface of the cisternae. (×176,000.)

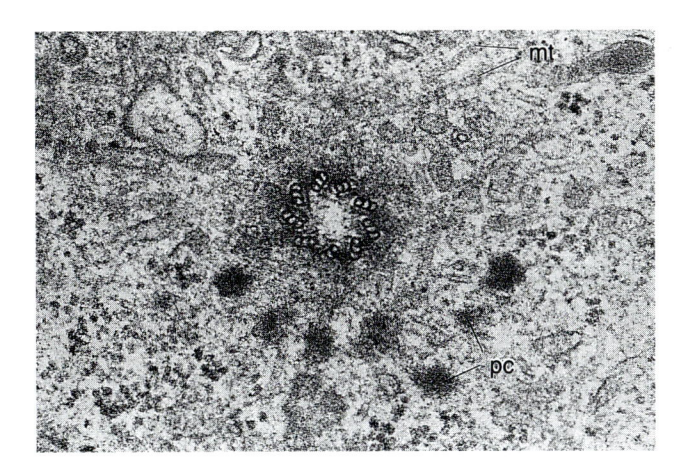

Fig. 1-24. TEM of a centriole showing the triplet arrangement of microtubules. Electron-dense pericentriolar satellites *(pc)* serve as nucleation sites for cytoplasmic microtubules *(mt)*. Cytoplasmic filaments and polyribosomes are also visible. (×87,000.)

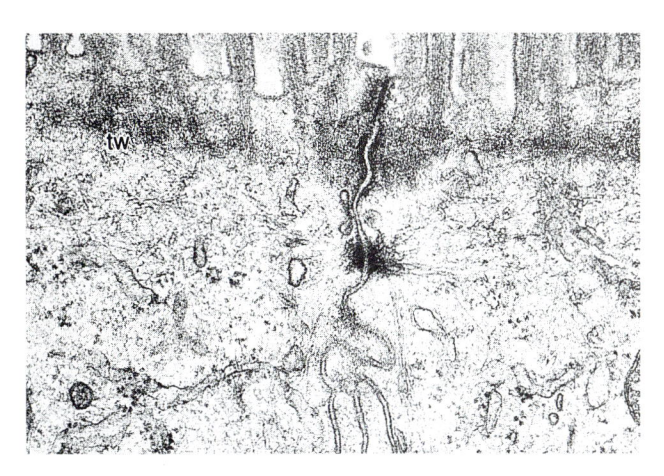

Fig. 1-25. TEM of the adluminal portions of two polarized intestinal epithelial cells showing the junctional complex (called terminal bar by LM) and the microfilaments of the terminal web (tw) just deep to the microvillous border. Note the desmosome with tonofilaments (keratin type of intermediate filaments) extending into the cytoplasm of each cell. Lateral borders of the cells interdigitate. (×36,000.)

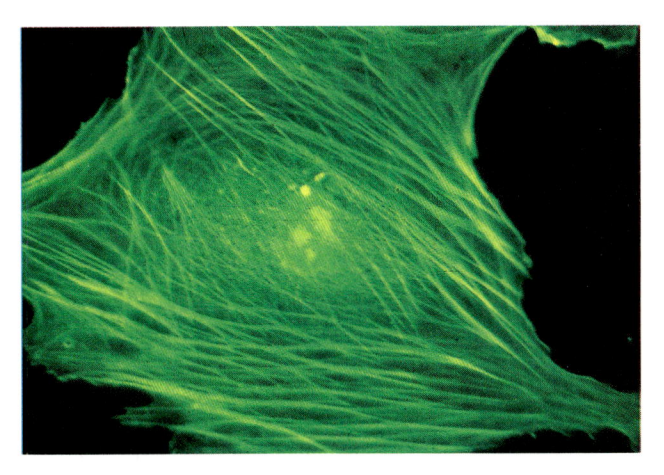

Fig. 1-26. An immunofluorescent micrograph demonstrating the localization of actin within NRK tissue culture cells. Bundles of actin filaments, sometimes called stress fibers, can be seen coursing in a diagonal pattern through the cytoplasm and around the periphery of the cell. (×500.)

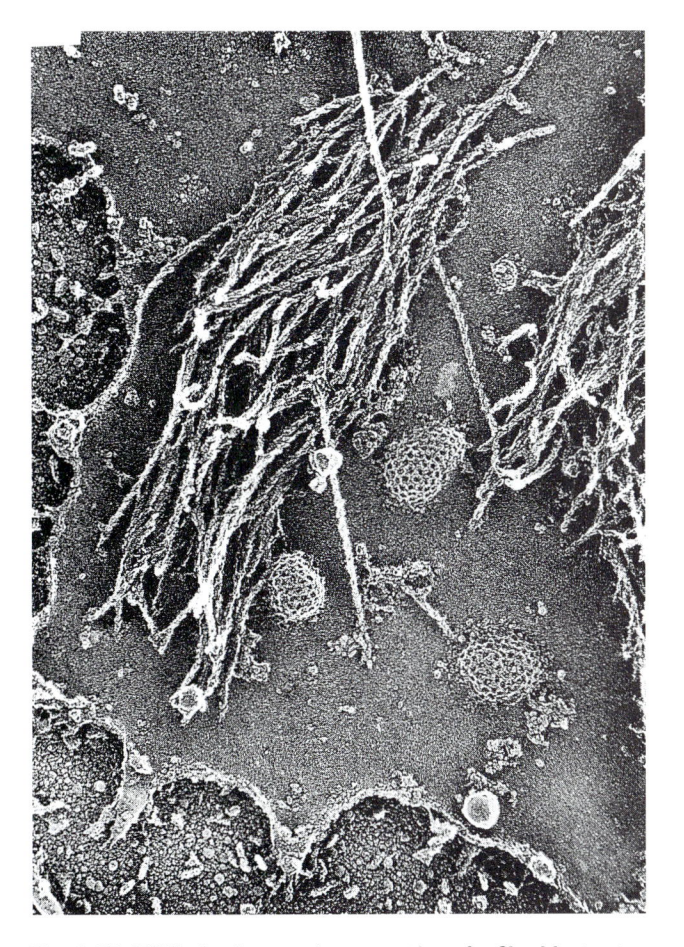

Fig. 1-27. TEM of a deep etch preparation of a fibroblast cytoskeleton showing several actin cables (stress fibers; see Fig. 1-26) attached to the cytoplasmic surface of the plasma membrane. The actin filaments have been decorated with the S1 fragment of myosin, resulting in the filaments having a barbed appearance. Coated vesicles, involved in receptor-mediated endocytosis, can be seen as honeycomb-shaped structures associated with the cytoplasmic surface of the membrane. (×52,500.)

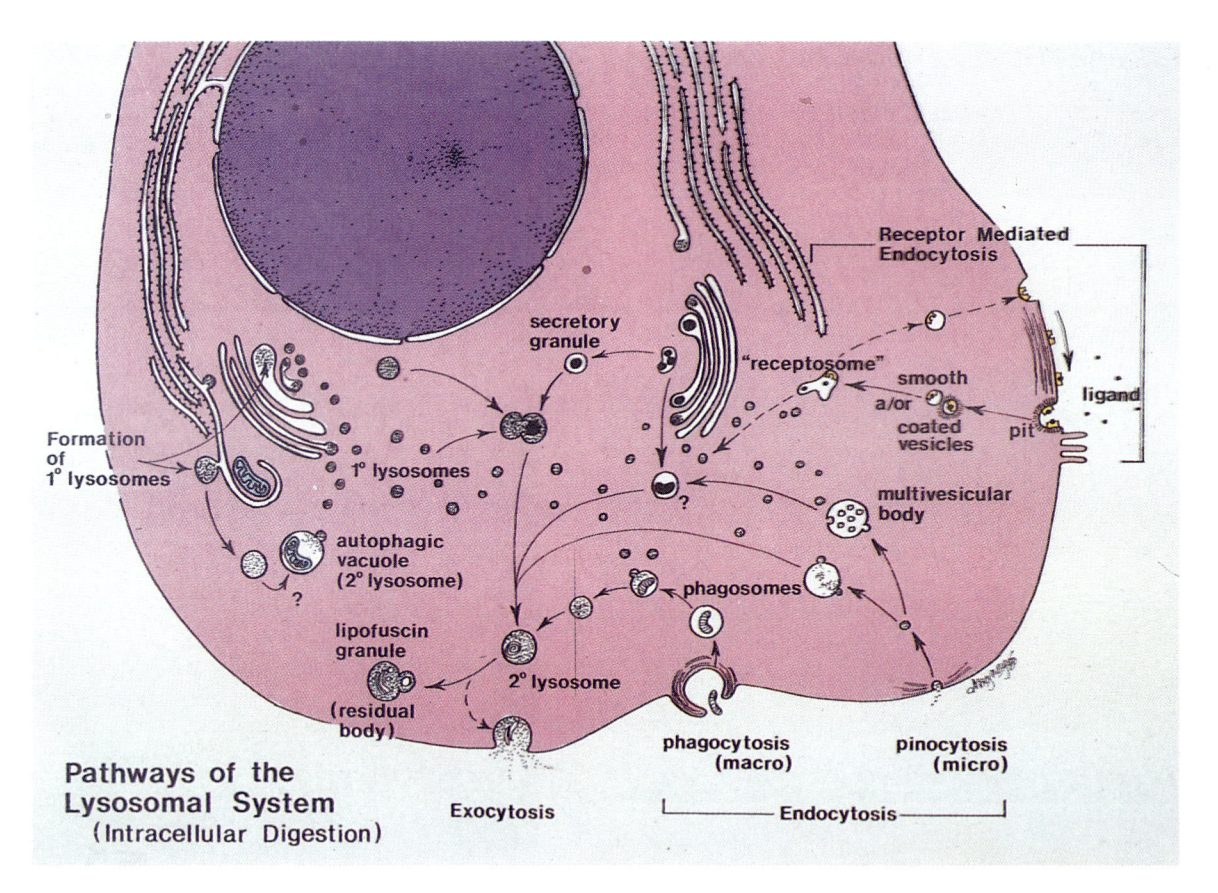

Fig. 1-28. Diagram of the pathways of the lysosomal system involved with endocytic uptake and intracellular digestion. Endocytic uptake or heterophagy includes phagocytosis and intracellular degradation of exogenous particles such as bacteria (see Figs. 1-29 and 1-30) as well as pinocytosis of fluid. Autophagy involves the degradation of endogenous intracellular organelles within lysosomal vacuoles (see Figs. 1-31 and 1-32). Receptor-mediated endocytosis involves the selective rapid uptake of molecules (hormones, growth factors, cholesterol, iron, etc.) from the extracellular fluid by specific protein receptors on the extracellular surface of the cell membrane (see Figs. 1-33 and 1-34). Following ingestion via clathrin-coated vesicles, receptosomes (endosomes) carry the ligand-receptor complexes into the cell where they may be delivered to the lysosomal system. In some instances, the receptors may be dissociated from the ingested ligand and recycled to the cell surface.

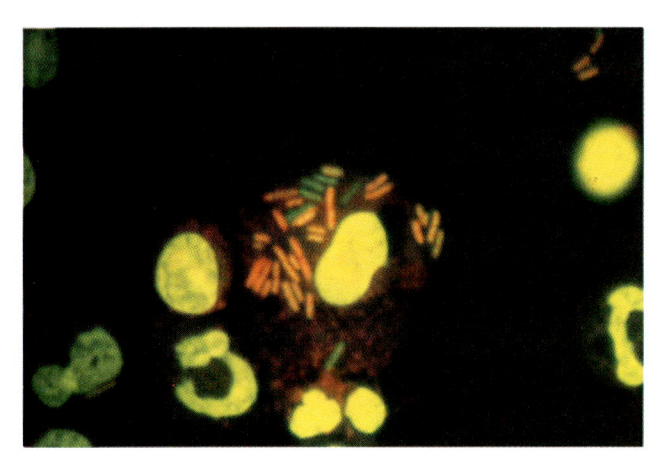

Fig. 1-29. Acridine orange stain of peritoneal exudate cells showing the phagocytosis of rod-shaped bacteria by a macrophage. Endocytosed bacteria in the phagolysosomal system that are dead stain orange, while viable bacteria are green. ($\times 700$.)

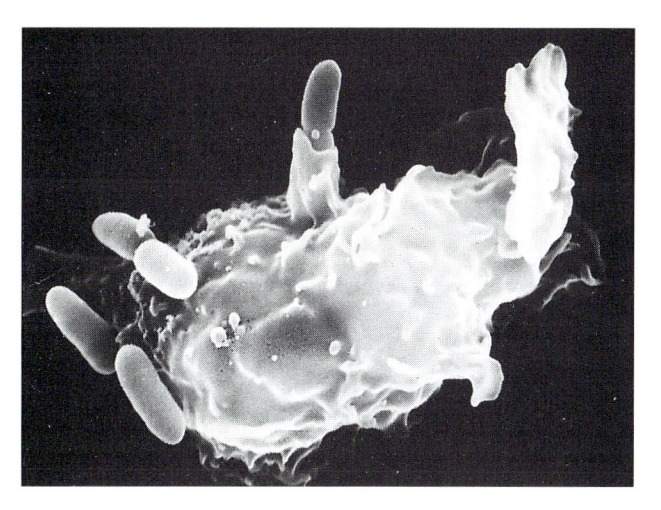

Fig. 1-30. SEM of peritoneal macrophage showing both membrane-adherent and partially ingested bacteria. Note the close adhesion of the macrophage membrane to the bacterium being endocytosed. ($\times 1000$.)

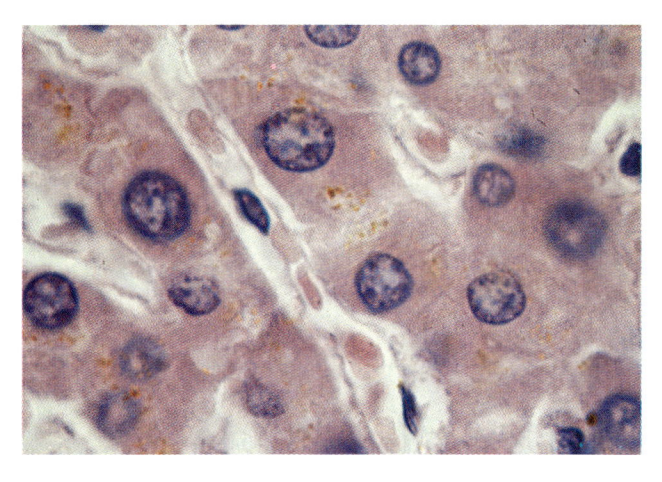

Fig. 1-31. LM of liver cell. Observe the golden brown lipofuscin pigment, which represents residual bodies (lysosomes) in the liver cell cytoplasm. (H&E; $\times 850$.)

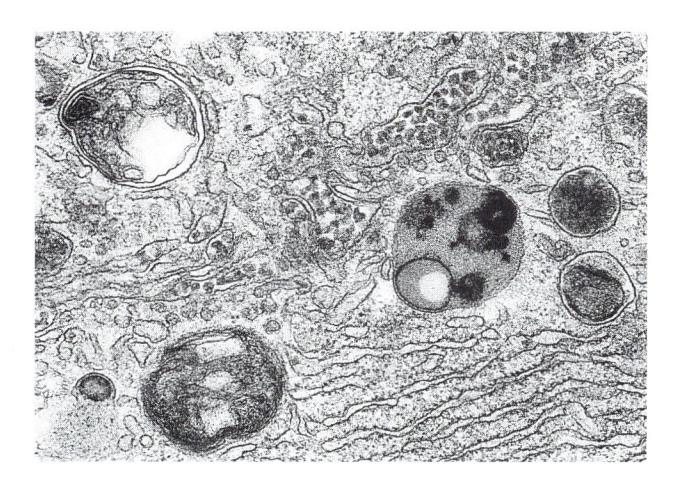

Fig. 1-32. TEM of liver cell cytoplasm containing several residual bodies (lysosomes) with undigested cytoplasmic residues scattered between elements of the RER and Golgi apparatus. The latter can be identified by the presence of lipoprotein particles within the lumen of the cisternae. ($\times 32,200$.)

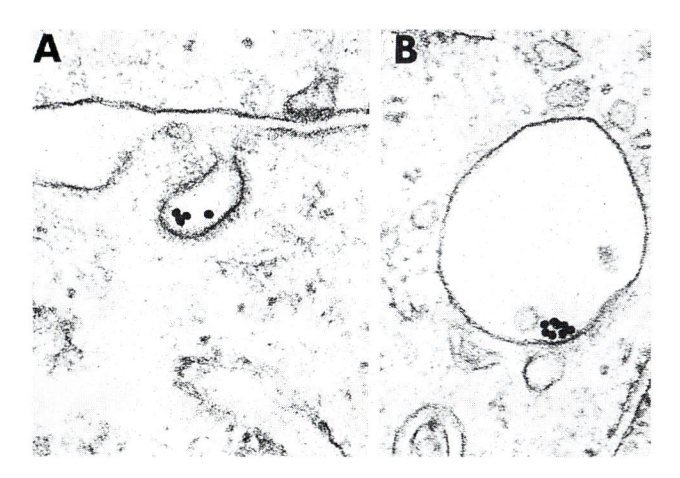

Fig. 1-33. TEM of receptor-mediated endocytosis in cultured human KB cells. **A,** A colloidal gold–labeled antitransferrin receptor antibody was used to localize the transferrin receptor within a clathrin-coated pit. **B,** After clustering of receptors, vesicles bud off from the surface and form receptosomes or endosomes, a process requiring about 20 seconds. The pH of the receptosome decreases, dissociating the ligand from the receptor and allowing the receptor to recycle to the cell surface, while the ligand eventually becomes degraded in the lysosomal apparatus. ($\times 81,500$.)

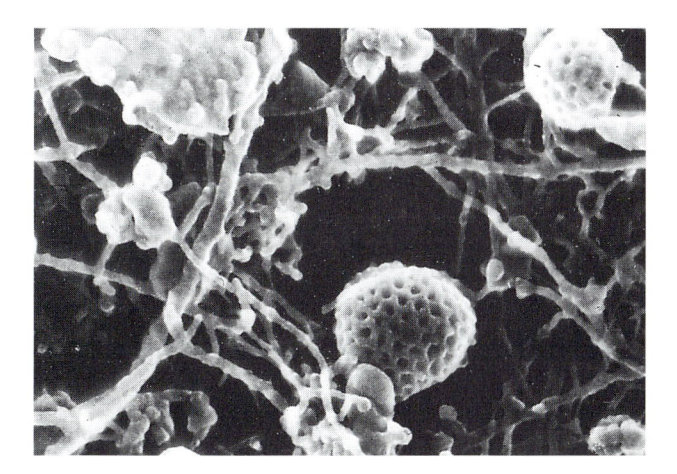

Fig. 1-34. SEM of the interior of a cell showing several different sizes of filaments of the cytoskeleton and clathrin-coated pit and vesicles. The coated pit *(center right)* has not yet detached from the plasmalemma. ($\times 82,000$.)

CHAPTER 2

EPITHELIUM

EPITHELIUM COVERS THE free surfaces of the body, lines body tubes and cavities, forms glands, and assumes many different arrangements to meet a variety of functions (i.e., protection, absorption, secretion, reproduction, excretion, digestion, lubrication, and sensory reception). The diversity of the epithelia associated with these functions can be linked to their use of surface modifications (of epithelial cells) and adaptation of cellular organelles to meet the unique functional requirement.

Classification of epithelia is based on the numbers of layers of cells (**simple,** one layer; **stratified,** two or more layers), the shape of the luminal or surface layer of cells **(squamous, cuboidal, columnar),** and the presence of surface specializations, such as **cilia** or **keratin.** Clusters of epithelial cells designed for secretion and connected to epithelial surfaces by ducts formed of epithelial cells are called **exocrine glands.** Masses of epithelial cells, or in some cases even individual cells, that in the absence of ducts release their secretory product into the vascular system are called **endocrine glands.**

Characteristics of epithelia include the presence of highly polarized contiguous cells, the absence of intercellular substance and blood vessels, and surface specializations of their intercellular, basal, and luminal surfaces. Depending on the function of the epithelium, epithelial cells may be attached to one another by specialized intercellular junctions associated with cellular adhesion (stratified epithelia), permeability (simple epithelia), cellular communication (glandular epithelia), or, in many instances, a combination of these. The **basement membrane** separates the basal surface of the epithelium from the underlying connective tissue and is composed of two elements, the **basal lamina** (type IV collagen) and a **reticular lamina** of variable thickness containing reticular fibers (type III collagen). The basal lamina of the epithelium serves both as a site of physical attachment for the epithelium and, in some instances, as a specialized permeable interface between the body and its environment (i.e., kidney and lung). The reticular lamina is bound to, and merges with, the underlying connective tissue, which serves as both a structural and a nutritional support for the avascular epithelium. Epithelial cells involved in ion transport may possess dramatic infoldings of the basal surface, which increase the surface area available for the movement of ions by membrane pumps.

Epithelial cells may possess two types of membrane specializations on the luminal surface: **microvilli** and **cilia.** Microvilli are finger-like projections of the luminal surface that amplify the surface area of the cell. Cells involved in membrane transport (i.e., small molecules such as sugars and amino acids) may have numerous densely packed microvilli, referred to by classical histologists as a **striate** or **brush border,** depending on their location in small intestine or kidney, respectively. Each microvillus contains a core of actin filaments whose state of polymerization may regulate its length and thereby the total area of the luminal surface. **Microvilli** are usually 0.1 μm in diameter and 0.5 to 1.0 μm in length. In the male reproductive tract, they are seen as exceedingly long projections called **stereocilia,** measuring up to 8 to 10 μm in length. **Cilia** are motile luminal specializations associated with the transport of extracellular materials such as mucus, debris, or cells. Each cilium is composed of nine double microtubules and a pair of central microtubules. Cilia are approximately 8 μm long and 0.2 μm wide and may be numerous on cellular surfaces, whereas a flagellum usually exceeds 30 or 40 μm in length and occurs only in sperm cells.

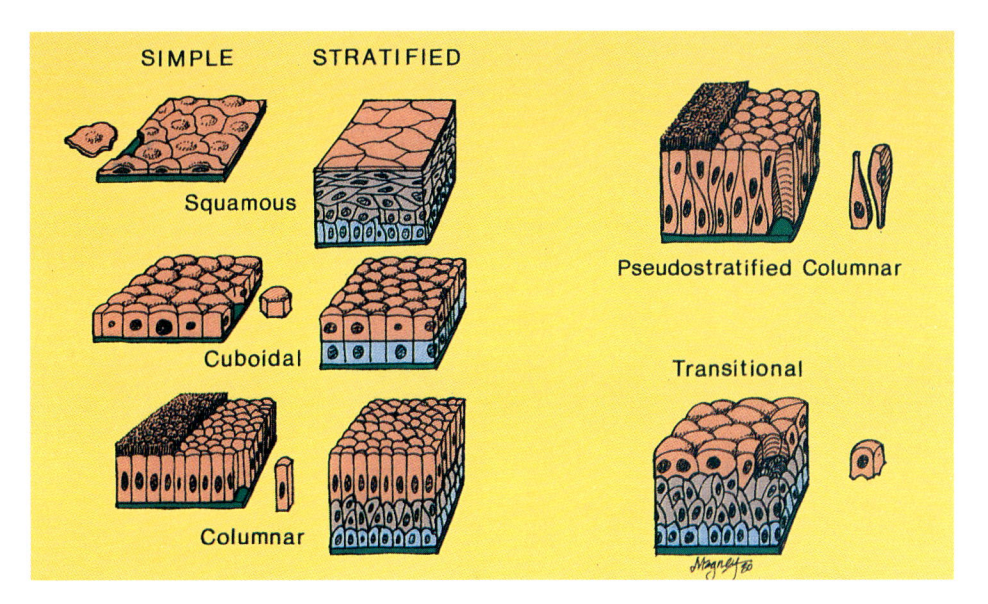

Fig. 2-1. Classification of the eight subdivisions of epithelia. Epithelium is a tissue that covers the free surfaces of the body. The cells are contiguous and rest on a basement membrane, which acts as an interface with the underlying connective tissue. Epithelia are classified as simple (containing one layer of cells), or stratified (multiple layers are present). The specific name of the epithelium reflects the shape of the cells lining the luminal surface (squamous, cuboidal, columnar, or transitional). Pseudostratified epithelium refers to the apparent presence of multiple cell layers; however, all cells are attached to the basement membrane, with only tall columnar cells reaching and forming the luminal surface. Transitional epithelia found in the urinary system are named for the changes in shape of surface cells during relaxed-stretched states related to storage of urine.

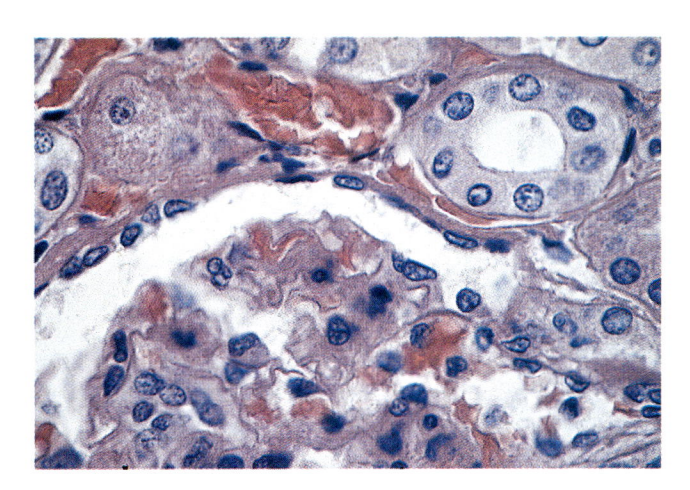

Fig. 2-2. LM showing a simple squamous epithelium lining Bowman's space of the renal corpuscle and a simple cuboidal epithelium forming the distal convoluted tubule in the kidney. (H&E; ×500.)

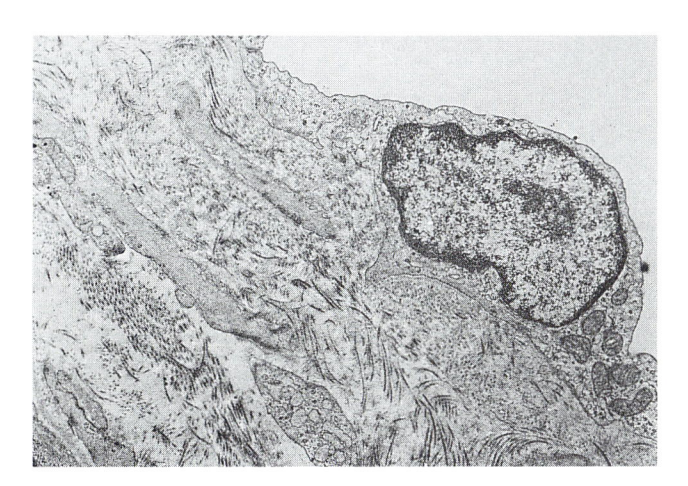

Fig. 2-3. A simple squamous cell seen by TEM. This cell is part of the mesothelium forming the visceral peritoneum of the intestine. Elements of connective tissue and smooth muscle are present beneath the basement membrane. (×4,600.)

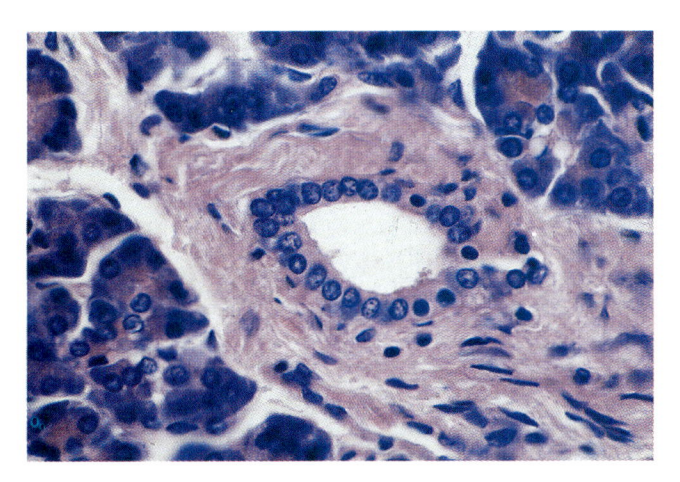

Fig. 2-4. Simple cuboidal epithelium of a pancreatic duct seen by LM. The duct is surrounded by connective tissue and pancreatic acini. (H&E; ×350.)

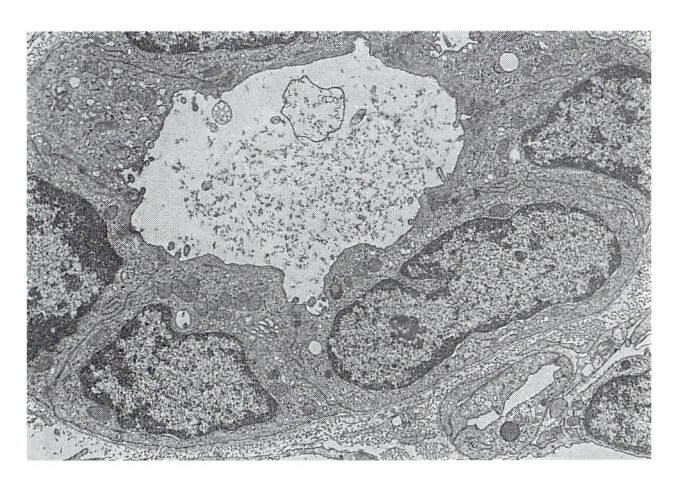

Fig. 2-5. Cross section of a pancreatic duct by TEM demonstrating simple cuboidal epithelium. Individual cells are approximately equal in height and width. (×3,400.)

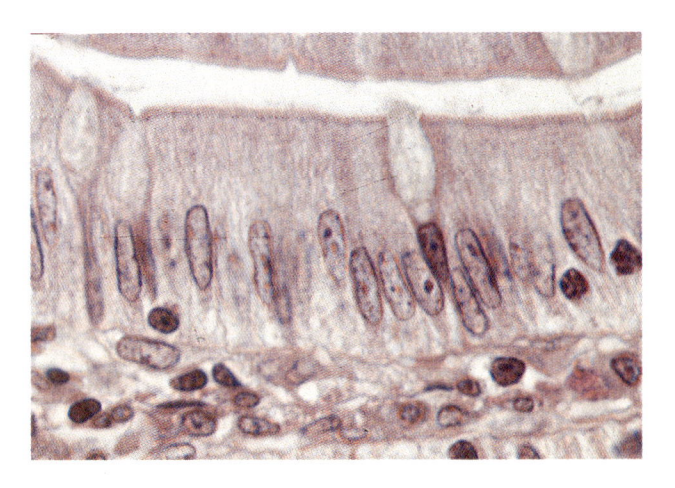

Fig. 2-6. LM of the small intestine revealing a simple columnar epithelium with goblet cells. Mucous granules in the goblet cells are unstained owing to the method used to fix the tissue. Intraepithelial lymphocytes are also present. (H&E; ×1,400.)

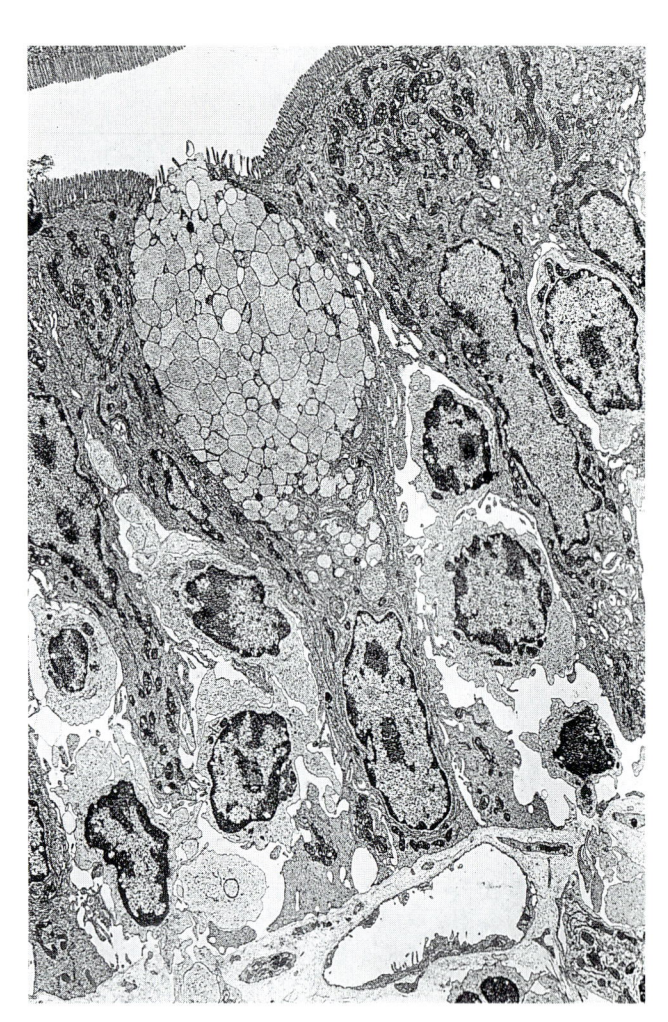

Fig. 2-7. TEM of the simple columnar epithelium in the small intestine. Note the goblet cell in the center of the micrograph and numerous intraepithelial lymphocytes between it and adjacent absorptive cells. A fenestrated capillary can be seen in the lamina propria beneath the goblet cell. (×4,000.)

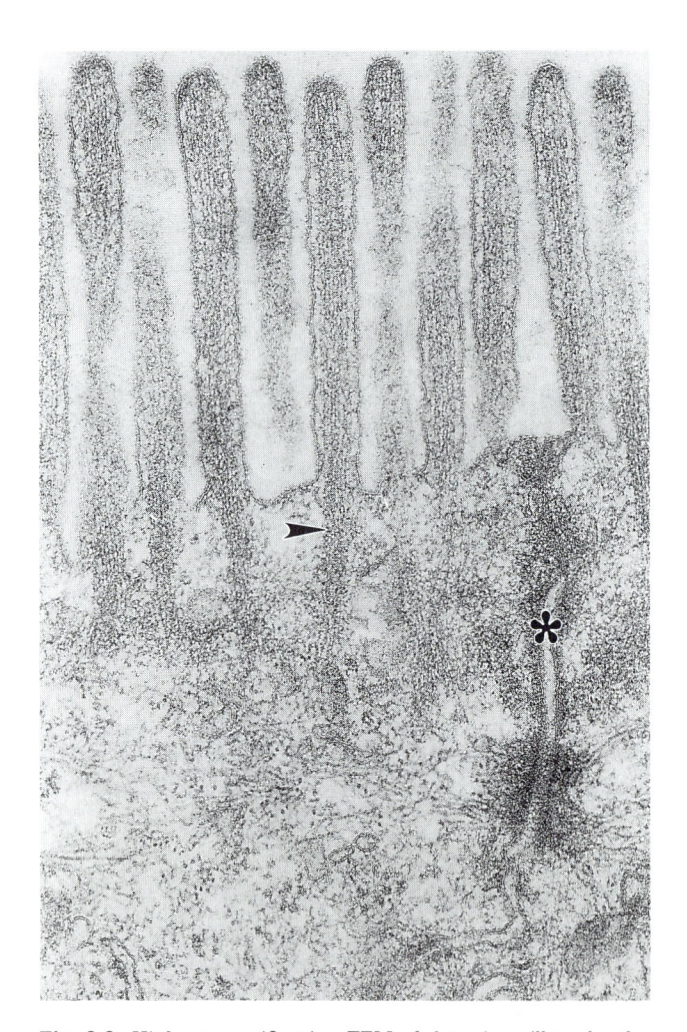

Fig. 2-8. Higher magnification TEM of the microvillous border of simple columnar epithelial cells in the small intestine. Bundles of actin filaments in the core of each microvillus (arrowhead) insert into the terminal web region, as do tonofilaments (intermediate filaments) from the desmosome (lower right) and actin filaments from the zonula adherens (asterisk) of the junctional complex. (×60,000.)

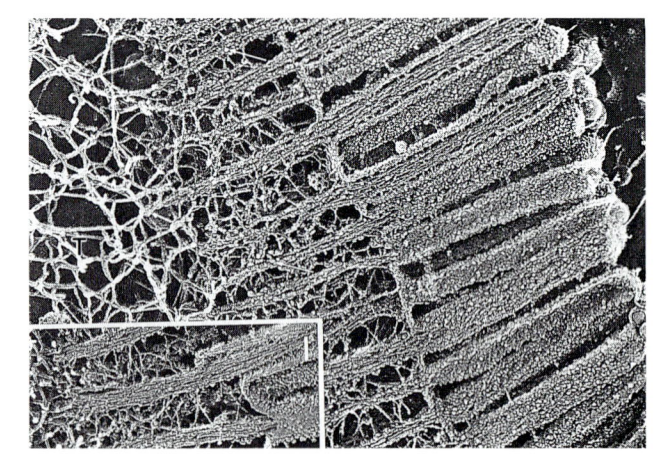

Fig. 2-9. TEM of a deep etch preparation of the terminal web region of a cell and its microvillous border. Note (as in Fig. 2-8) the relationships between actin in the core of each microvillus and the network of intermediate filaments in the terminal web (T). Inset (lower left) shows that tightly packed bundles of actin filaments in each microvillus are enmeshed by a fine network of cross-linked filaments. (×38,800.)

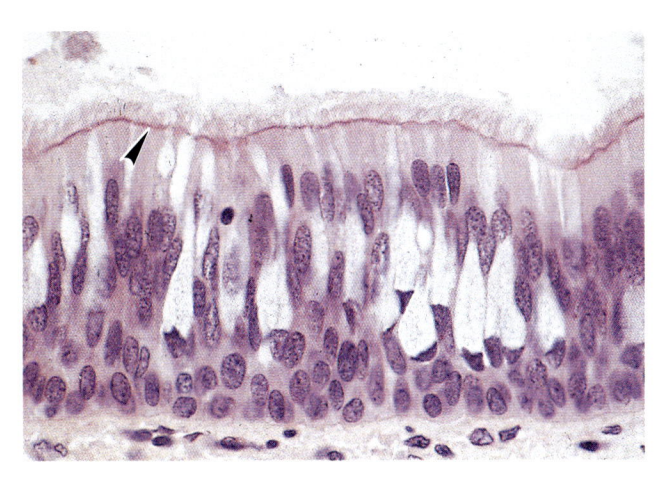

Fig. 2-10. LM of pseudostratified columnar epithelium with goblet cells and cilia. The basal bodies at the root of the cilia appear as a thin eosinophilic line *(arrowhead)* at the apex of the cells. (H&E; ×460.)

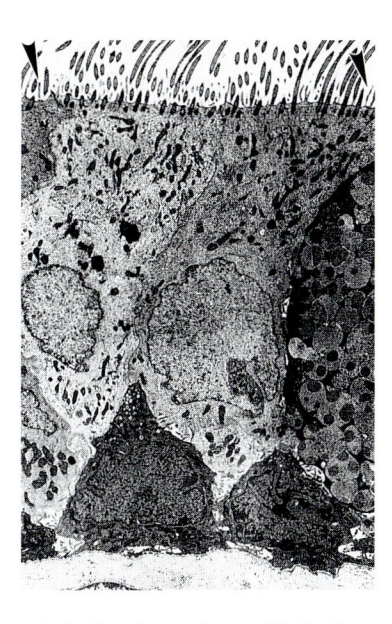

Fig. 2-11. TEM of ciliated pseudostratified columnar epithelium of the tracheal mucosa. Observe the presence of both cilia and microvilli *(arrowheads)* on the apical surfaces of the cells. (×1,600.)

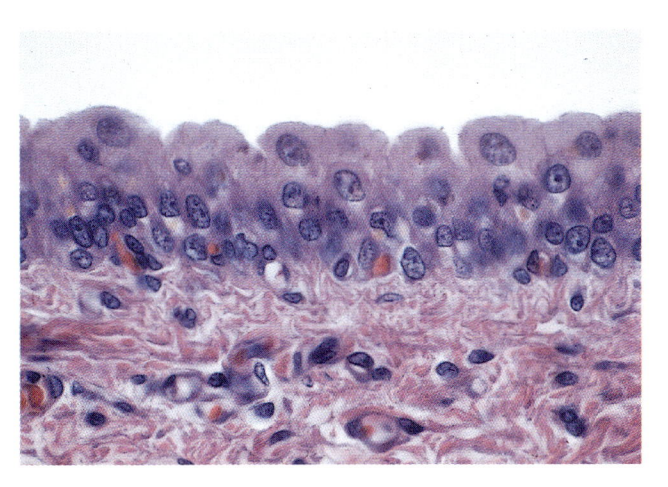

Fig. 2-12. Transitional epithelium of the urinary bladder seen by LM. Umbrella cells, at the lumen, will stretch and flatten as the bladder fills. Red blood cells within capillaries are separated from the epithelium by the basement membranes of both the epithelium and the capillary endothelium. (H&E; ×500.)

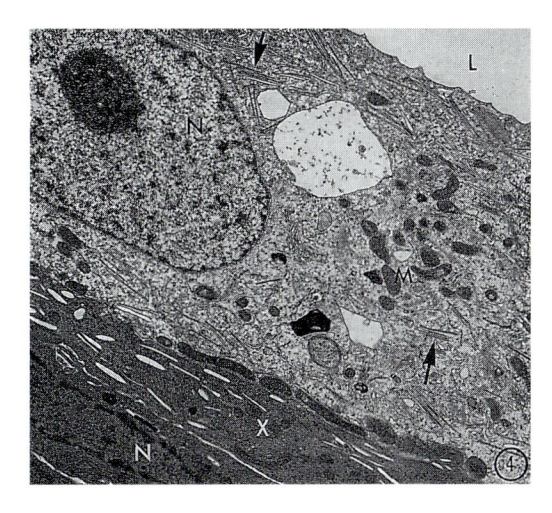

Fig. 2-13. TEM of transitional epithelium from the bladder. Umbrella cells form the luminal surface of the epithelium but do not contact the basement membrane. These cells contain discoidal vesicles *(arrow)* associated with endocytosis/exocytosis of luminal membrane when the cell undergoes shape change (squamous-cuboidal-squamous, etc.) because of stretch or relaxation of the bladder. (×3,100.)

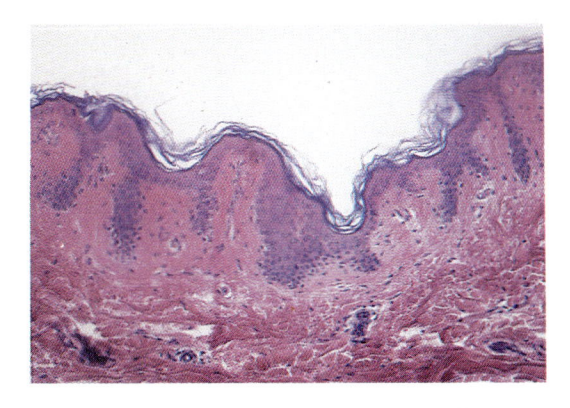

Fig. 2-14. LM of thin skin demonstrates stratified squamous keratinized epithelium. Acidophilic connective tissue underlies the epithelium, and basophilic squames of dead keratinized epithelial cells border the free surface. (H&E; ×200.)

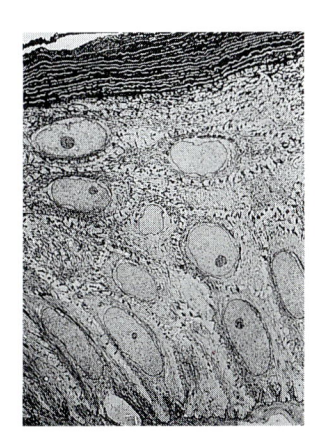

Fig. 2-15. TEM of stratified squamous keratinized epithelium from thin skin. The basement membrane is seen at the bottom right. Note the change in cell shape as the cells migrate from the basement membrane toward the surface. Desmosomes can be seen as dense spots at the cell margins. (×1,500.)

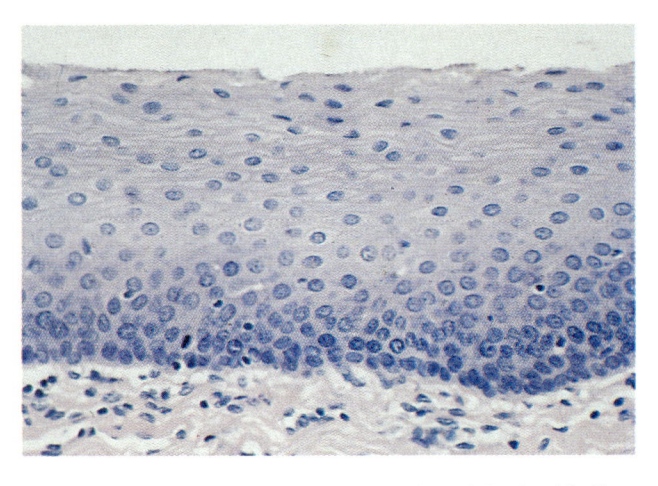

Fig. 2-16. LM of stratified squamous nonkeratinized epithelium of the esophagus. This thick epithelium contains many layers of cells. The long axes of the surface cells are parallel to the basement membrane, while those of basal cells are perpendicular to it. The nuclei of cells of the upper layers are ovoid, not flattened, and the luminal surface lacks keratinized squames. (H&E; ×350.)

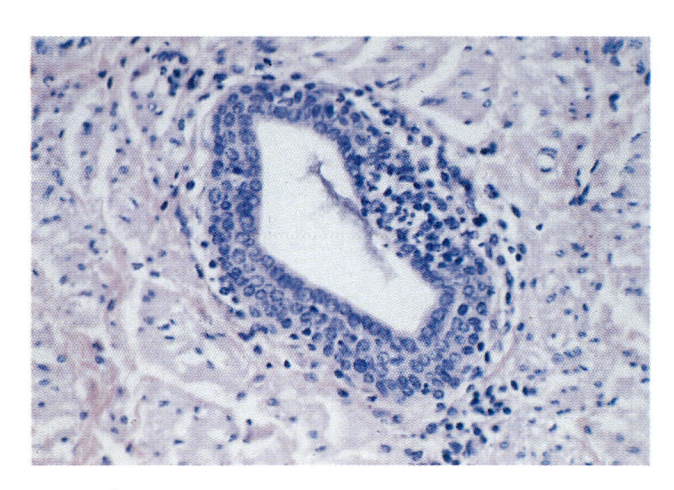

Fig. 2-17. LM of a duct lined by stratified cuboidal epithelium. Small lymphocytes are present in the epithelium and the adjacent connective tissue. (H&E; ×250.)

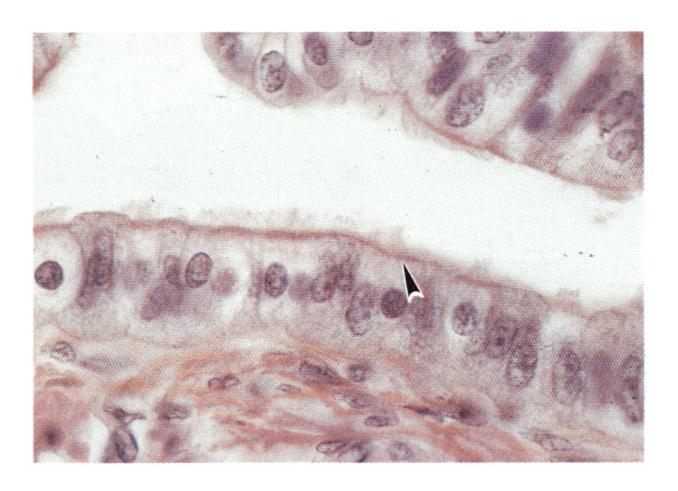

Fig. 2-18. LM of simple columnar ciliated epithelium from the uterine tube. The basal bodies of the cilia form an acidophilic band in the apical cytoplasm *(arrowhead)*. At this magnification, the cilia look like thin filaments extending into the lumen. (H&E; ×600.)

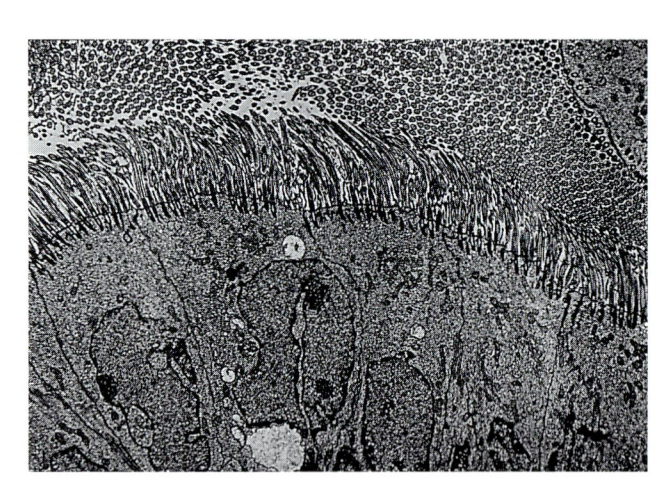

Fig. 2-19. TEM of simple columnar epithelium in the uterine tube showing the apical surface of ciliated cells bordering the lumen. The cilia arise from basal bodies located immediately beneath the cell surface. (×2,100.)

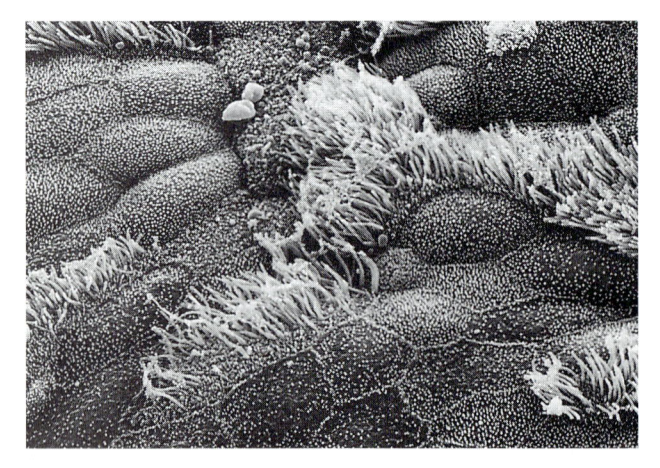

Fig. 2-20. SEM of cilia and microvilli on the luminal surface of rat trachea. Note that the apical surfaces of cells with microvilli or cilia may be distinguished from one another because of the greater length of cilia (about 8 to 10 μm) versus that of microvilli (about 1 μm). (×1,450.)

EPITHELIUM 17

Glycocalyx - Cell Membrane
sialic acid ▲
sulfated proteoglycans
Basement Membrane
Intrinsic Molecules

lamina rara (20nm)

sulfated proteoglycans
chondroitin sulfate
heparin sulfate

lamina densa
(30 - 100 nm)
(basal lamina)

type IV collagen
laminin
entactin/nidogen
and minor proteins

anchoring fibrils
reticular lamina

type V-VI-VII collagen?
type III collagen (reticular fibers)

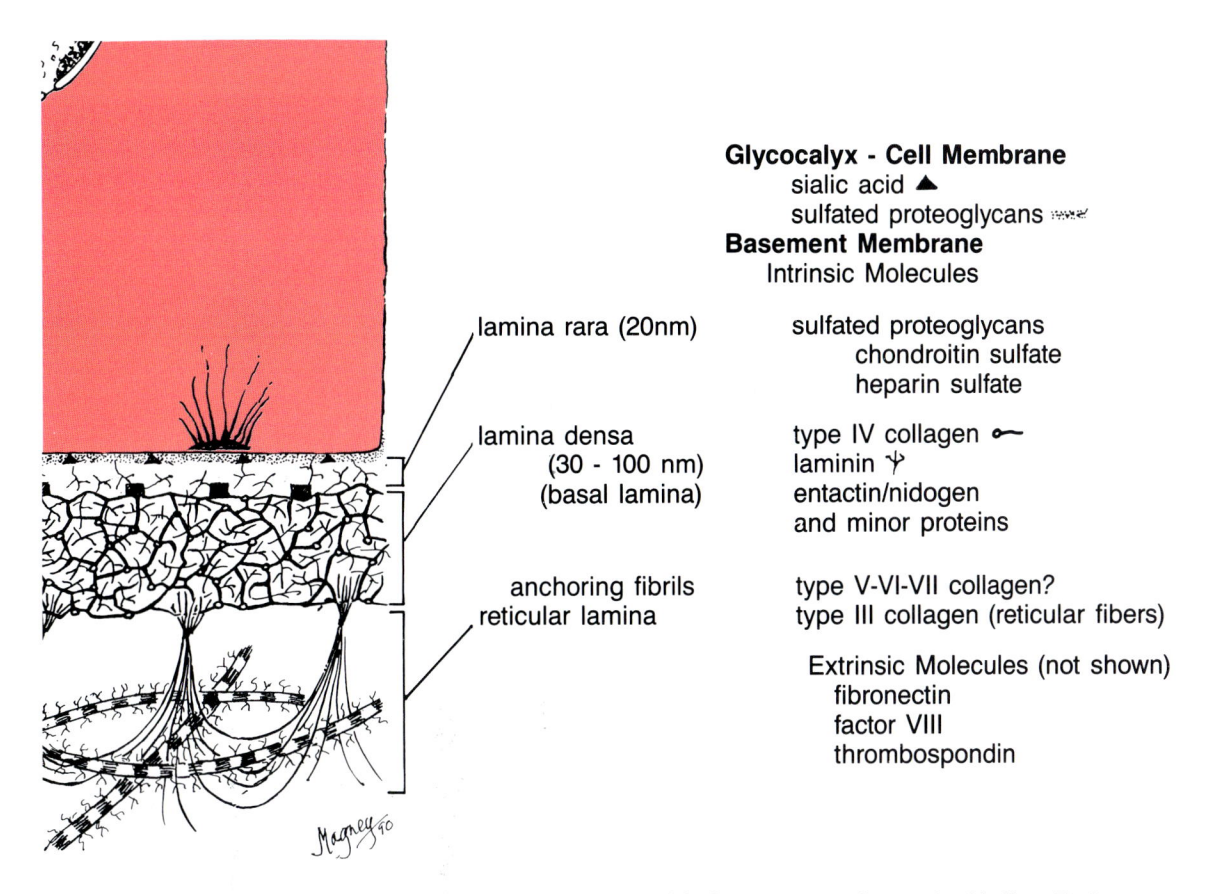

Extrinsic Molecules (not shown)
fibronectin
factor VIII
thrombospondin

Fig. 2-21. Drawing of the structural components of the basement membrane of epithelium. Each cell has an anionic charge on its surface from the presence of charged groups of carbohydrates in the glycocalyx (cell coat). The basement membrane consists of three components. The lamina rara, an electron-lucent zone rich in polysaccharides, is located between the cell membrane and the second component, the lamina densa (basal lamina). The lamina densa consists of a lattice of type IV collagen and laminin to which are bound sulfated proteoglycans and other minor proteins. The third component, the reticular lamina, consists of type III collagen fibrils and anchoring fibrils that strengthen the interface between the lamina densa and underlying reticular lamina.

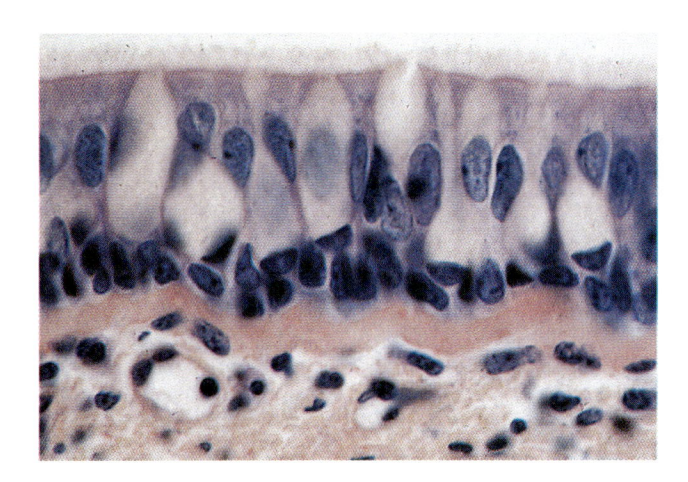

Fig. 2-22. Pseudostratified columnar epithelium with cilia and goblet cells seen by LM. The basement membrane is thick, smooth, and pink and lies immediately below the epithelium. (H&E; ×450.)

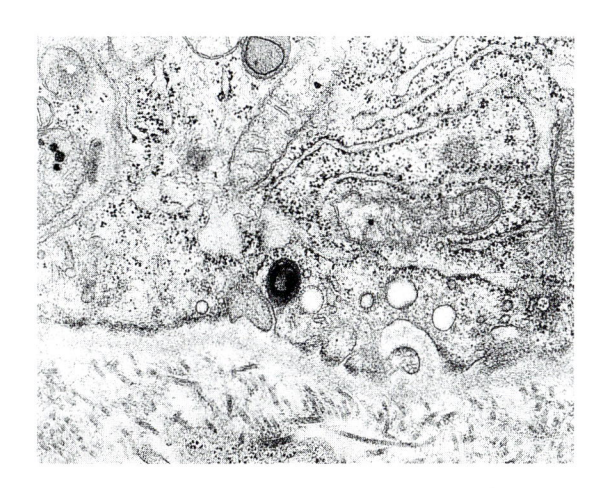

Fig. 2-23. TEM of the basal region of a stratified squamous epithelium showing the basement membrane and underlying connective tissue. Immediately below the plasmalemma of the epithelial cell, the lamina rara and lamina densa (basal lamina) of the basement membrane are clearly seen. Anchoring fibrils extend from the lamina densa into the adjacent connective tissue, where they intercalate with reticular fibers. (×13,000.)

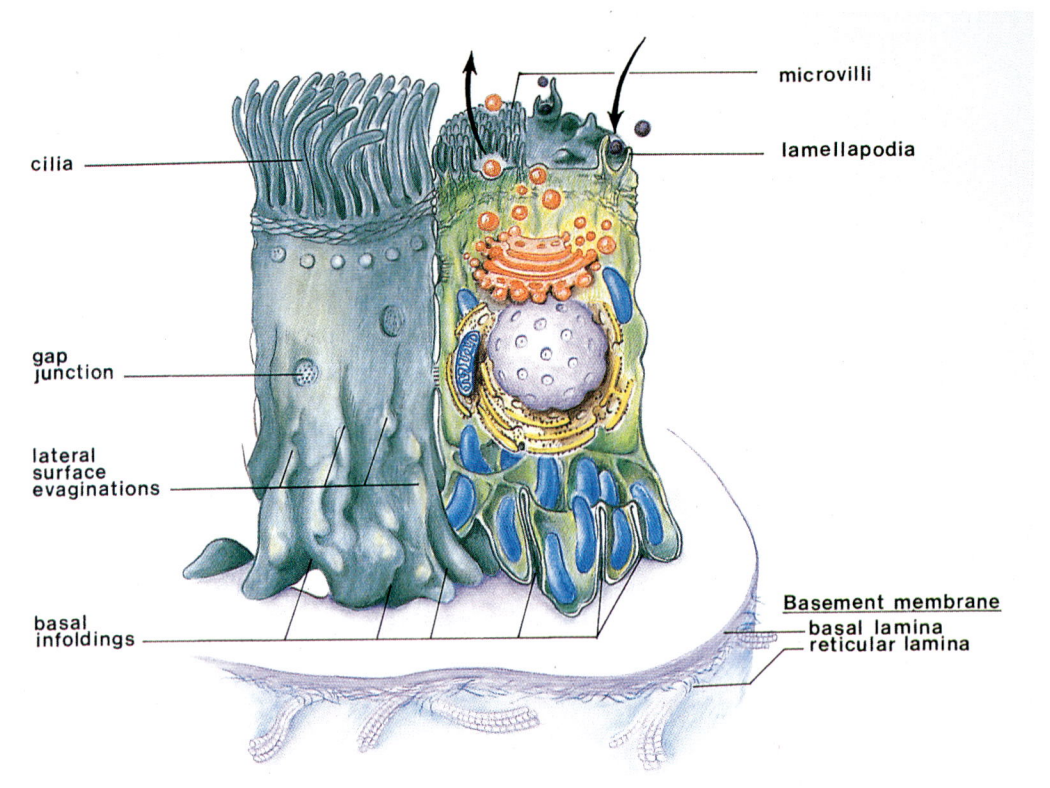

Epithelial Cell Surface Specializations

Fig. 2-24. Surface specializations characteristically found in epithelial cells include luminal surface projections such as cilia or microvilli, junctions to regulate permeability (zonula occludens), adhesion (desmosome), communication (gap), amplification of basal membrane related to ion transport (parietal cell in stomach and proximal or distal tubule cells in kidney), and modifications of the basal surface to facilitate attachment to the basement membrane.

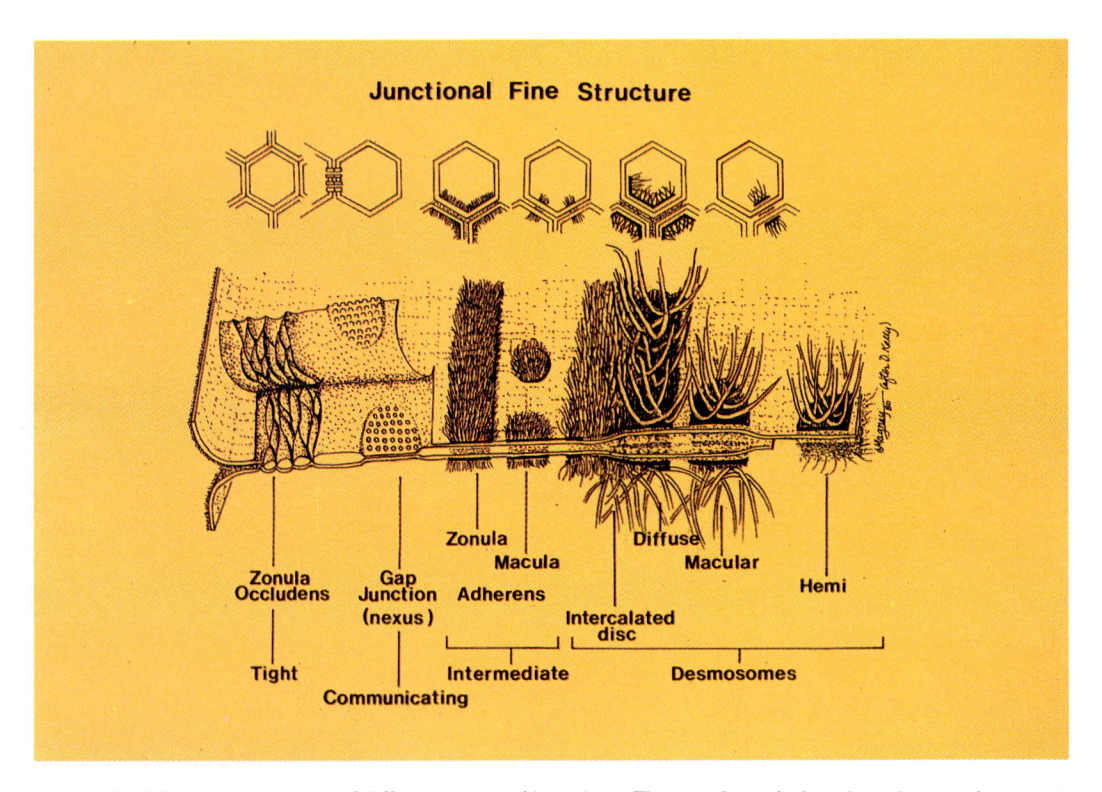

Junctional Fine Structure

Fig. 2-25. Fine structure of different types of junctions. The zonula occludens junction regulates permeability between adjacent epithelial cells in most epithelia, except for stratified squamous where permeability is regulated by an intercellular lipid barrier. Gap junctions facilitate the intercellular passage of small molecules and are found in excitable cells (e.g., nerve and cardiac or smooth muscle cells) as well as nonexcitable cells (e.g., osteocytes, Sertoli cells, granulosa cells, intestinal epithelial cells). A variety of junctions using either actin (zonula adherens) or intermediate filaments have been described in different cell types.

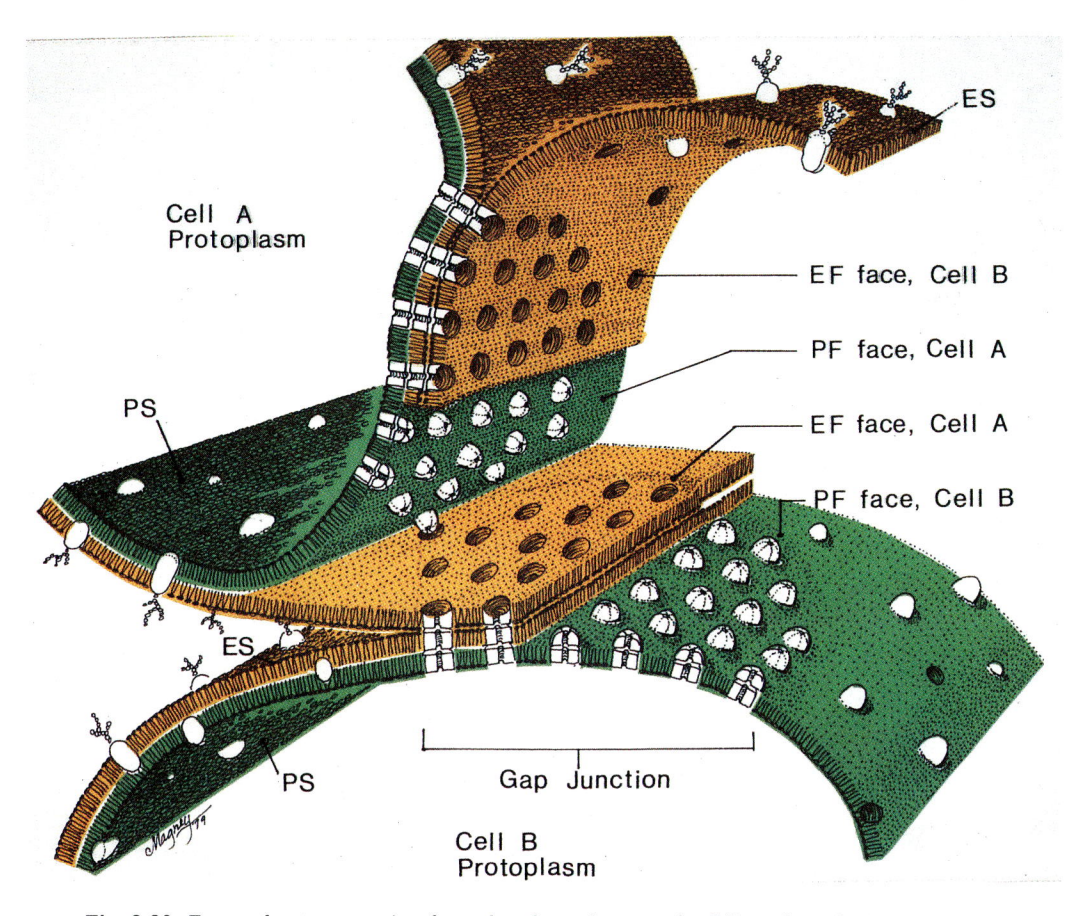

Fig. 2-26. Freeze fracture passing from the plasmalemma of cell B to that of cell A. Note that the fracture plane occurs within the lipid bilayer of each cell membrane. Intramembranous particles are usually more numerous in the protoplasmic fracture membrane face (PF face), where they are often seen as groupings of hexagonally packed intramembranous particles forming gap junctions. Gap junctions control transport of ions and small molecules between adjacent coupled cells, resulting in the communication of electrical and metabolic signals. Such ionic or molecular transport via gap junctions is thought to occur through the central channel formed by opposing connexons in each cell membrane.

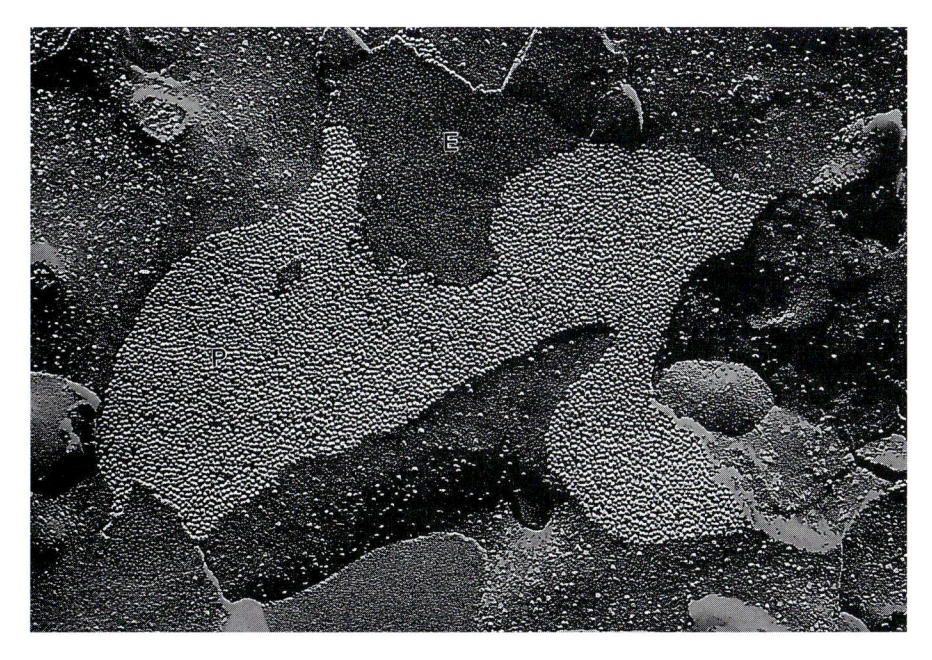

Fig. 2-27. FF of a gap junction between tumor cells. Both the protoplasmic (*P*) and extracellular (*E*) faces are seen, and gap junctions appear in both. ($\times 25,000$.)

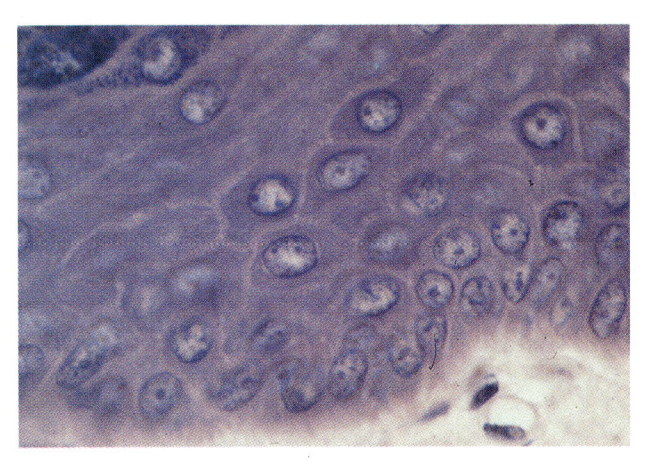

Fig. 2-28. Stratified squamous epithelium of skin. By LM the cells of this layer appear to have spiny borders, which, by TEM, are seen to be points of intercellular adhesion called desmosomes. However, the impression gained by LM resulted in the name of "stratum spinosum" for this layer of skin. (H&E; ×900.)

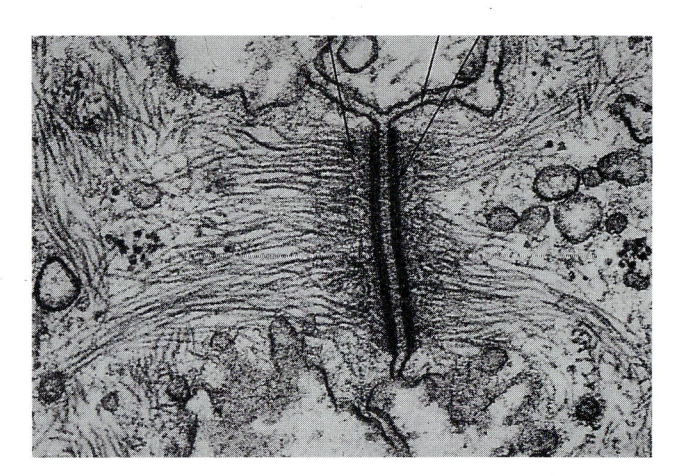

Fig. 2-29. Desmosomes, as viewed by TEM, exhibiting tonofilaments embedded in electron-dense plaque at the junction and extending into the cytoplasm. Tonofilaments do not cross intercellular space, although recent studies suggest that some particles called membrane linkers may somehow be attached to intramembranous particles (see Fig. 2-30). (×56,700.)

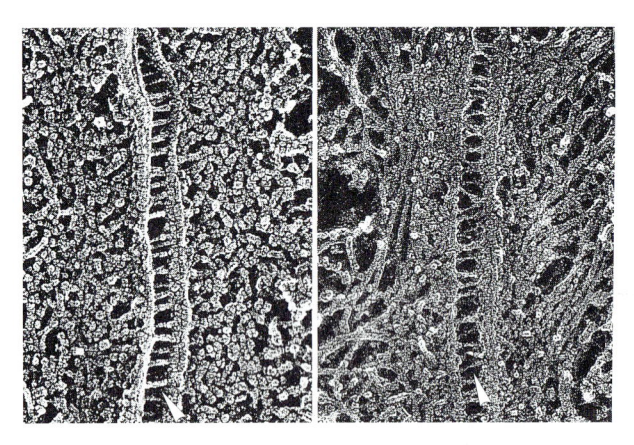

Fig. 2-30. Deep etch TEM of desmosomes revealing tonofilaments in a cross fracture of cytoplasm. Dense masses of filaments can be seen near the plasmalemma, as can the presence of membrane linkers *(arrowheads)* crossing the extracellular space between the adjacent cells. (×90,000.)

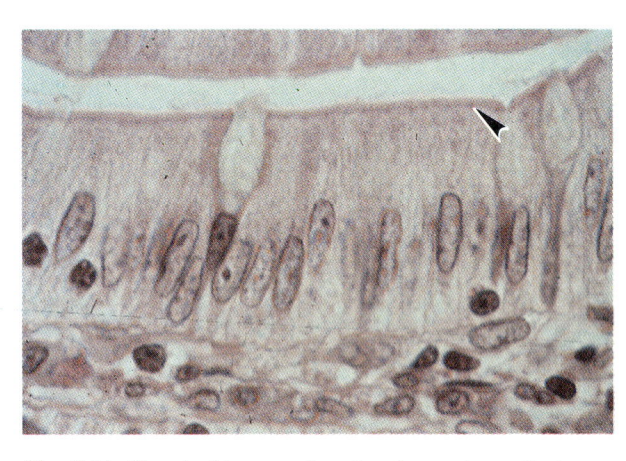

Fig. 2-31. Terminal bars, or junctional complexes that prevent luminal contents from penetrating lateral intercellular space. They are seen here by LM as darkly stained spots *(arrowhead)* at the lateral cell membranes immediately below the microvillous border. (H&E; ×1,300.)

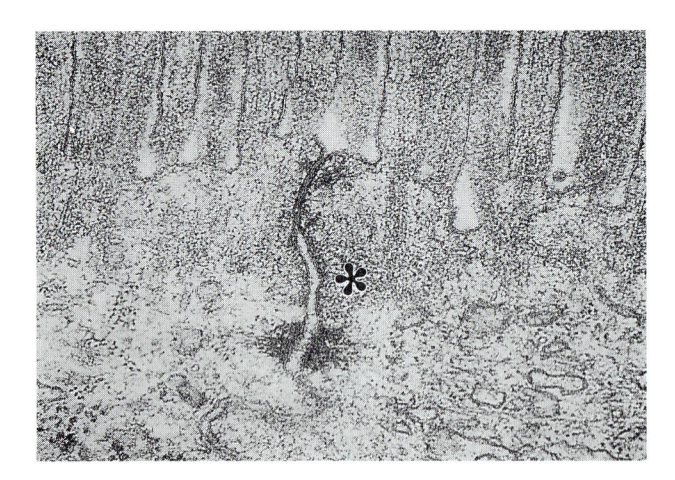

Fig. 2-32. TEM of a terminal bar. It is made up of a zonula occludens (reduced intercellular space and punctate membrane fusion) and a zonula adherens (slightly increased intercellular space and microfilaments [*asterisk*] of the terminal web associated with a moderate density of cytoplasm). A desmosome (macula adherens), which functions in intercellular adhesion, is also seen below this junctional complex. Microvilli containing actin filaments appear at the top (see Figs. 2-8 and 2-9). (×49,500.)

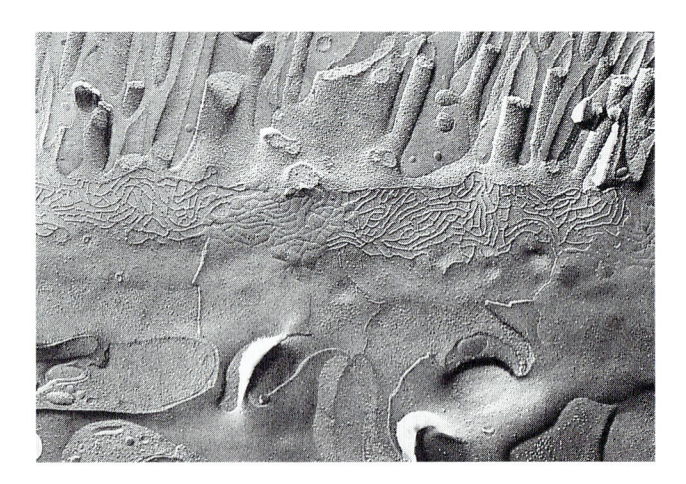

Fig. 2-33. A zonula occludens (tight junction) seen here by FF. It appears as an anastomosing web (representing membrane fusion) that encircles the luminal end of the lateral membranes of each cell, attaching it to adjacent cells and sealing off the lumen from the interstitium. In the protoplasmic fracture face the web appears as protruding ridges (composed of intramembranous particles), whereas the extracellular fracture face shows the presence of the web as linear depressions (see Figs. 2-24 and 2-25). (×40,000.)

CHAPTER 3
CONNECTIVE TISSUE

CONNECTIVE TISSUE IS composed of three components; **cells, fibers,** and **ground substance.** The fibers and ground substance together are known as the **extracellular matrix.** The functions of connective tissue are multiple and varied, including structural support, an immunologic barrier, storage and metabolism of fat, and conservation of water.

Two broad categories of connective tissue cells exist. The first includes those found only in connective tissues—**fibroblasts, adipocytes, macrophages, plasma cells, reticular cells,** and, in the embryo, **mesenchymal cells.** The second category consists of **hematogenous cells** that move from the vascular system (i.e., marrow, spleen) into connective tissue. It includes **lymphocytes, monocytes, granulocytes,** and developing **blood cells,** which are discussed in later chapters.

Fibers found in the extracellular matrix include **collagen** and **elastin.** Collagen is the most abundant protein in the human body and the principal type of fiber found in connective tissue. Based on their morphology, amino acid composition, and physical properties, 10 to 12 different types of collagen have been identified, although the exact functions of many of them remain to be defined. **Type I collagen** has high tensile strength, comprises about 90% of the total body collagen, and is found in skin, tendon, bone, dentin, and loose connective tissue. By LM, bundles of type I collagen are seen as eosinophilic fibers, while at the TEM level the fibers are seen to be composed of individual fibrils with 64 nm periodicity. **Type II collagen** forms fibrils with 64 nm periodicity that can be detected by TEM, but it does not form eosinophilic bundles by LM and is found in cartilage, the nucleus pulposus, the vitreous body, and cornea. **Type III collagen,** also known as reticular fibers, consists of fibrils with 64 nm periodicity that have a high content of carbohydrate. This explains their staining with silver and the periodic acid Schiff method. Type III collagen does not form large bundles visible by LM and is distributed widely in the body, including skin, blood vessels, and the stroma of lymphoid, liver, and other organs. **Type IV collagen** does not form fibrils with 64 nm periodicity, but it comprises a fine filamentous meshwork known as the basal lamina of the basement membrane associated with epithelial cells and the basal lamina (external lamina) of muscle cells, Schwann cells, and adipocytes. **Type V collagen** is similar to type IV collagen in that it does not form fibrils. Although found in small amounts throughout the body, its structure and function still remain to be determined. Recently **type VII collagen** has been identified in anchoring fibrils connecting the basement membrane of epithelia to underlying connective tissue, and **type X collagen** has been detected in the epiphyseal plate of bone. However, their functional roles and structure must still be determined. Besides the fibroblast, many types of collagen can be produced by a number of different connective tissue cell types (adipocytes, chondrocytes, osteocytes, and reticular cells). Type IV collagen found in the basal lamina is produced by epithelial cells, muscle cells, and Schwann cells of the peripheral nervous system.

Elastic fibers in the extracellular matrix have two structurally distinct components at the TEM level. The first is an amorphous substance composed of **elastin,** a special protein rich in nonpolar amino acids, which accounts for its staining with the dye orcein (Verhoeff stain) at the LM level. The second component consists of **microfibrils** that incompletely surround strands of the amorphous component and may serve to orient the elastin. Like collagen, elastin can be produced by numerous cell types including fibroblasts, smooth muscle cells, and chondrocytes in elastic cartilage.

The ground substance of the extracellular matrix is composed of **glycosaminoglycans** (previously called mucopolysaccharides) and **structural glycoproteins.**

Glycosaminoglycans, or **GAGs,** are linear, unbranched polysaccharide chains composed of repeating disaccharide units. Because of their high content of acidic side groups (hydroxyl, carboxyl, and sulfate), they bind large amounts of water as a shell of hydration. GAGs in turn are covalently attached to a larger core protein and thus constitute a **proteoglycan molecule.** These proteoglycan molecules are usually connected via noncovalent bonds by a link protein to long chain-like molecules of hyaluronic acid (the only nonsulfated GAG molecule), which then form large molecular aggregates that gives connective tissue its semifluid gel-like properties. **Structural glycoproteins,** such as **fibronectin** (abundant in all connective tissue; referred to as cold insoluble globulin in blood), **chondronectin** (cartilage), and **osteonectin** (bone), are composed chiefly of protein with attached branched carbohydrate side chains. They possess specialized regions for attachment to cellular surfaces and various GAGs in the extracellular matrix. Because of their bivalent symmetry, structural glycoproteins may play an important role in the adhesion of cells to one another and to components of the extracellular matrix, such as collagen, or GAGs bound to the surface of fibers or cells.

The general macroscopic classification of connective tissues is based on the relative abundance of cells, extracellular fibers, and ground substance:
1. **Mucous**—contains large amounts of ground substance and few cells or fibers and found in the umbilical cord and embryonic tissues.
2. **Reticular**—composed of reticular fibers (type III collagen) and present in the stroma of liver, adipose tissue, and lymphoid organs.
3. **Loose or areolar**—made up of equivalent amounts of cells, fibers, and ground substance and found in subcutaneous regions and mesenteries and as an interface between adjacent tissues.
4. **Adipose**—composed of adipocytes arranged in loose clusters or dense masses of cells, as seen in subcutaneous fat, epiploic appendages of the large intestine, or the omenta.
5. **Dense connective**—comprised mainly of either collagen or elastin with few intervening cells. Regular dense connective tissue consists of fibers arranged in one plane (i.e., tendons), whereas irregular dense connective tissue has fibers traveling in multiple planes (i.e., dermis of the skin).
6. **Specialized connective**—includes those designed for support (bone and cartilage) or transport (blood), which are discussed in separate chapters.

COMPOSITION OF GROUND SUBSTANCE

1. Proteoglycan (PG) – protein core + GAG

PG AGGREGATE

0.3μ

Glycosaminoglycan (GAG)

Chondroitin sulfate
Keratan sulfate
also
Heparan sulfate
Dermatan sulfate
Hyaluronic acid

Link protein
Hyaluronic acid (HA)
PG MONOMERE (M)
Core protein

2. Glycoprotein

Fibronectin
Laminin
Chondronectin

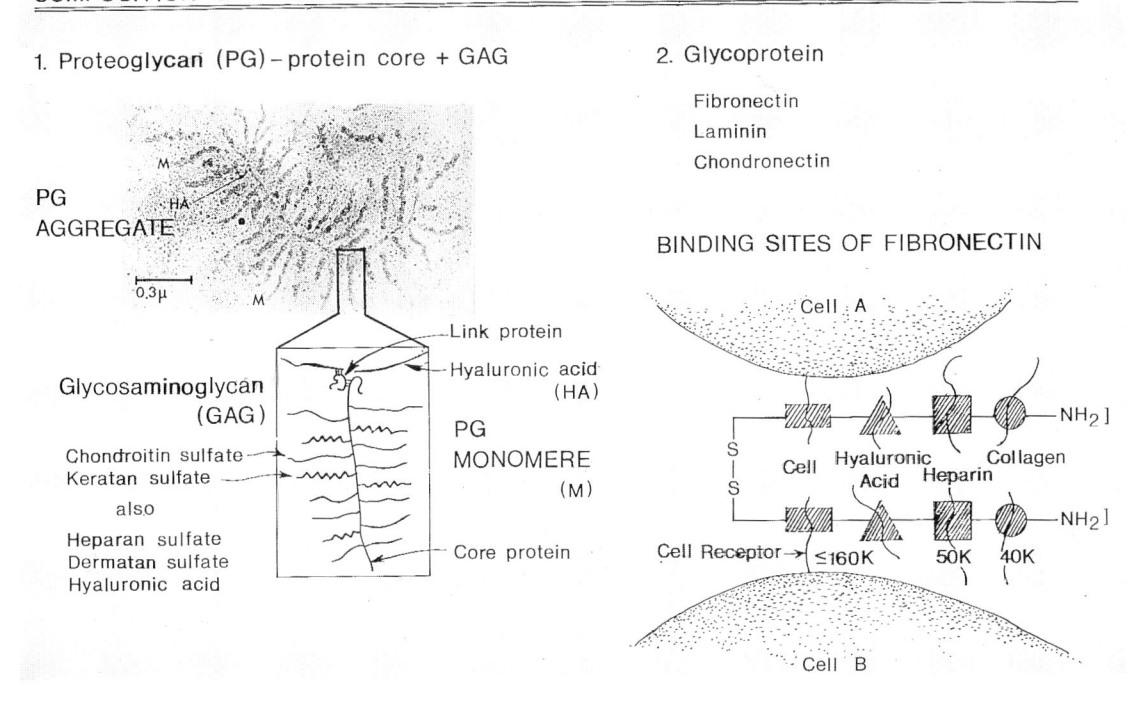

BINDING SITES OF FIBRONECTIN

Cell A

Cell — Hyaluronic Acid — Heparin — Collagen — NH_2]

Cell Receptor → ≤160K   50K   40K — NH_2]

Cell B

Fig. 3-1. Diagram illustrating the composition of ground substance in the extracellular matrix. Considerable heterogeneity in proteoglycan size and structure exists between different tissues owing to variations in the number, size, or degree of sulfation of GAG chains. The proteoglycan aggregate illustrated in this frame is from cartilage. Recently fibronectin, chondronectin, and laminin (all glycoproteins) have been identified as structural elements of the connective tissue matrix. Fibronectin is a major surface glycoprotein of the fibroblast, but it may be produced by other mesenchymally derived cells, by epithelial and endothelial cells, and by some marrow-cell types. It is also found in plasma and is sometimes called cold-insoluble globulin. Laminin is a constituent of basement membranes; chondronectin is found within the matrix of cartilage.

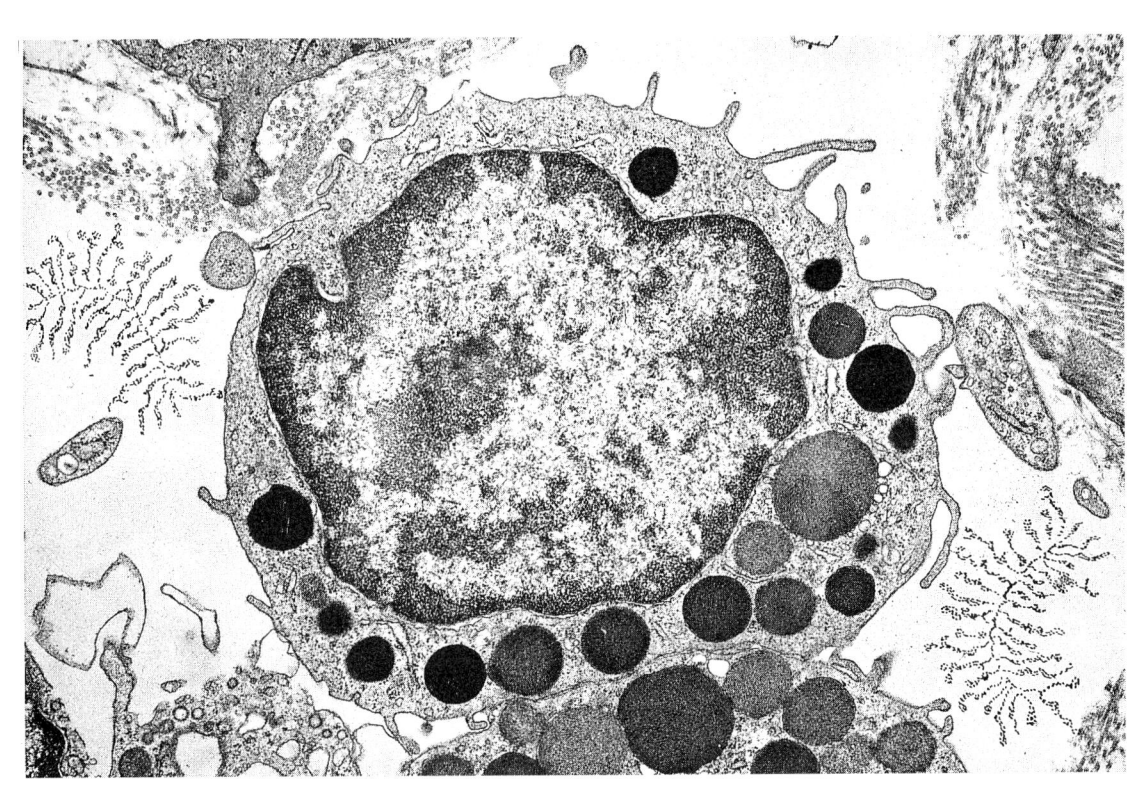

Fig. 3-2. TEM of a mast cell in connective tissue. Note the presence and size of proteoglycans (drawn in ink) in the extracellular space. Examples of collagen fibrils and fibers can also be seen in the extracellular space. (×10,000.)

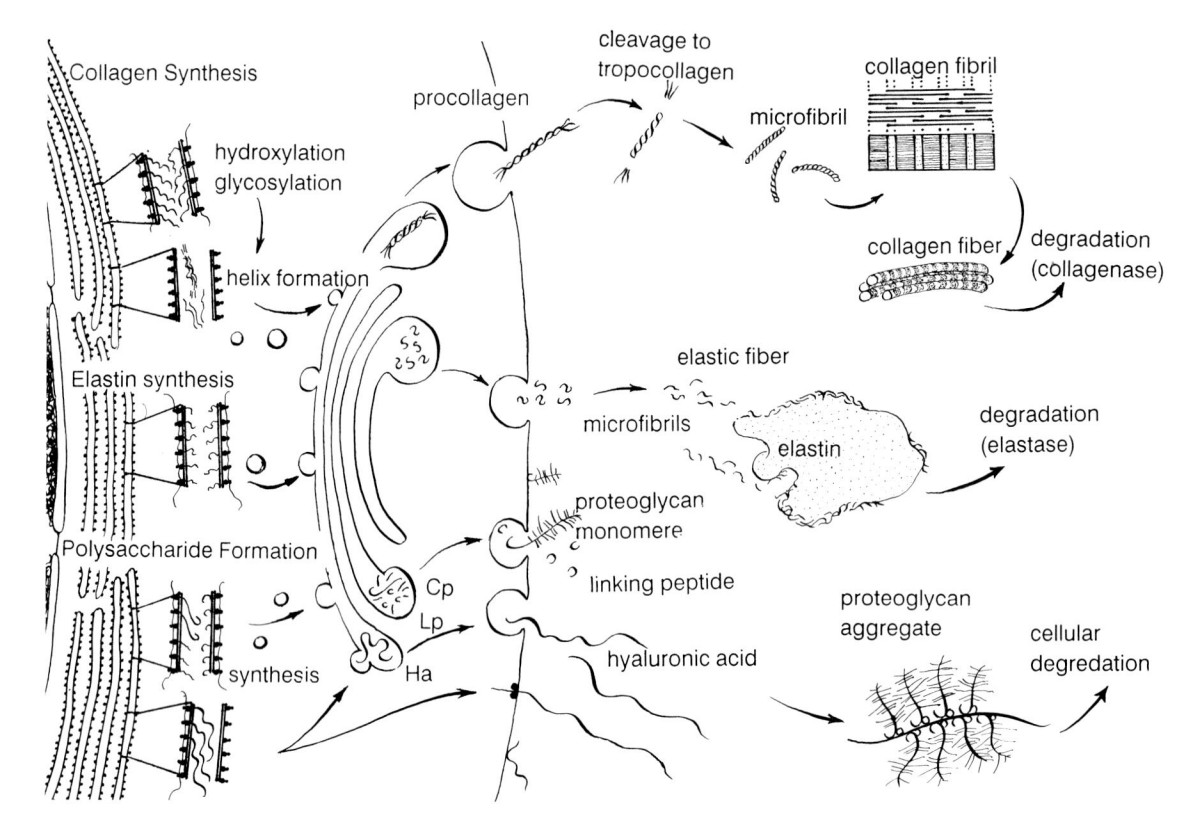

Fig. 3-3. Drawing of a fibroblast illustrating steps in the intracellular synthesis and extracellular formation of collagen, elastic fibers, and proteoglycans. The intracellular formation of both collagen and elastin results in the secretion of a *pro* form of the molecule. Procollagen or proelastin are modified extracellularly to permit formation of fibers. Exopeptidases clip off the amino- or carboxyl- termini of procollagen, thereby making the molecule more insoluble. Cross-linking of adjacent tropocollagen molecules is facilitated by lysyl oxidase, and in the case of elastin, lysine residues are cross-linked to form the unusual amino acids, desmosine and isodesmosine. Glycosaminoglycans are secreted by vectorial transport through the Golgi apparatus, whereas hyaluronic acid may follow a similar pathway or possibly may be released via a transporter molecule as occurs in microorganisms. Small amounts of proteoglycans and hyaluronic acid may also be associated with the extracellular surface of cell membranes.

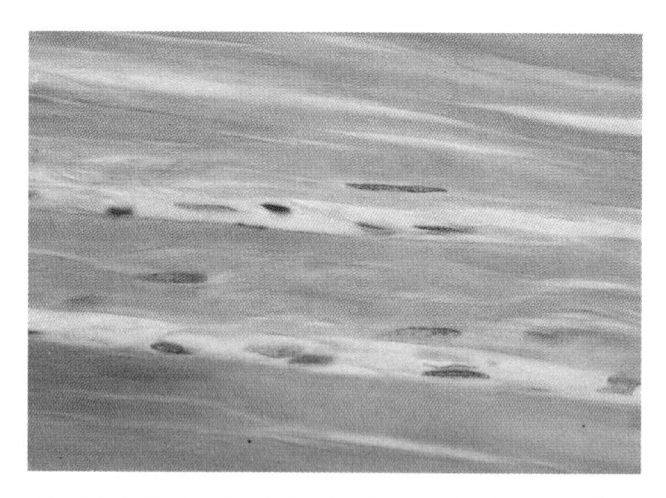

Fig. 3-4. LM of tendon in longitudinal section demonstrating a dense array of collagen fibers and interspersed fibroblasts. (H&E; ×500.)

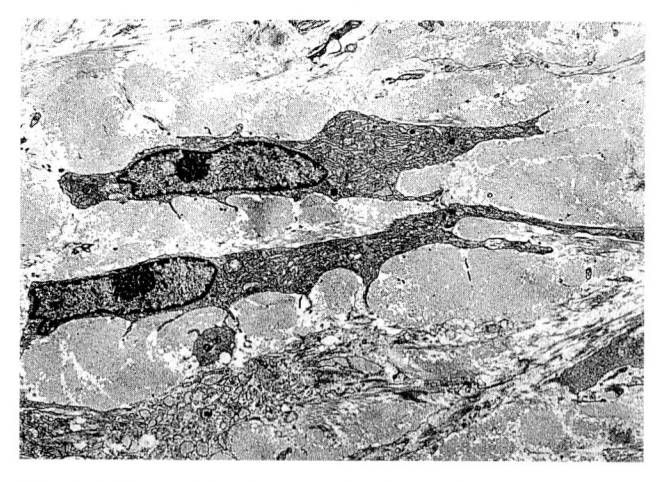

Fig. 3-5. TEM of fibroblasts and collagen. Note the size and plane of section of the collagen fibers. (×3,600.)

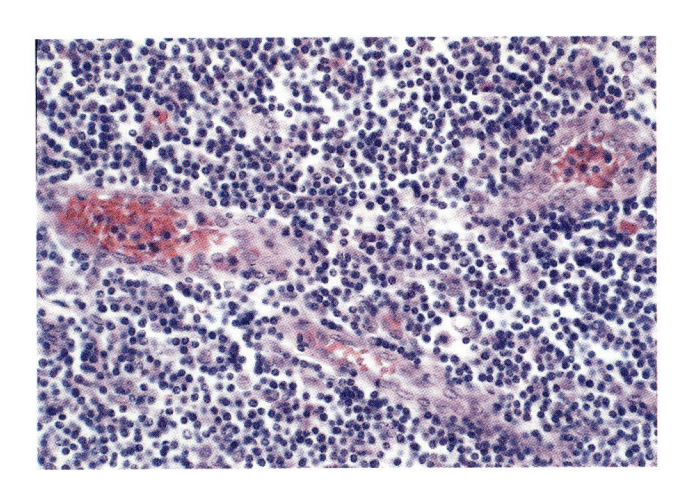

Fig. 3-6. LM of a section of lymph node stained with H&E. The lymph node is an organ composed mainly of lymphocytes, which make up the parenchyma or functional part of the organ, suspended in a net or framework of reticular fibers called the stoma. Reticular fibers are unstained in this section and therefore are not seen. (H&E; ×250.)

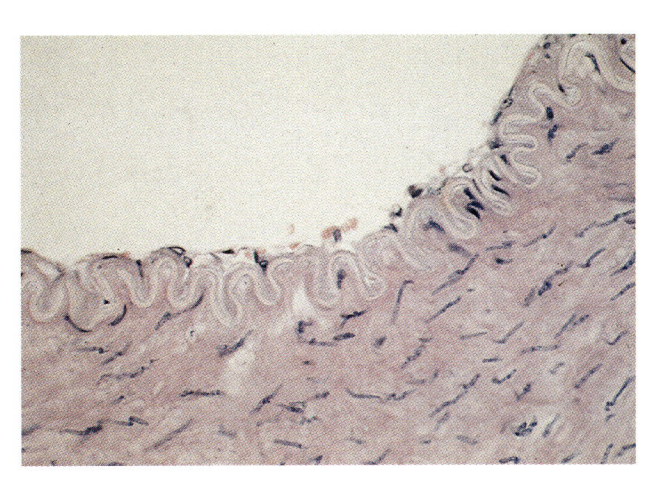

Fig. 3-7. LM of a muscular artery. These arteries have an internal elastic lamina made up of elastic fibers produced by fibroblasts and smooth muscle cells. The lamina is located near the lumen where, in fixed tissue, it has a folded, ribbon-like configuration and is glassy or translucent (hyaline) in appearance. (H&E; ×250.)

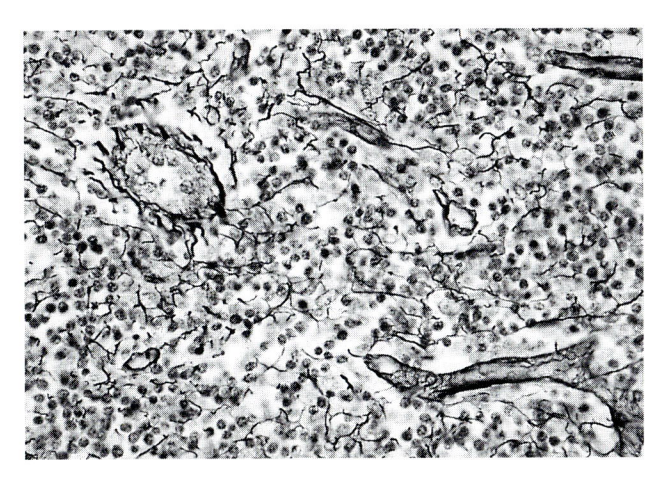

Fig. 3-8. LM of a lymph node permitting visualization of the reticular fibers produced by reticular cells (compare to Fig. 3-6). Note the arrangement of reticular fibers around smooth muscle cells in small blood vessels. (Silver stain; ×250.)

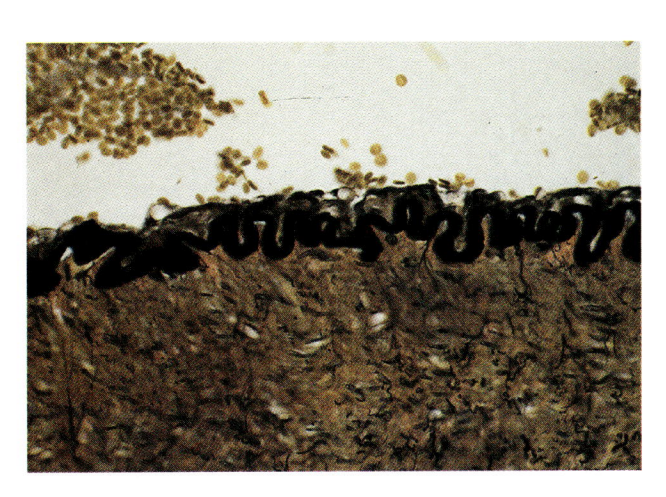

Fig. 3-9. LM of a muscular artery. The internal elastic lamina is selectively stained black. Compare it with the image directly above. (Verhoeff stain) (×250.)

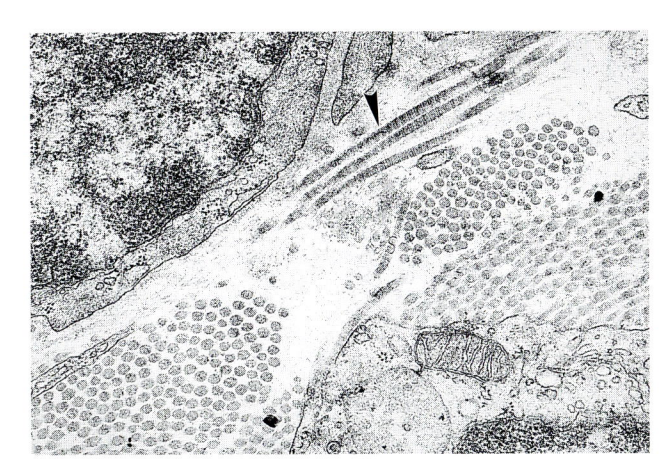

Fig. 3-10. TEM of the extracellular matrix subtending epithelial cells and basal lamina. Reticular fibers are generally smaller in diameter than collagen fibers but also possess 64 to 67 nm periodicity. Observe reticular fibers in longitudinal section adjacent to the basal lamina *(arrowhead)*, and compare them with the cross sections of larger collagen fibers seen in the bundles below. The basal lamina of an epithelial cell *(upper left)* is composed of collagen type IV. (×11,000.)

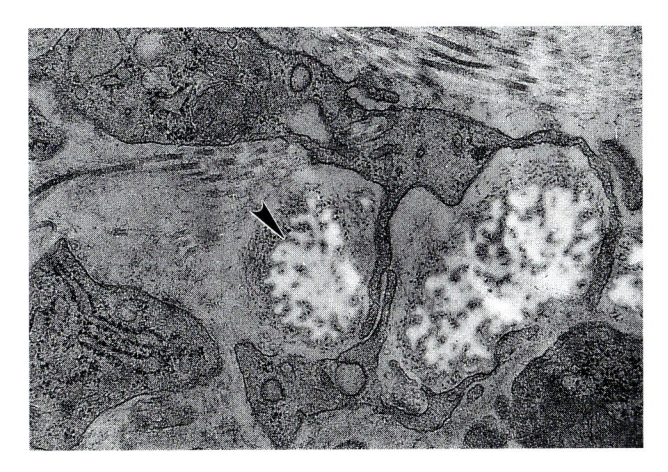

Fig. 3-11. Higher-magnification TEM showing the microfibrillar component *(arrowhead)* of elastic fibers and their arrangement around amorphous elastin (nonstaining in this fixation). Collagen fibers are also seen. (×9,500.)

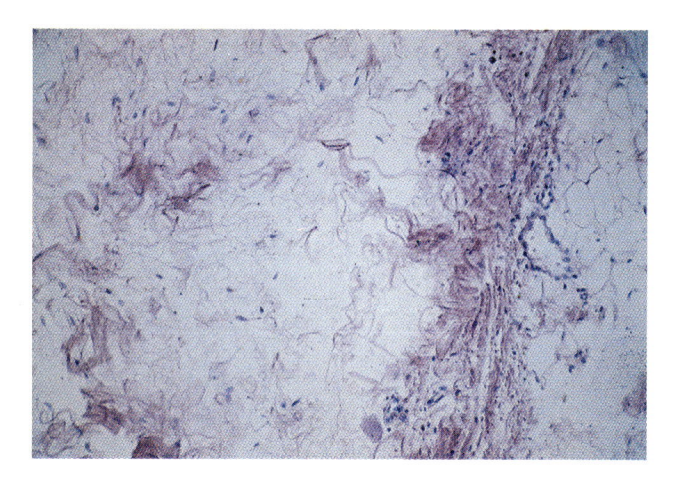

Fig. 3-12. LM of loose connective tissue. Cells and collagen fibers are equally abundant in loose connective tissue. It serves as the interface or packing substance between all other tissues or organs in the body. Compare this to other types of connective tissue on this page. Contrast the relative abundance of cells and fibers and their arrangement. (H&E; ×100.)

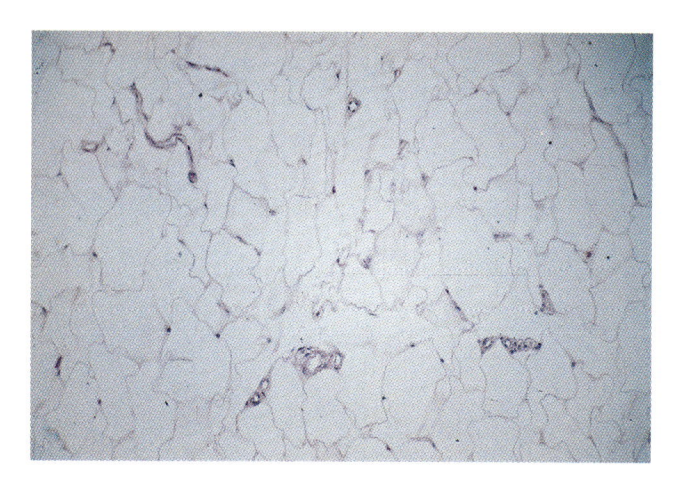

Fig. 3-13. LM of adipose connective tissue. The predominant cell is the adipocyte, or fat cell, surrounded by a delicate network of reticular fibers that attaches it to neighboring cells or tissues. Large bundles of collagen are absent. (H&E; ×100.)

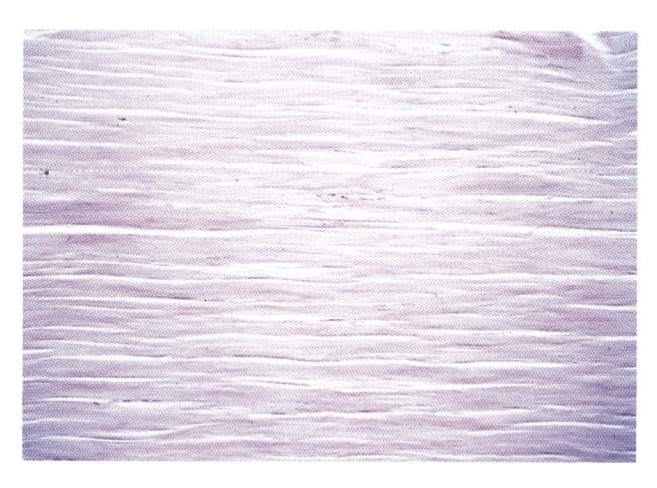

Fig. 3-14. LM of tendon, which is dense regular connective tissue. Large bundles of collagen (type I) fibers are oriented in the same plane. Cellular elements are few and consist mainly of fibroblasts. (H&E; ×100.)

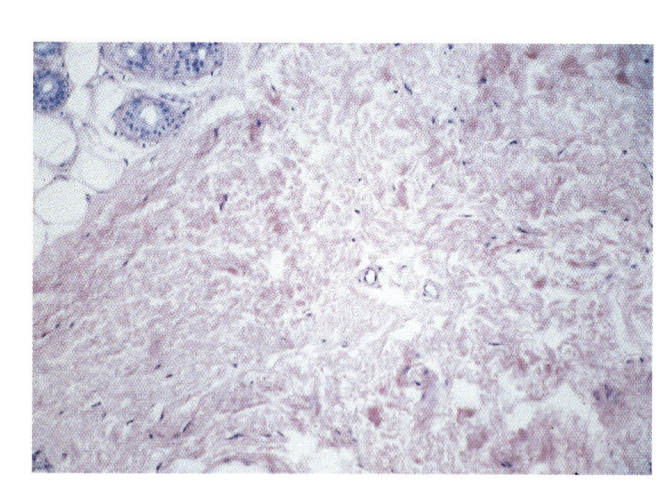

Fig. 3-15. LM showing the dermis of skin, which is dense irregular connective tissue. Collagen bundles predominate but are oriented in several different planes, giving the appearance of an irregular arrangement. (H&E; ×100.)

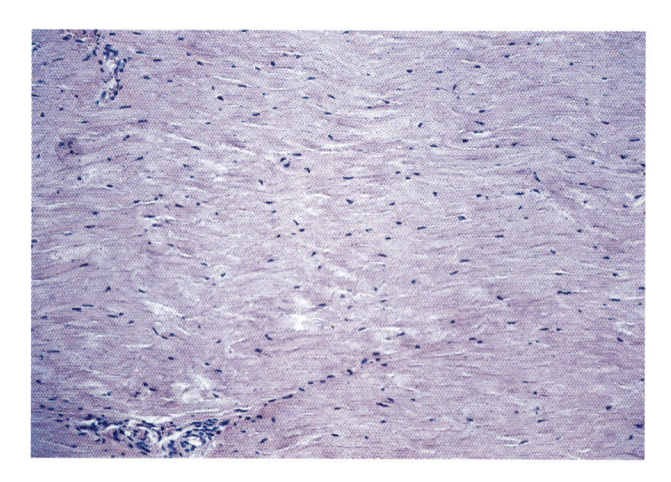

Fig. 3-16. LM of the ligamentum nuchae (interspinous ligament) showing that it consists of a dense regular arrangement of connective tissue fibers with compact masses of elastic fibers predominating. The presence of elastic fibers is masked by the eosinophilic staining of collagen. (H&E; ×100.)

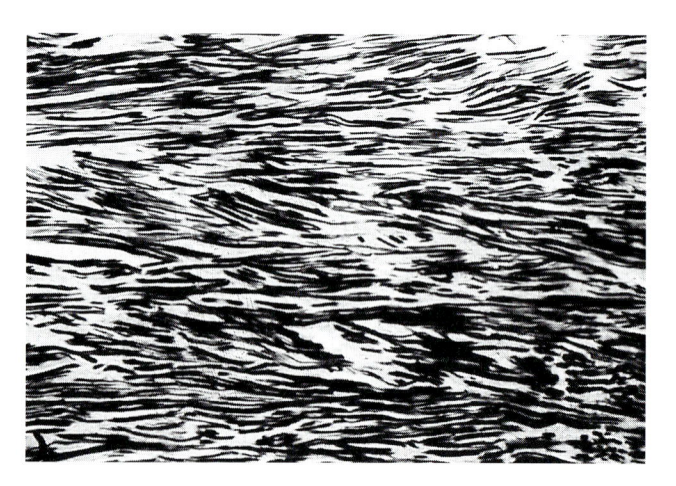

Fig. 3-17. LM of the ligamentum nuchae with an elastin stain, which reveals the presence of large masses of elastic fibers oriented in the same plane. Compare this to Fig. 3-16. (Verhoeff stain; ×100.)

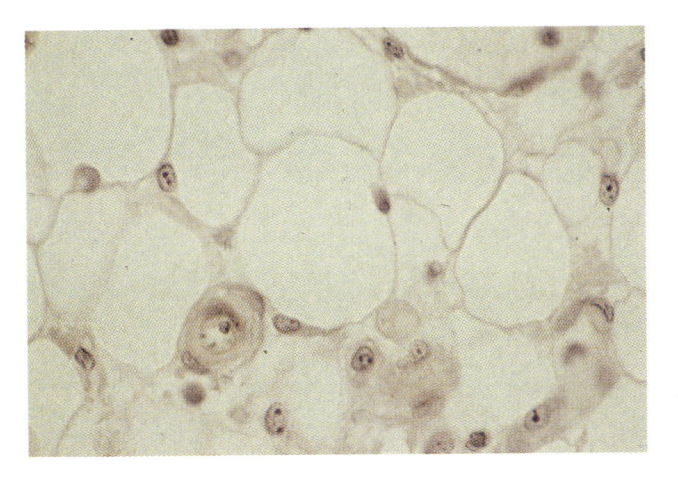

Fig. 3-18. LM of adipocytes. The nuclei are eccentrically placed in an attenuated cytoplasm that surrounds a lipid inclusion. (H&E; ×500.)

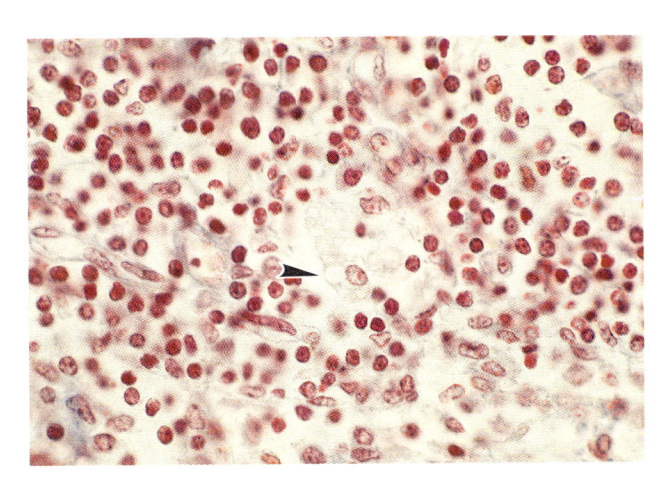

Fig. 3-19. A fixed macrophage *(arrowhead)* by LM in lymph node exhibiting frothy, vacuolated cytoplasm. (Azan stain; ×400.)

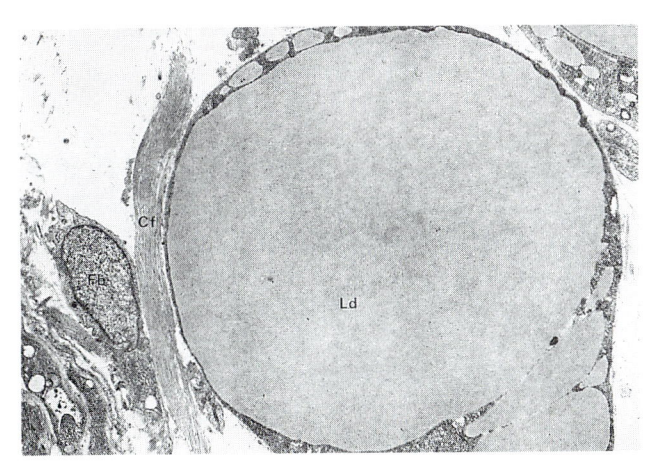

Fig. 3-20. TEM of an adipocyte from the subcutaneous tissue of a 6-month-old fetus. The nucleus *(N)* is pressed to one side of the cell by the large lipid droplet *(Ld)*. The cytoplasm is reduced to a thin rim containing small Golgi complexes and mitochondria. Collagen fibers *(Cf)* and fibroblasts *(Fb)* are seen at left. (×1,600.)

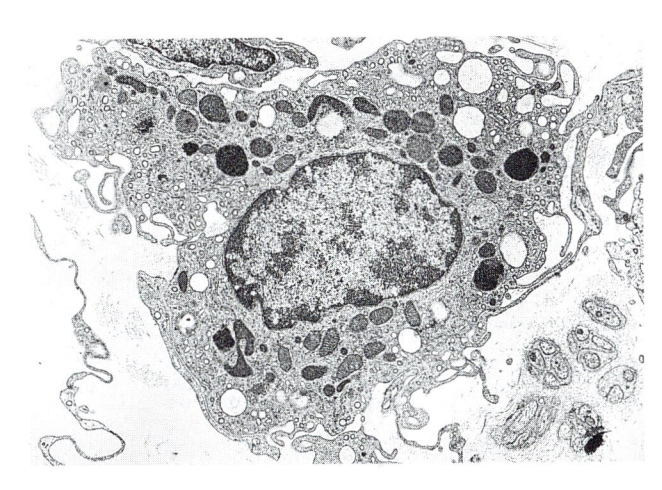

Fig. 3-21. A free macrophage (TEM) exhibiting numerous cytoplasmic infoldings, vacuoles, coated vesicles, and residual bodies. Examples of collagen fibers and unmyelinated nerve fibers are also seen in the extracellular matrix. (×6,000.)

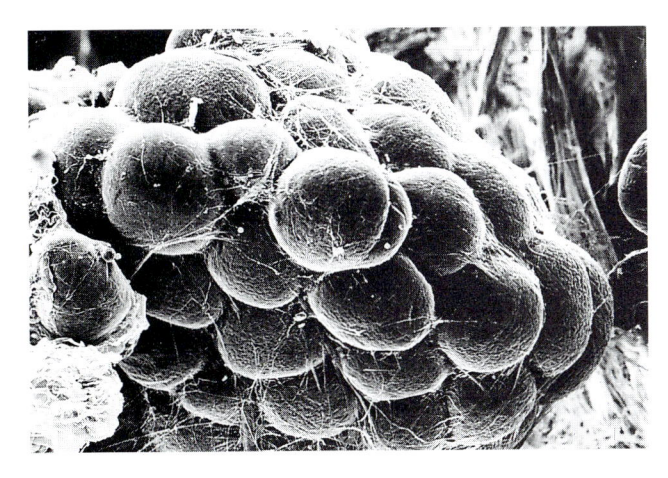

Fig. 3-22. SEM of a cluster of adipocytes. Fibrous strands represent part of the supportive network of reticular fibers. (×150.)

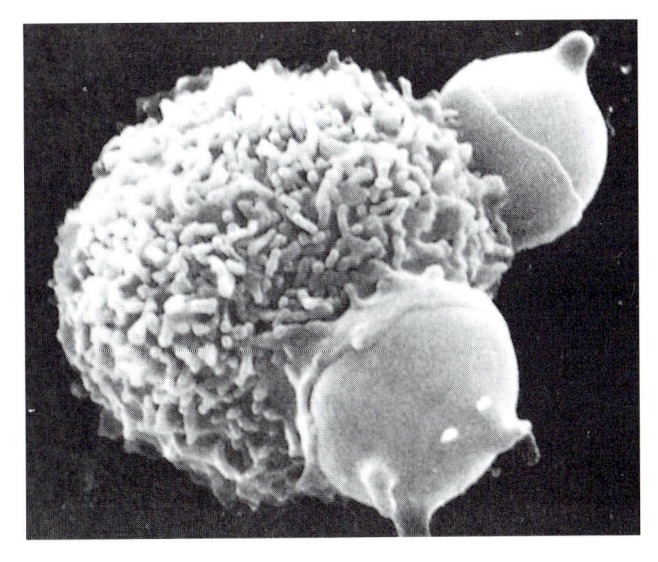

Fig. 3-23. SEM of a mouse macrophage ingesting opsonized red blood cells. (×3,700.)

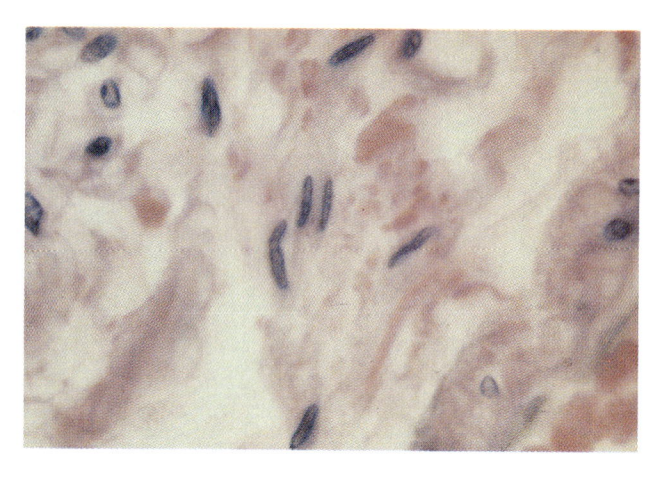

Fig. 3-24. Fibroblasts (in the center of this LM) produce the precursors of the extracellular fibers of connective tissue: collagen, elastin, and reticular fibers. (H&E; ×1,000.)

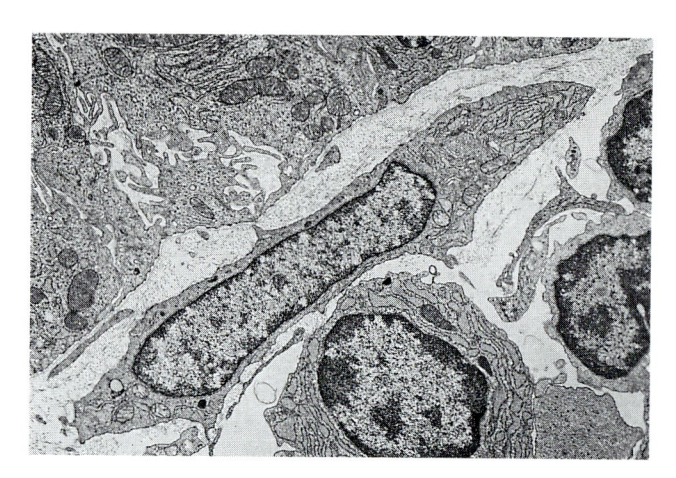

Fig. 3-25. TEM demonstrating an elongate, spindle-shaped fibroblast and, in contrast, a rounded plasma cell below it. The basal portion of a simple columnar epithelial cell is seen at the upper left. (×3,900.)

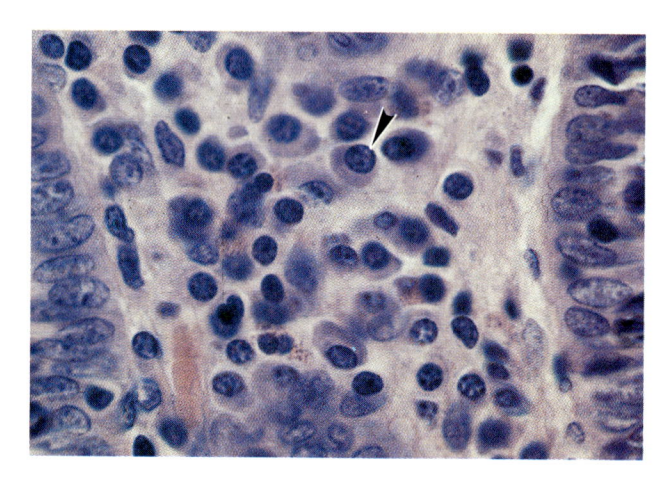

Fig. 3-26. Plasma cells with eccentric nuclei *(arrowhead)* within connective tissue. These cells contain nuclei with a "clock-face" configuration of condensed chromatin and basophilic cytoplasm. By LM, plasma cells are often seen beneath mucosal surfaces (as here, in the intestine) and in lymphoid tissue. (H&E; ×500.)

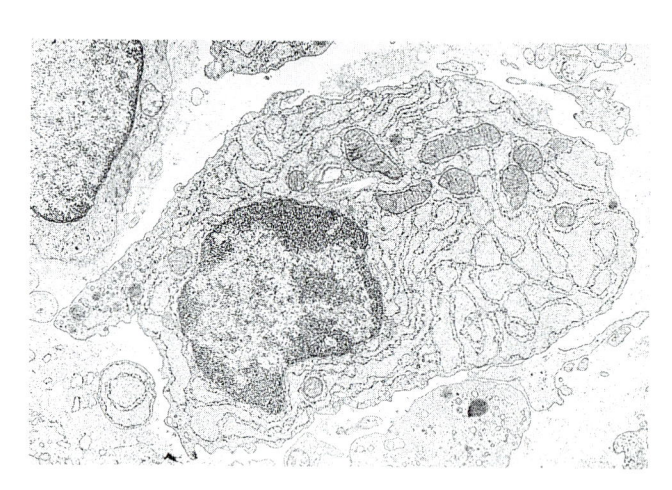

Fig. 3-27. A plasma cell by TEM exhibiting dilated cisternae of rough endoplasmic reticulum. This cell is active in secretion of protein (antibody). Nuclear patterns of euchromatin and heterochromatin are evident. (×3,200.)

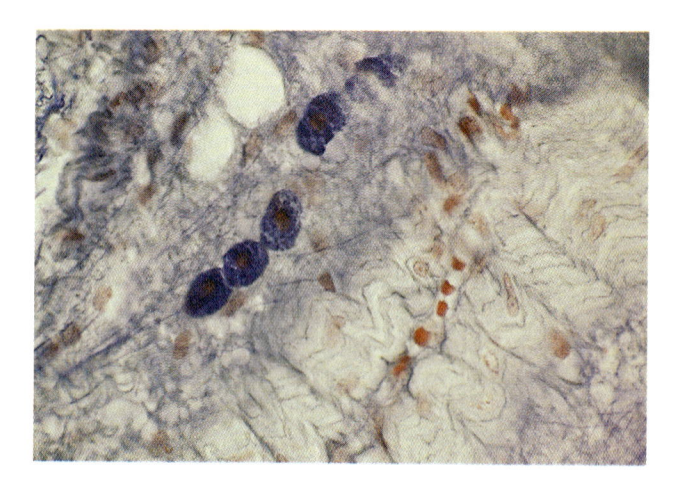

Fig. 3-28. LM of four mast cells in connective tissue. Note large, densely packed granules within the cytoplasm and the central nucleus. (Aldehyde fuchsin stain; ×500.)

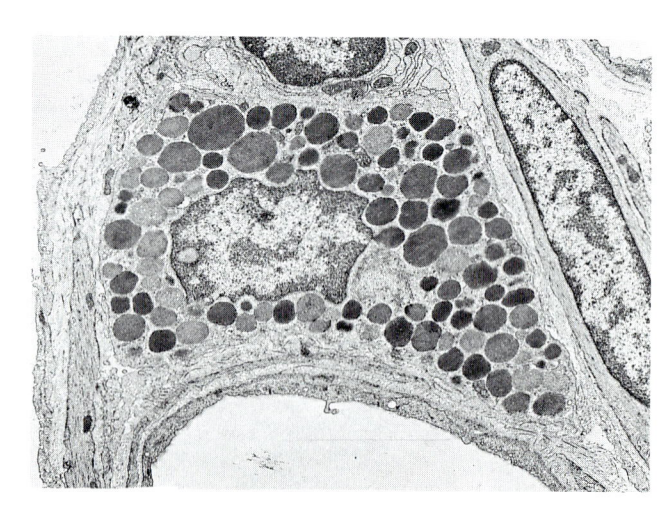

Fig. 3-29. TEM of a mast cell. Granules contain histamine, which increases the permeability of small venules producing edema, and heparin, an anticoagulant. A portion of a capillary is seen at upper right. (×3,200.)

CHAPTER 4

CARTILAGE

CARTILAGE IS A specialized form of connective tissue designed for tissue support and weight bearing. Like other connective tissues, it consists of cells and extracellular matrix. Unlike other connective tissues, the extracellular matrix is modified to form a semirigid gel. Cells embedded within the matrix occupy spaces called **lacunae** and are called **chondrocytes,** whereas peripheral, formative cells are called **chondroblasts.**

The extensive extracellular matrix is produced by **chondrocytes/chondroblasts** and consists of connective tissue fibers, proteoglycans, and chondronectin. Depending on the type of cartilage, connective tissue fibers in the matrix may include type II collagen fibrils exhibiting 64 nm periodicity but not aggregating to form bundles visible by LM, elastic fibers, or type I collagen. Nonfibrous components of the extracellular matrix include **sulfated proteoglycans** and **hyaluronic acid,** which together form **proteoglycan aggregates** and **chondronectin.** The abundant proteoglycans in cartilage are responsible for the high water content and, together with collagen for reinforcement, give cartilage its solid, yet resilient properties. **Chondronectin,** a structural glycoprotein, enhances the adherence of chondrocytes to the extracellular matrix. Production of extracellular matrix results in a peripheral zone surrounding each chondrocyte that is rich in proteoglycans and deficient in collagen. This zone is called the **capsular** or **territorial matrix** because of its intense basophilic staining with hematoxylin and eosin. Located between adjacent chondrocytes is the **interterritorial matrix,** which exhibits less basophilic staining because of its lower content of proteoglycans.

Variations in the cellular and fibrous components of the extracellular matrix result in the classification of three different types of cartilage. The most common type, **hyaline cartilage,** contains type II collagen and a high proportion of sulfated proteoglycans that, because of their similar refractive index, make the collagen fibrils undetectable by LM. Hyaline cartilage serves as a temporary skeleton in the embryo and forms the epiphyseal plate during the growth of long bones. It is also present in the supporting cartilages of the respiratory tract, the costal cartilages of ribs, and the articular surfaces of bones.

Elastic cartilage contains an abundance of elastic fibers within the matrix in addition to type II collagen. Elastic cartilage is more pliable and deformable than hyaline cartilage. It is located in the external ear, auditory tube, epiglottis, and larynx. Both hyaline and elastic cartilage arise from mesenchymal precursors and are therefore surrounded by an interface of dense connective tissue called a **perichondrium.** Cartilage is a unique connective tissue; it is avascular because of its production of factors inhibiting angiogenesis, and therefore it must derive its nutritional support by diffusion from blood vessels located in the perichondrium.

Fibrocartilage, unlike hyaline or elastic cartilage, does not differentiate from mesenchymal cells but, instead, differentiates in areas of dense connective tissue subjected to stress of the demands of weight bearing. Thus fibrocartilage lacks a perichondrium, and the extracellular matrix of fibrocartilage contains a dense network of coarse, eosinophilic, type I collagen fibers easily visible by LM. Both the cell density and the amount of proteoglycans in fibrocartilage are less than that of either hyaline or elastic cartilage. Fibrocartilage can be found in intervertebral disks, pubic symphysis, menisci and ligaments of joints, and at the insertion of tendons or ligaments into bone.

Cartilage undergoes growth by two different mechanisms: **appositional growth,** a result of the differentiation of osteoprogenitor cells in the perichondrium into chondroblasts, and **interstitial growth,** the mitotic division of chondrocytes. Clusters of cells derived from a single chondrocyte within matrix may be designated as **isogenous cell nests or groups.** In cartilage of the epiphyseal plate cell the cells are arranged in rows.

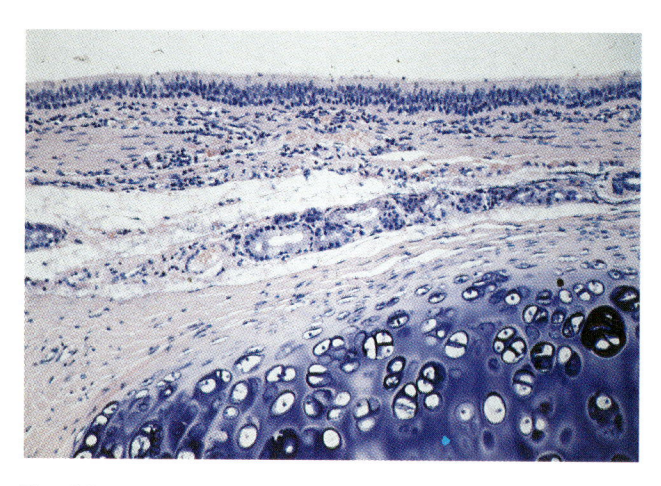

Fig. 4-1. A portion of hyaline cartilage (c) is seen beneath the tracheal epithelium in this LM. An eosinophilic perichondrium surrounds the matrix of the cartilage, which appears basophilic. (H&E; ×300.)

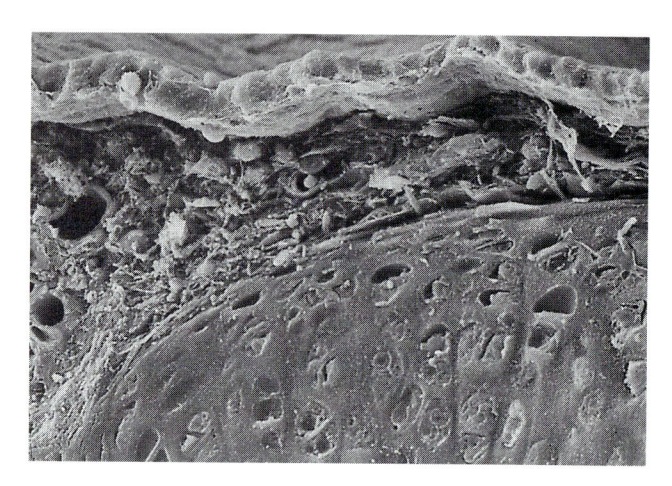

Fig. 4-2. Compare this SEM of tracheal cartilage to the previous LM of the same tissue (Fig. 4-1). Identify the perichondrium, the cartilage matrix, and cavities within the matrix called lacunae that house chondrocytes. (×400.)

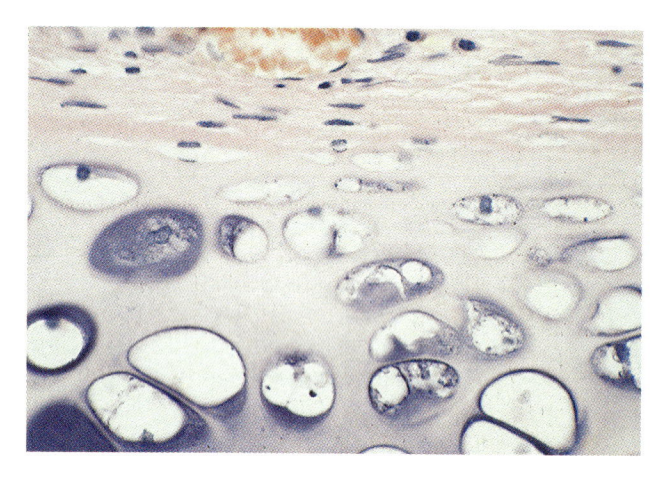

Fig. 4-3. Chondrogenic cells and chondroblasts are located in the basal portion of the perichondrium of hyaline cartilage. (H&E; ×750.)

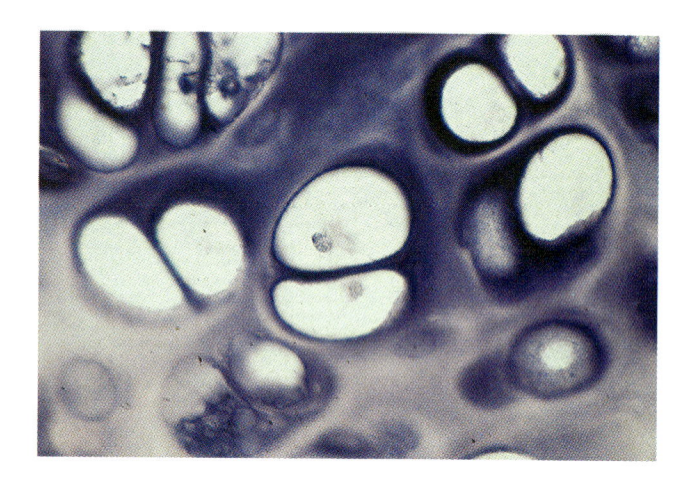

Fig. 4-4. In hyaline cartilage, chondrocytes or groups of chondrocytes called isogenous cell nests are housed in lacunae that are surrounded by basophilic territorial matrix. The chondrocytes have shrunk away from the lacuna walls as a result of the process of fixation. (H&E; ×1,200.)

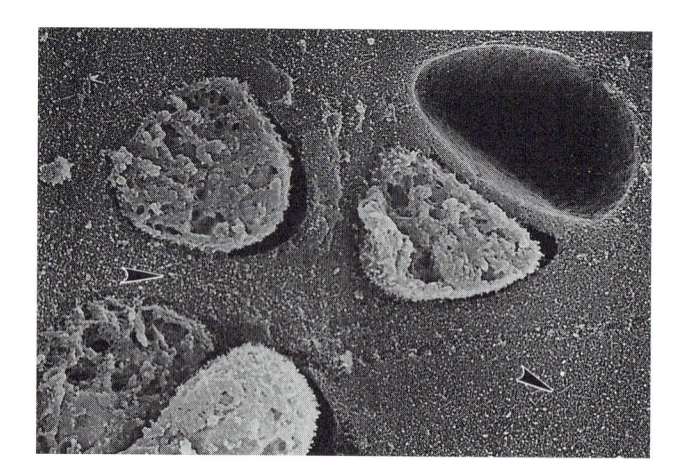

Fig. 4-5. SEM of isogenous cell nests shows chondrocytes covered by short microvilli occupying the entire lacuna. The interterritorial matrix contains thin collagen fibrils (arrowheads). (×3,000.)

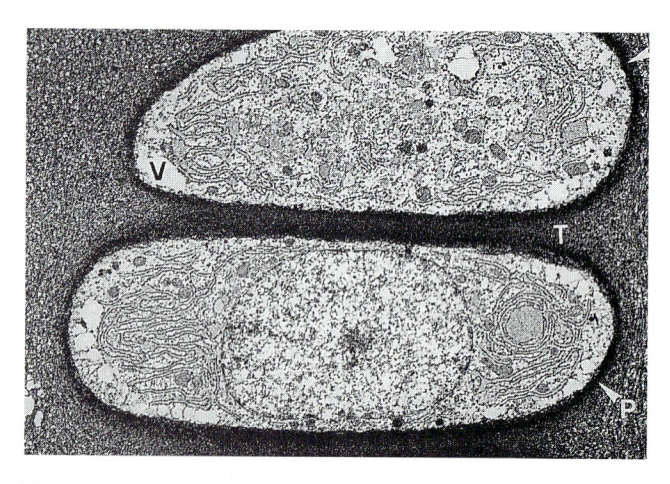

Fig. 4-6. This electron micrograph (TEM) of hyaline cartilage reveals proliferating chondrocytes that were fixed in the presence of ruthenium hexamine trichloride to stabilize proteoglycans in the matrix. P, Pericellular (capsular) matrix; T, interterritorial matrix; V, artifactual vacuoles created by fixation. (×3,900.)

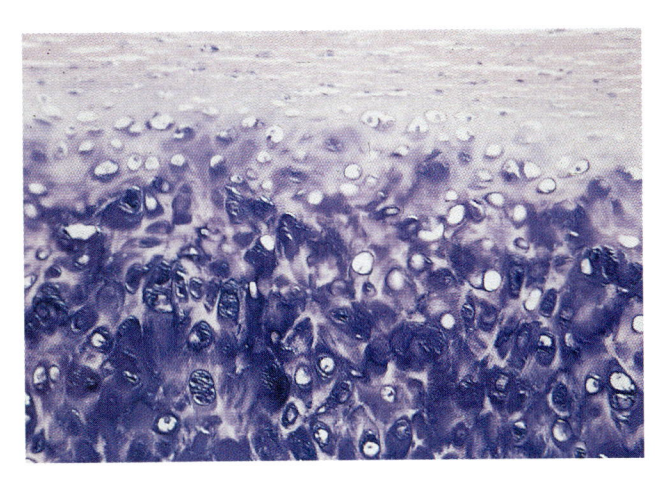

Fig. 4-7. This LM shows elastic cartilage from the epiglottis. Elastic fibers look unstained (or light pink in older specimens) and weave between lacunae. The basophilia of the matrix is due to sulfated glycosaminoglycans. Perichondrium is at the top of the section. (H&E; ×300.)

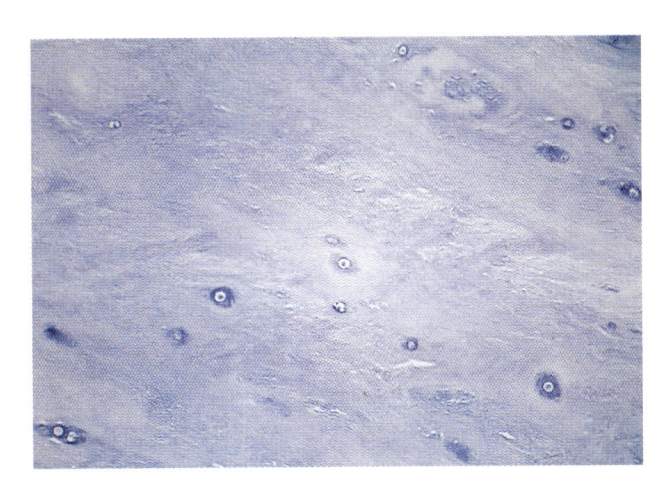

Fig. 4-8. In this LM of fibrocartilage observe the shape of the cells, their relative numbers, and the presence of fiber bundles. (H&E; ×300.)

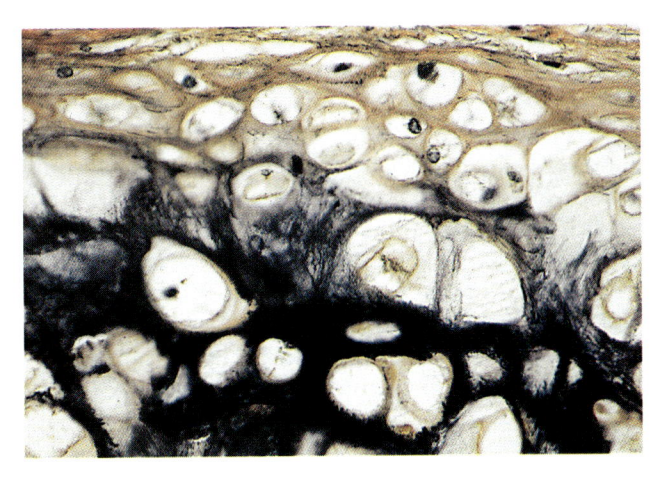

Fig. 4-9. In this high-magnification LM of elastic cartilage and perichondrium the elastic fibers are selectively stained black. Compare it to Fig. 4-7. (Verhoeff stain; ×750.)

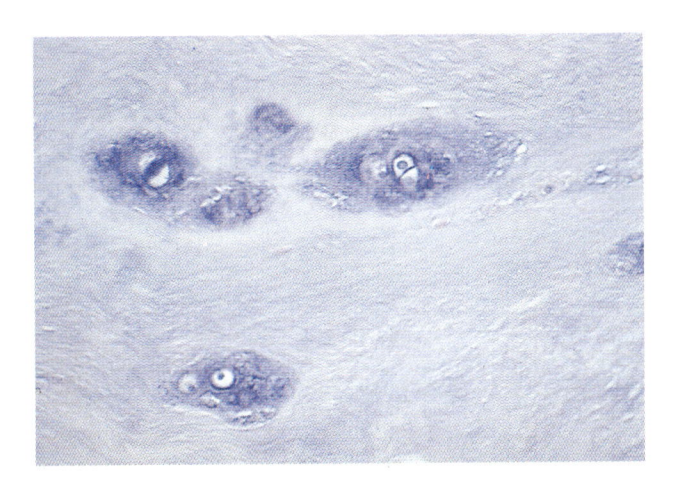

Fig. 4-10. A high-magnification LM of fibrocartilage demonstrates cell nests and their territorial matrix. (Compare to Fig. 4-8.) (H&E; ×750.)

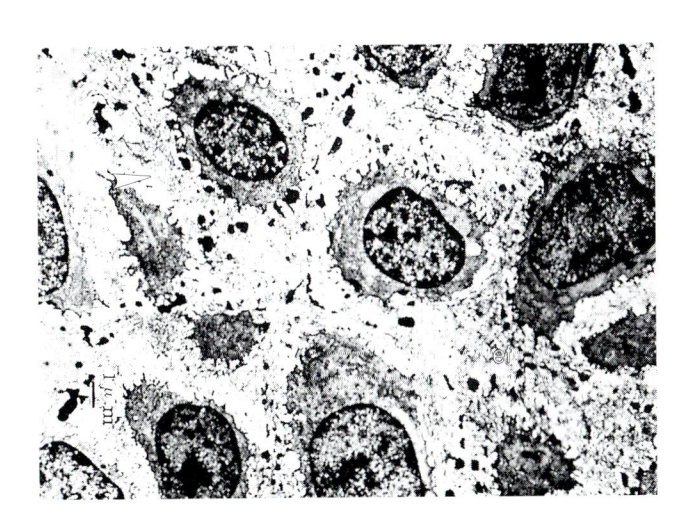

Fig. 4-11. TEM of chondrocytes in elastic cartilage. The interterritorial matrix contains slender collagen fibrils *(arrowhead)*, proteoglycan particles, and strongly electron-dense elastic fibers *(ef)*, some of which are associated with the surfaces of chondrocytes. (×3,200.)

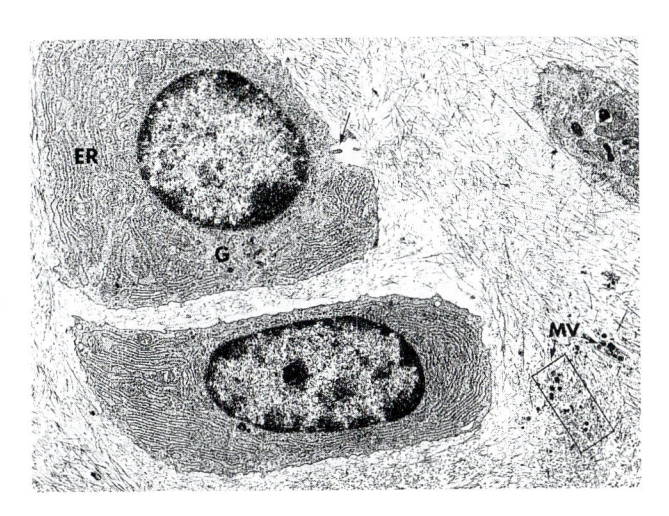

Fig. 4-12. By TEM note the presence of aggregations of collagen fibers in the matrix of fibrocartilage. Compare this image with the TEM of hyaline cartilage (Fig. 4-6) showing dispersed collagen fibrils. *ER*, Endoplasmic reticulum; *G*, Golgi; *Mv*, matrix vesicles. (×5,600.)

CHAPTER 5

BONE

BONE IS A specialized connective tissue that has a calcified extracellular matrix designed to provide a rigid framework for support and protection of soft tissues of the body. Bones also form a lever system that, when combined with skeletal muscle, makes locomotion possible. In addition to these functions, bone serves as a reservoir for developing blood cells and for ions (i.e., calcium phosphate) that can be stored or released in a regulated manner to maintain homeostasis of body fluids.

Cells embedded within the calcified matrix occupy spaces called **lacunae** and are called **osteocytes,** whereas cells on peripheral surfaces of bone are called **osteoblasts.** Processes of adjacent osteocytes occupy thin channels in the calcified matrix called **canaliculi** that allow the cells to communicate via gap junctions. Cells involved in the remodeling of calcified bone matrix are called **osteoclasts.** Osteoclasts are often seen within surface depressions in the matrix known as **Howship's lacunae.**

The extracellular matrix of bone consists of both inorganic components—hydroxyapatite crystals and amorphous calcium phosphate—and organic components—including type I collagen, proteoglycans, and glycoproteins (sialoprotein and osteocalcin).

The surfaces of bone are completely covered by layers of **osteoprogenitor cells. Periosteum** covers the external surface of bone and consists of osteoprogenitor cells and fibroblasts embedded in a dense fibrous connective tissue layer. Bundles of collagen in the periosteum called **Sharpey's fibers** penetrate the bone and anchor the periosteum to the bone matrix. The internal surfaces of bone are lined by **endosteum,** which consists of a single layer of osteoprogenitor cells and delicate connective tissue.

Two types of bone can be distinguished by gross examination: **compact bone** and **cancellous** or **spongy bone.** Compact bone consists of consecutive layers or lamellae that are laid down parallel to one another or of lamellae in concentric circular arrays around a vascular channel. The former constitute **inner** and **outer circumferential lamellae** in long bones, whereas the concentric lamellae surrounding blood vessels form a microscopic unit referred to as a **Haversian system** or **osteon.** Collagen fibers within individual lamellae are parallel to one another but are laid down perpendicular (or in orthogonal array) to those in adjacent lamellae, thereby giving greater strength to the bone as additional lamellae are formed. Surrounding each osteon is an amorphous layer called **cementing substance,** which consists mainly of ground substance and a few collagen fibers. **Interstitial lamellae** are irregularly shaped groups of parallel lamellae that lie between adjacent osteons as a result of incomplete removal of osteons during growth and remodeling of bone.

Compact bone forms the surfaces of all bones and therefore surrounds cancellous or spongy bone that is found inside the epiphyses (ends of long bones), or within flat bones. Spongy bone consists of a three-dimensional array of spicules or trabeculae made up of parallel lamellae. In long bones, spongy bone serves to transmit the load of weight bearing from the larger articular surface to the narrower diaphyseal shaft.

During the formation of each bone, two types of bone tissue appear. The first is called **primary, woven,** or **immature bone.** It is identified by an irregular orientation of collagen fibers, a low mineral content, and a high proportion of osteocytes. Immature bone tissue is temporary and is replaced, in the adult, by **secondary bone** tissue, which shows a characteristic lamellar arrangement, a higher mineral content, and a lower proportion of osteocytes.

The formation of bone tissue occurs by either **intramembranous** or **endochondral ossification.** Intramembranous bone formation takes place within richly vascularized condensations of mesenchymal tissue, where mesenchymal cells differentiate into osteoblasts and produce primary or immature bone matrix. This deposition of immature bone is followed by remodeling with the formation of secondary or mature bone. In endochondral bone formation, condensations of mesenchymal cells first give rise to a hyaline cartilage model of the bone. Calcification of the peripheral diaphyseal region in the cartilagenous model leads to formation of a periosteal collar followed by degeneration of internal chondrocytes. An osteogenic bud containing blood vessels penetrates the periosteal collar and brings osteoblasts into the degenerating cartilagenous matrix, thereby forming the **primary ossification center.** Later in embryonic development, **secondary ossification centers** develop at the epiphyseal ends of each long bone. As growth of the long bone continues, the remaining hyaline cartilage becomes restricted either to the articular surfaces (which persist throughout adult life) or to the epiphyseal plate, which serves as a region permitting growth in bone length until adulthood. At this time a boney union of the diaphysis and epiphyses occurs, and no further increase in growth of the long bone can take place.

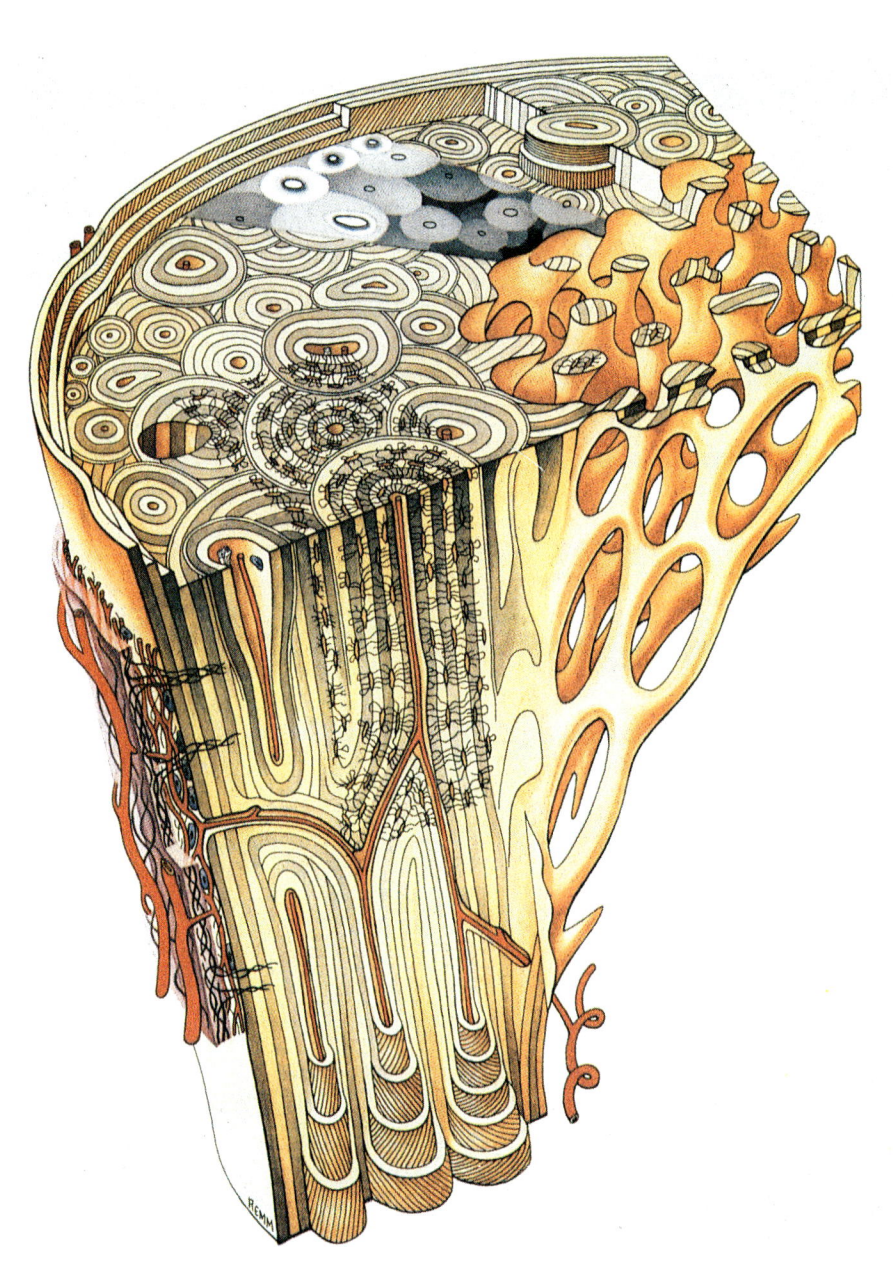

Fig. 5-1. Microstructure of mature bone in both transverse section *(top)* and longitudinal section and areas of compact and cancellous bone. Central area in transverse section simulates a microradiograph, with densities reflecting variations in mineralization. Note general construction of osteons, distribution of osteocyte lacunae, Haversian canals and their contents, resorption spaces, and different views of structural basis of bone lamellation.

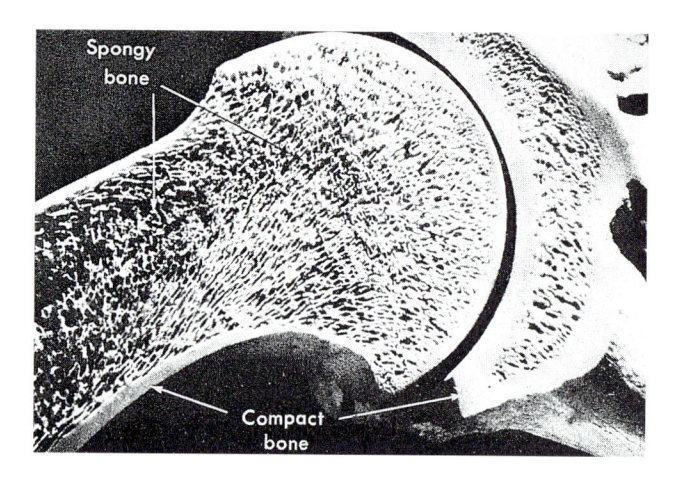

Fig. 5-2. Macrophotograph of head of humerus demonstrating spongy (cancellous) bone in marrow cavity and compact bone externally.

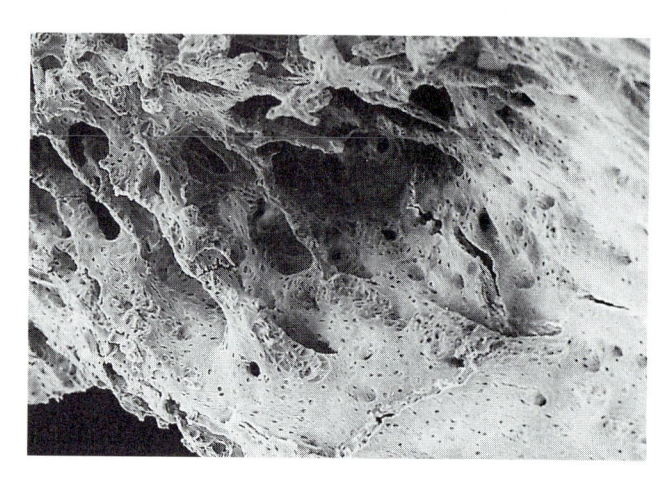

Fig. 5-3. SEM of long bone showing endosteal surface adjoining marrow cavity and demonstrating junction between cancellous bone with trabeculae *(upper left)* and adjacent compact bone *(lower right)*. (×30.)

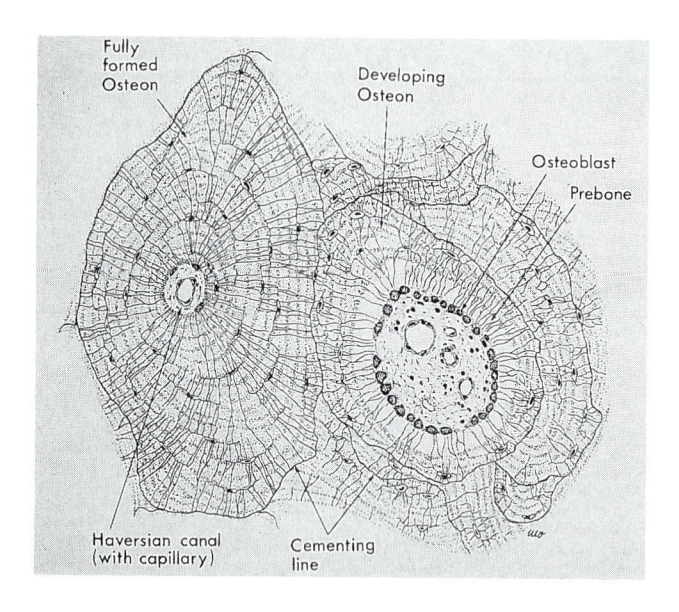

Fig. 5-4. A drawing of osteons illustrating organization of mature and developing Haversian systems. Observe arrangement of lamellae and radial distribution of canaliculi between lacunae in adjacent lamellae.

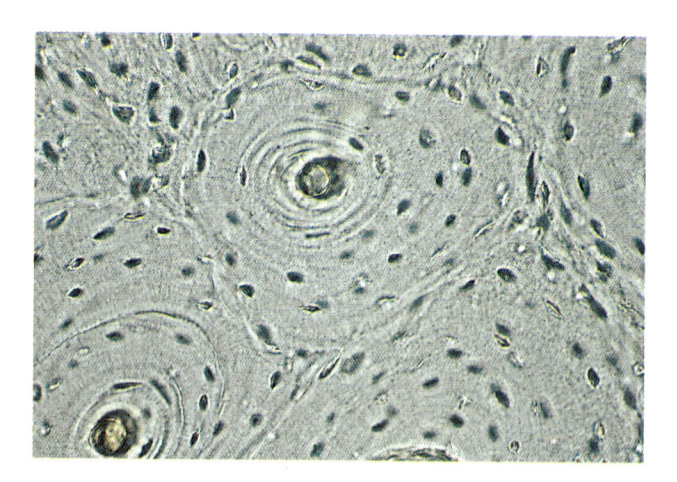

Fig. 5-5. LM of ground bone showing osteon in cross section. Compare it to Fig. 5-4, then locate lacunae of osteocytes, Haversian canal, lamellae, and cementing line surrounding osteon. (×150.)

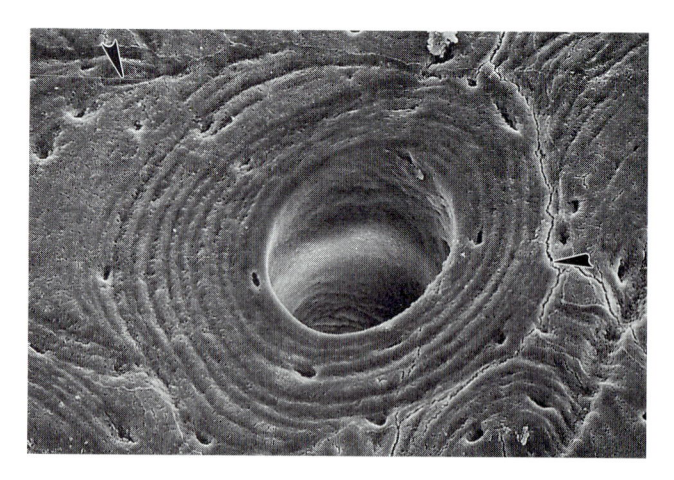

Fig. 5-6. SEM of osteon in cross section. Lamellae, lacunae, and cementing line *(arrowheads)* of the osteon are clearly seen. (×450.)

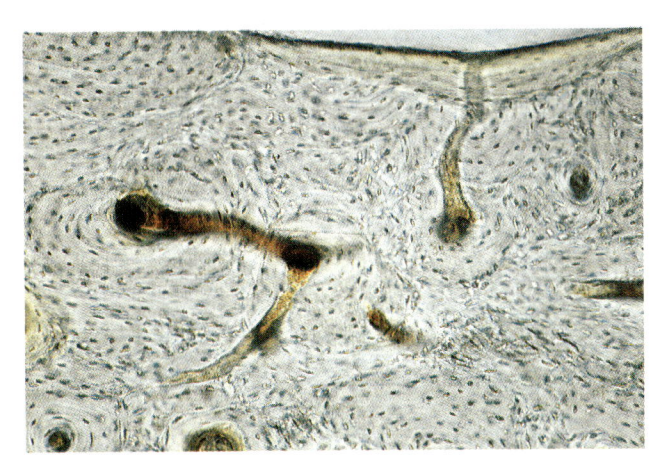

Fig. 5-7. LM of ground bone (from diaphysis of long bone) seen in cross section. Marrow cavity bordered by inner circumferential lamellae is seen at top. Identify Haversian canals, osteons, Volkmann's canals, and osteocytes in lacunae. (×100.)

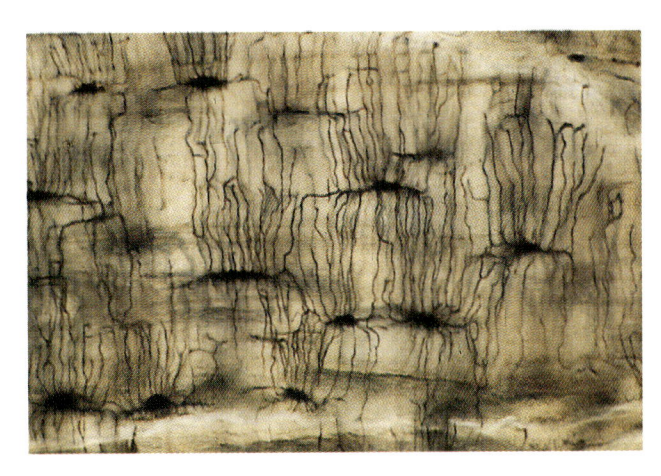

Fig. 5-8. LM section of ground bone. Observe that lacunae (containing osteocytes) are joined by canaliculi through which osteocytes may maintain physiologic and anatomic contact with each other. (×650.)

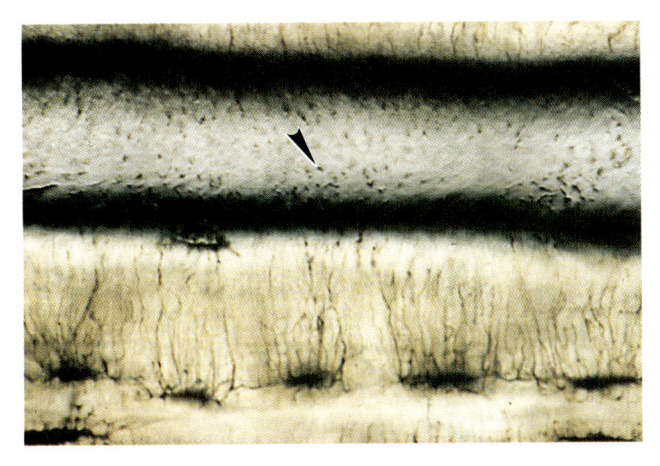

Fig. 5-9. High-magnification LM of Haversian canal in longitudinal section (top) of ground bone revealing openings of canaliculi (arrowhead). Osteocytes in lacunae (below) receive metabolites from vessels in Haversian canal by way of diffusion and intercellular coupling (gap junctions) of osteocytic processes within canaliculi. (×650.)

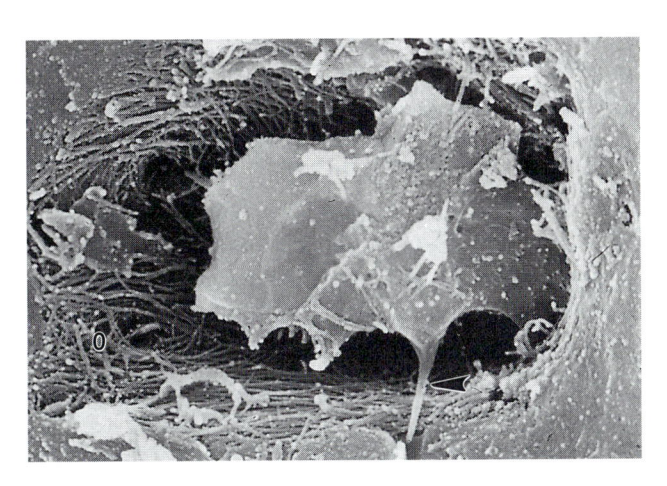

Fig. 5-10. Osteocyte within lacuna (SEM) extending a cytoplasmic process (arrowhead) into canaliculus below. Observe unmineralized collagen, called osteoid (o), surrounding cell body. (SEM; ×9,000.)

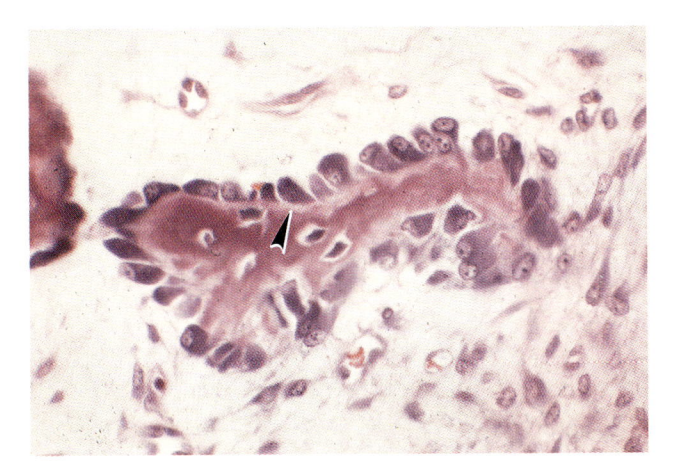

Fig. 5-11. Columnarlike osteoblasts in pig embryo arrayed on bone spicule during intramembranous bone formation (LM). Osteoblasts are very basophilic because of production and secretion of protein (collagen, etc.). Osteoid (arrowhead) appears as lightly stained areas beneath osteoblasts. (H&E; ×400.)

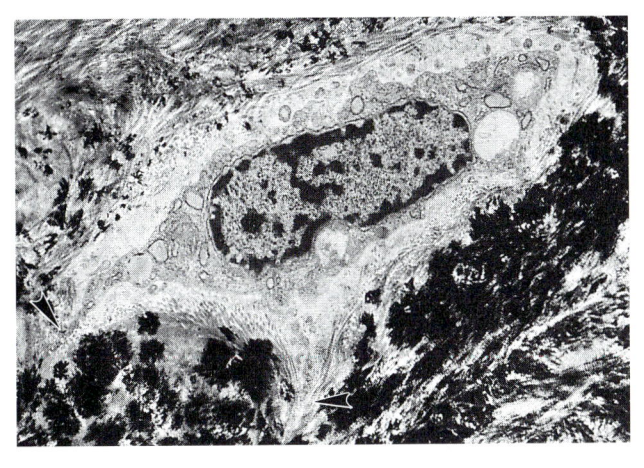

Fig. 5-12. Bone formation by osteoblasts seen by TEM. Unmineralized periosteum is at upper left. Electron-dense bone matrix (mineralized) surrounds cytoplasmic processes (arrowheads) extending into canaliculi. (×6,300.)

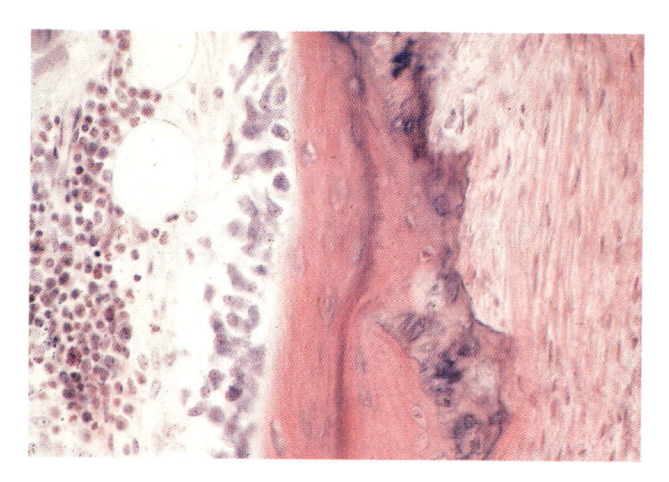

Fig. 5-13. LM showing compact bone *(center)* with osteocytes in lacunae. To left of bone are osteoblasts, elongate basophilic cells involved in secretion of bone matrix. Periosteum covers bone *(on right)*. (H&E; ×250.)

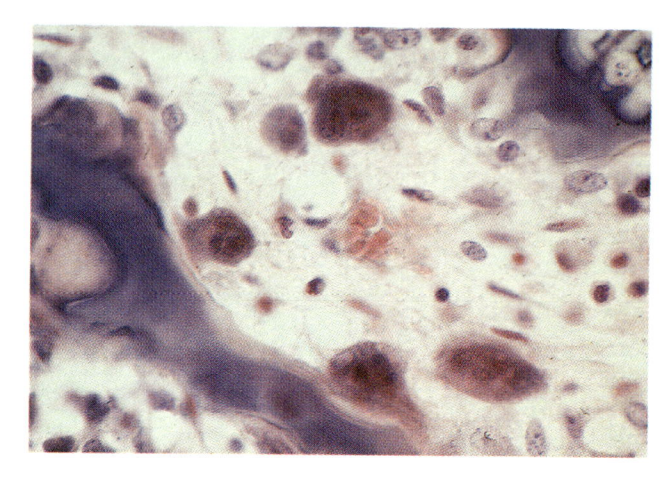

Fig. 5-14. Multinucleated, eosinophilic osteoclasts seen by LM. One osteoclast *(lower center)* is in a Howship's lacuna, a cavity or depression in bone caused by cell's action in resorbing bone matrix. (H&E; ×400.)

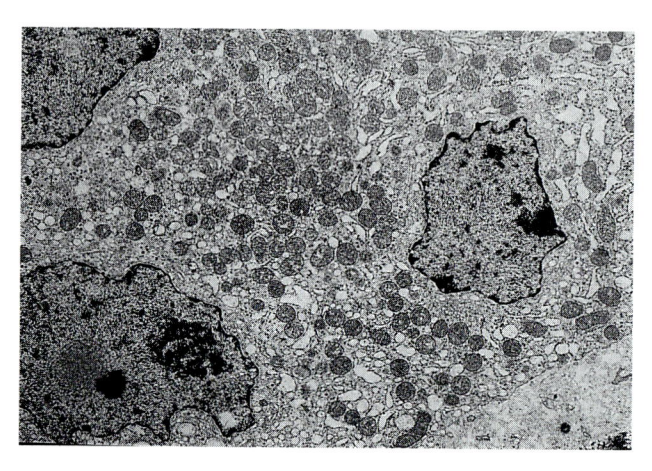

Fig. 5-15. Osteoclast as seen by TEM. Notice numerous mitochondria and multiple nuclei. Bone matrix is at upper left. (×4,200.)

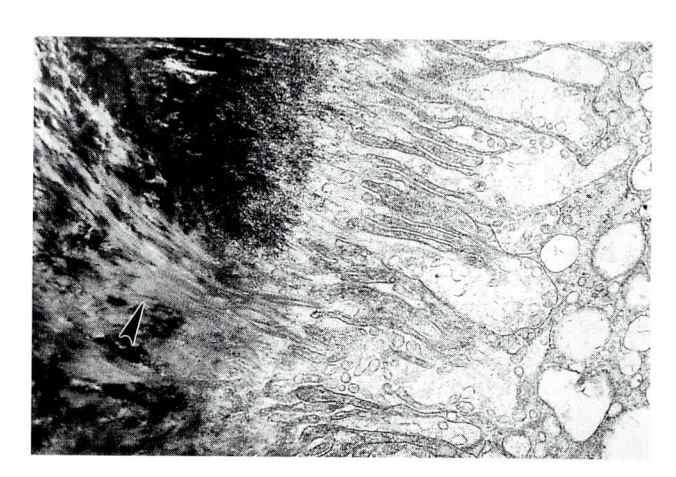

Fig. 5-16. TEM of part of an osteoclast in contact with bone *(left)*, which it is resorbing. Folds of osteoclast plasmalemma, called "ruffled border," serve to increase surface area of cell, which is active in resorption. Note collagen fibers *(arrowhead)* in bone matrix. (×8,300.)

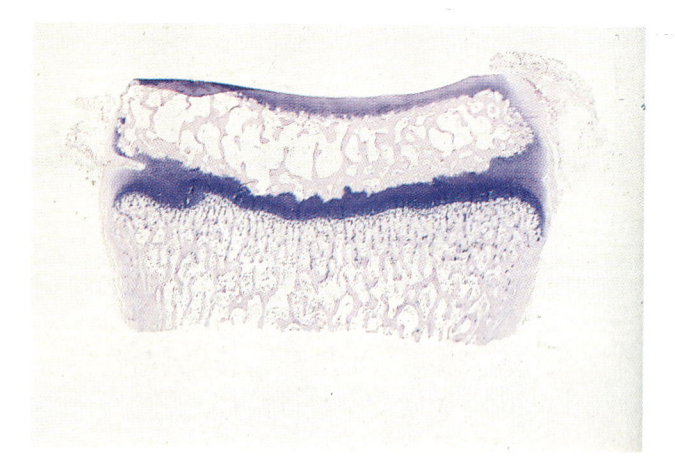

Fig. 5-17. Macrophotograph of long bone. Thin articular cartilage covering epiphysis is seen above, while deeply basophilic cartilage of epiphyseal plate separates epiphysis from metaphysis. (H&E; ×4.)

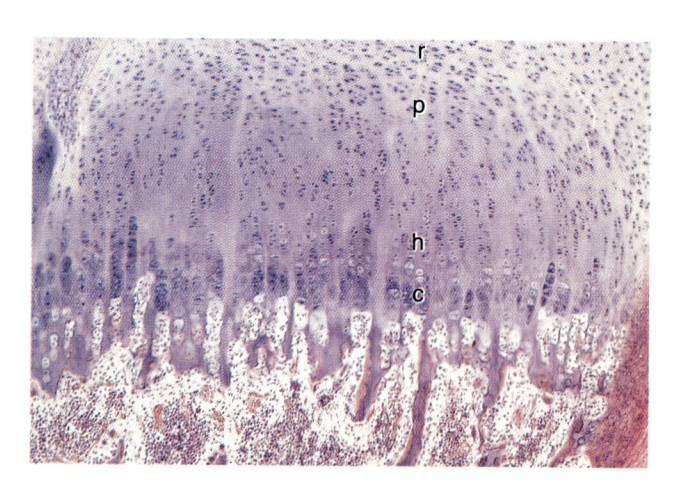

Fig. 5-18. LM of epiphyseal plate. Zone of resting cartilage *(r)* is seen at top and marrow cavity at bottom. Spicules of calcified cartilage matrix with thin depositions of newly formed bone on their surfaces project into marrow cavity. *p*, Zones of proliferation; *h*, hypertrophy; *c*, calcification. (H&E; ×100.)

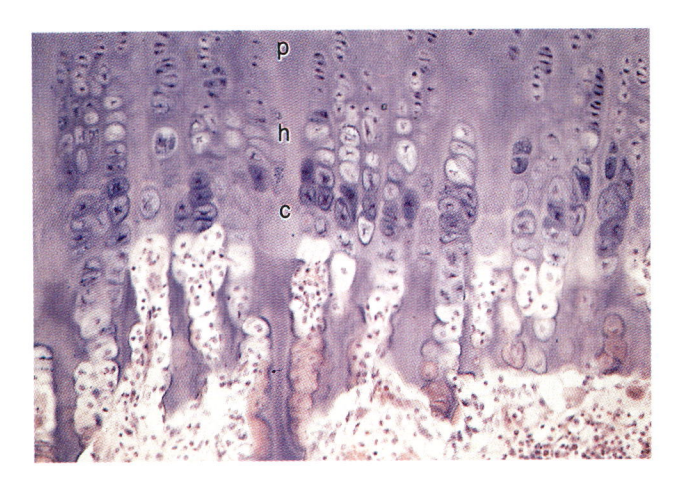

Fig. 5-19. LM of epiphyseal plate showing *(top to bottom)* zone of proliferation *(p)*, where chondrocytes in lacunae divide, producing growth of cartilage; zone of hypertrophy *(h)*, where cells accumulate glycogen; and zone of calcification *(c)*, where chondrocytes die and matrix calcifies. Newly formed (eosinophilic) bone is seen on some spicules of calcified cartilage. (H&E; ×200.)

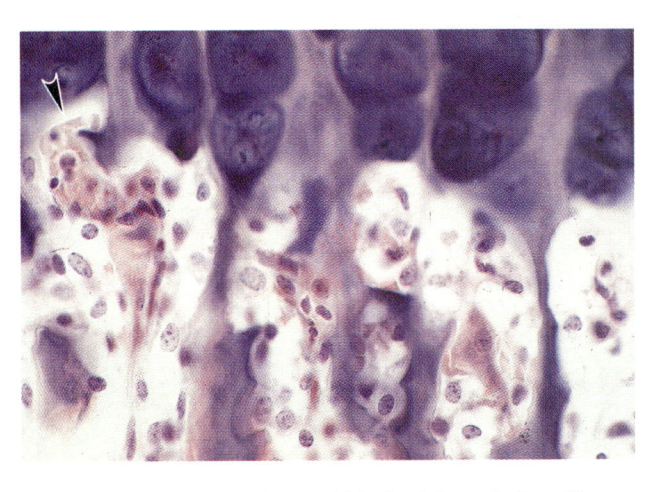

Fig. 5-20. Higher magnification LM of epiphyseal plate. Hypertrophied chondrocytes have died in zone of calcification, and invading vascular buds *(arrowhead)* from marrow have opened lacunae in calcified cartilage. Bone is deposited by osteoblasts on remaining spicules of cartilage. Remodeling of bone/cartilage matrix by osteoclasts is an active process in this region. (H&E; ×300.)

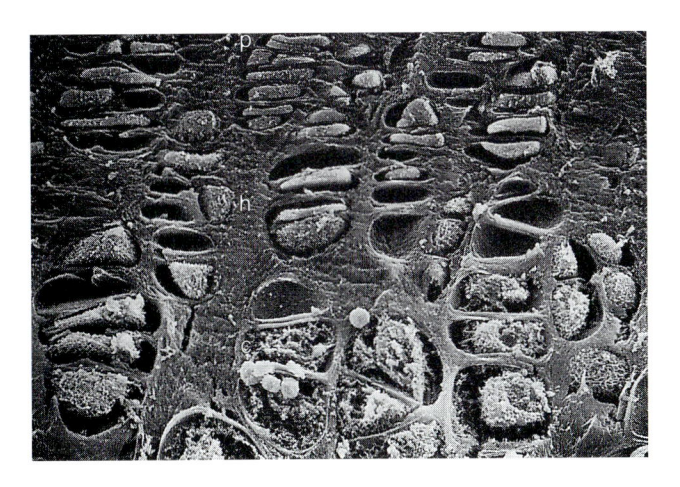

Fig. 5-21. SEM of cartilage of epiphyseal plate showing zones of proliferation *(p)*, hypertrophy *(h)*, and calcification *(c)*. Compare with Fig. 5-19. (×500.)

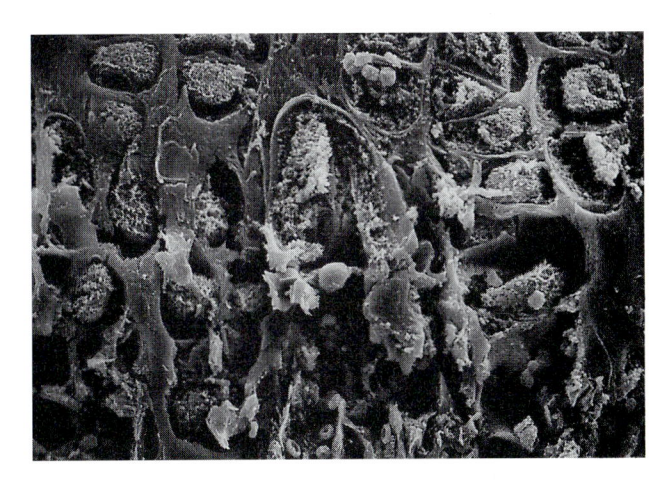

Fig. 5-22. SEM of epiphyseal plate showing zone of calcification and adjacent marrow *(below)*. Compare with Fig. 5-20. (×500.)

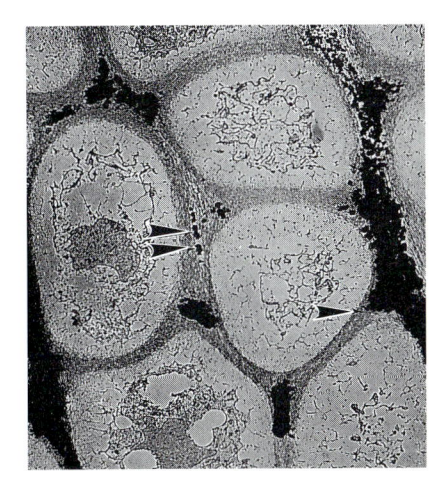

Fig. 5-23. TEM of hypertrophied chondrocytes in the epiphyseal plate. Deposits of hydroxyapatite crystals *(arrowheads)* are located at periphery of lacunae, which contain remnants of degenerating chondrocytes. (×1,350.)

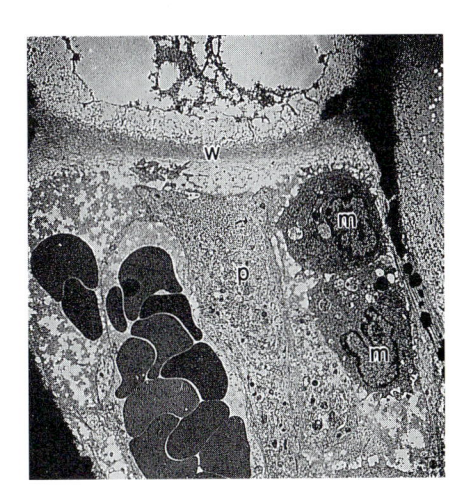

Fig. 5-24. TEM of zone of calcification of epiphyseal plate. When chondrocytes die as a result of changes in matrix, osteoclasts and capillaries in the vicinity break down noncalcified collagenous crosswalls between lacunae. Osteogenic cells then migrate into resulting cavities in calcified cartilage and begin deposition of new bone. *w*, Lacuna crosswall decalcified; *p*, osteoprogenitor cell; *m*, monocytes. (×1,750.)

CHAPTER 6
PERIPHERAL BLOOD

BLOOD is a unique connective tissue in that the extracellular matrix forms a circulating fluid compartment called **plasma** (55% by volume) in which are suspended the cellular elements (45% by volume). The fluid plasma compartment contains proteins (i.e., globulins, albumins, fibrinogen, and assorted enzymes), hormones, metabolites, various salts in solution, and colloidal substances such as chylomicrons in dispersed form. The extracellular matrix of typical connective tissues usually contains formed connective tissue fibers such as collagen or elastin; however, in peripheral blood, fibrous proteins are not normally formed unless clotting has initiated the polymerization of the soluble monomeric blood protein, fibrinogen, into insoluble fibrin fibers. **Serum** is equivalent to plasma after removal of fibrinogen and other elements of clotting.

The cellular elements of blood include **erythrocytes** (red blood cells), **leukocytes** (white blood cells), and circulating cytoplasmic fragments known as **platelets**, all of which are formed by hemopoiesis in bone marrow and lymphoid tissues. **Red blood cells** are anucleate biconcave disks that mainly function within the cardiovascular system through their efficient transport of oxygen and carbon dioxide to and from different tissues/organs in the body. Platelets are cytoplasmic fragments derived from megakaryocytes, and like red blood cells, they are anucleate. They play an important role in the clotting of blood and also serve as the source of platelet-derived growth factor, an important cytokine in the body.

Two distinct categories of **white blood cells** have been identified based on their nuclear morphology and the presence of characteristic specific granules within their cytoplasm. The first category, **agranular** or **mononuclear leukocytes,** includes **lymphocytes** and **monocytes,** which possess round or slightly indented nuclei and small lysosomes known as azure granules. Lymphocytes can be subdivided into two important groups based on their function. **T lymphocytes** are long-lived cells involved in **cellular immunity,** including delayed hypersensitivity, graft rejection, and, for some antigens, the modulation of antibody responses. Subsets of T cells regulating these processes are referred to as T helper cells, T suppressor cells, cytotoxic T cells, and memory T cells. **B lymphocytes** are primarily involved in **humoral immunity** and are responsible, after appropriate stimulation, for the formation in various tissues of plasma cells that secrete immunoglobulins.

Monocytes circulate for brief periods in peripheral blood and then migrate into tissues where they differentiate into macrophages. Their primary role is the phagocytosis and digestion of microorganisms or substances recognized as nonself, as well as the processing of antigens for stimulation of immunocompetent lymphoid cells. The monocyte may also give rise to actively phagocytic cells distributed throughout the body, known as the **mononuclear phagocytic system** (i.e., connective tissue macrophages [histiocytes], foreign body giant cells, Kupffer cells, alveolar macrophages, peritoneal macrophages, microglia, osteoclasts, and free or fixed macrophages in lymphoid tissues).

The second category of white blood cells are the **granular leukocytes,** which have lobulated nuclei and specific granules in their cytoplasm that stain with components of the Romanovsky-based stains and from which these cells draw their names **(neutrophils, eosinophils,** and **basophils). Neutrophils** are also known as **PMNs** (polymorphonuclear cells) because of the presence of two to five nuclear lobes. Specific granules of neutrophils contain lysozyme, lactoferrin, collagenase, and bactericidal cationic proteins, while the azure granules (lysosomes) found in most white blood cells contain acid hydrolases, myeloperoxidase, lysozyme, elastase, and neutral proteases. Neutrophils play a major role in bacterial phagocytosis.

Eosinophils contain a complex group of substances in their specific granules including acid phosphatase, arylsulfatase, histaminase, beta-glucuronidase, cathepsin, phospholipase, eosinophilic peroxidase, major basic protein, and RNAase. Eosinophils are drawn into connective tissue by factors released by mast cells during allergic reactions and parasitic infections. The eosinophil neutralizes agents secreted by mast cells (i.e., leukotrine C, histamine), thereby modulating the allergic reaction enhanced by mast cells, and also participates in the phagocytic disposal of antigen-antibody complexes formed in allergic responses, such as hayfever or asthma.

Basophils contain specific granules rich in heparin, histamine, chemotactic factors for eosinophils and neutrophils, leukotrines, platelet-activating factor, and enzymes capable of degrading connective tissue elements. These cells, like mast cells, have immunoglobin E bound to receptors on their surface, and immunologic triggering of them results in secretion of specific granules leading to immediate hypersensitivity reaction. In its extreme form this is referred to as anaphylactic shock.

The differential count in peripheral blood, size, shape, cytoplasmic characteristics, and life span of the different blood cells are shown in the following table.

TYPES OF PERIPHERAL BLOOD CELLS

	RBC	PLATELET	LYMPHOCYTE	MONOCYTE	PMN	EOSINOPHIL	BASOPHIL
No/mm³ or percent in differential count	$4.5\text{-}5 \times 10^6$	$1.5\text{-}4 \times 10^5$	20%-25%	4%-8%	60%-70%	1%-4%	0.5%-1%
Diameter (μm)	7-8	2-5	7-12	9-12	10-12	10-12	10-12
Nuclear shape	——— Anucleate ———		——— Mononuclear ———		——— Lobulated ———		
					2-5 lobes	2-3 lobes	2-3 lobes
Cytoplasmic granules							
Azure	−	−	+	+	+	+	+
Specific	−	−	−	−	+	+	+
Life span (days)	120	7-12	Days-months	Months-years	Hours-days	8-12 days	?

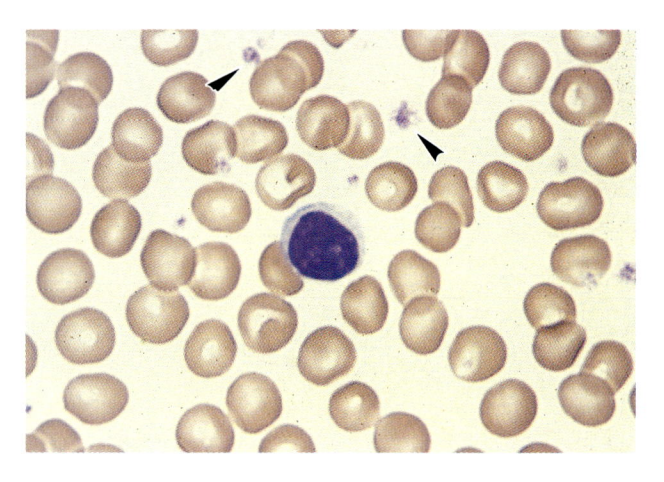

Fig. 6-1. LM of red blood cells, platelets *(arrowheads)*, and a lymphocyte in peripheral blood. Note thin, lightly basophilic rim of cytoplasm surrounding nucleus of lymphocyte. (Wright's stain; ×1,100.)

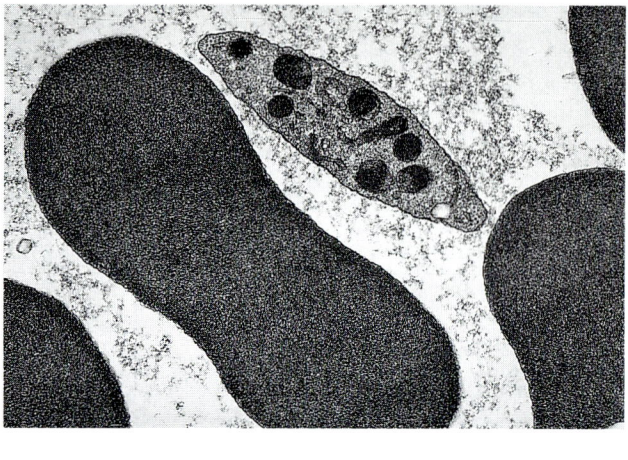

Fig. 6-2. Erythrocytes and platelet seen by TEM. Erythrocyte has dense, homogeneous appearance because of presence of hemoglobin and absence of cell organelles. Locate cisternae of platelet's dense tubular system, dense granules, and microtubules. Compare platelet to those seen in Fig. 6-1 by LM. (×9,000.)

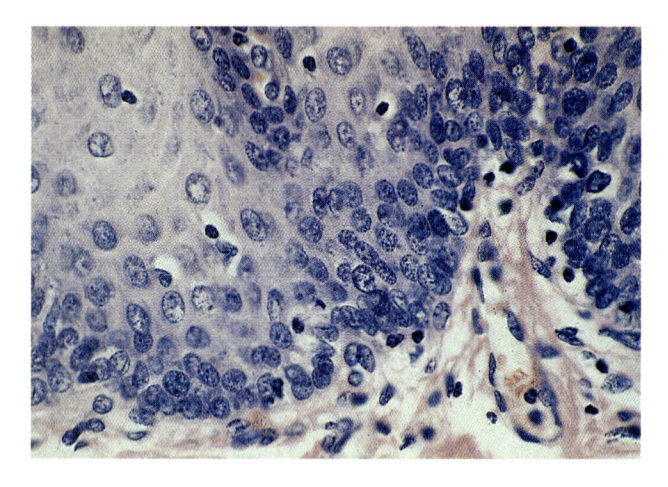

Fig. 6-3. LM of esophageal mucosa. Lymphocytes are identified by small, dense nuclei lying between epithelial cells and within underlying connective tissue. (H&E; ×250.)

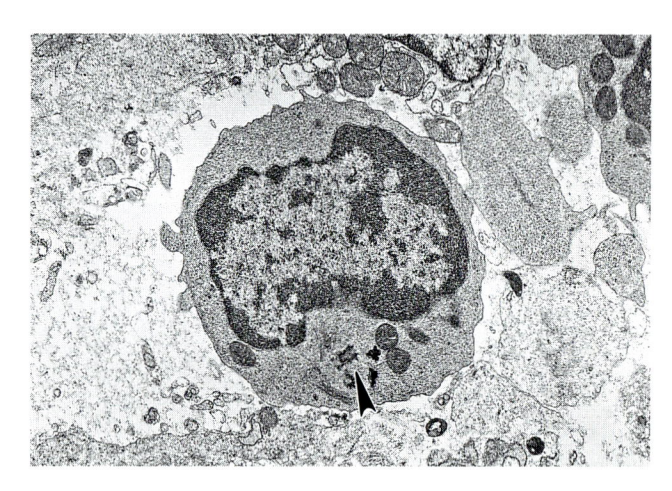

Fig. 6-4. TEM of lymphocyte. Membranous organelles are few, but there are abundant free ribosomes in surrounding cytoplasm. A pair of centrioles *(arrowhead)* and several mitochondria are seen. (×5,100.)

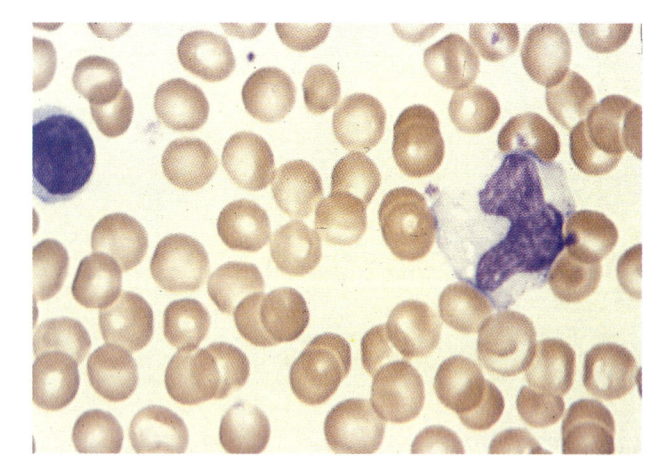

Fig. 6-5. LM of peripheral blood. Compare monocyte *(right)* with lymphocyte *(left)* and red blood cells, which are scattered throughout field. Monocyte is a large cell with gray, vacuolated cytoplasm, a few azure granules, and indented nucleus in which chromatin has a "raked" appearance. In contrast, the smaller lymphocyte possesses condensed chromatin and is surrounded by thin rim of basophilic cytoplasm. (Wright's stain; ×1,100.)

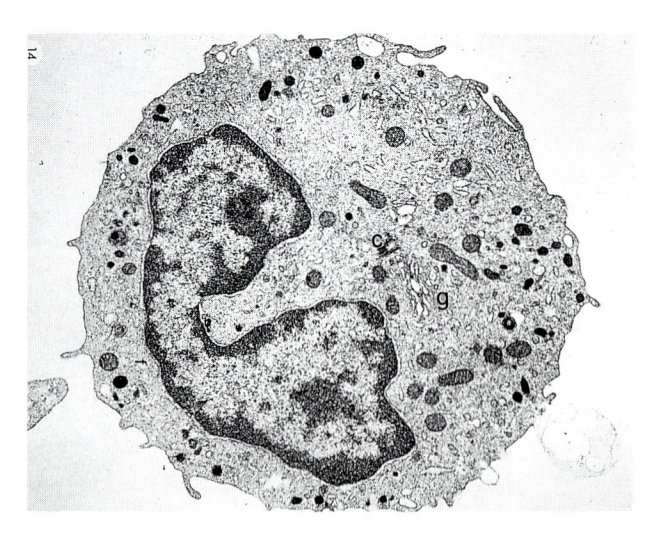

Fig. 6-6. Monocyte (TEM) exhibiting small lysosomal granules (azure granules) and indented nucleus. Monocytes are precursors of tissue macrophages. *g*, Golgi; *c*, centriole. (×6,500.)

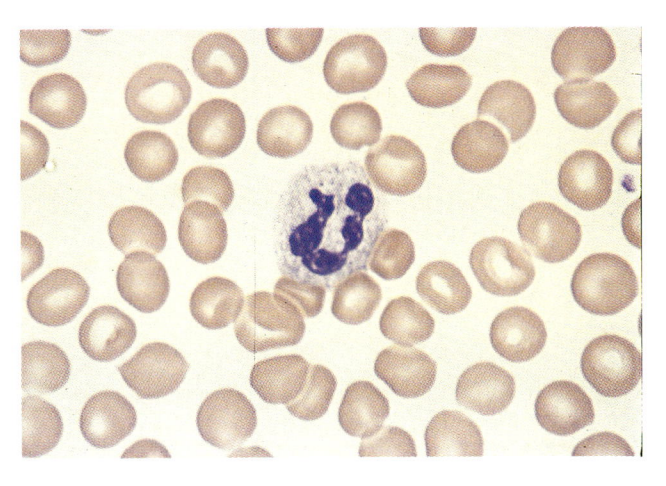

Fig. 6-7. LM of polymorphonuclear leukocyte (also known as PMN or neutrophil) in peripheral blood. Notice multilobed nucleus and azure and specific granules. Compare in size with red blood cells. (Wright's stain; ×1,100.)

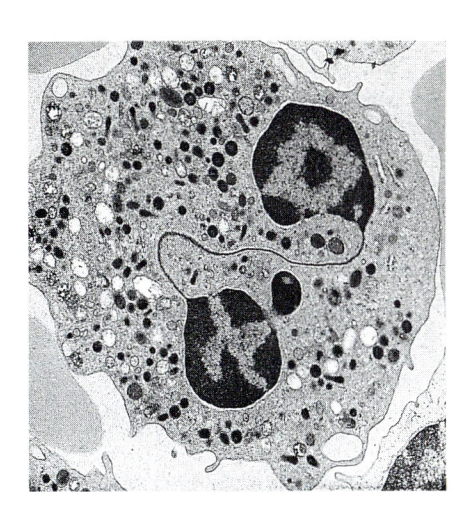

Fig. 6-8. TEM of polymorphonuclear leukocyte. Observe multilobed nucleus and specific granulation. (×5,200.)

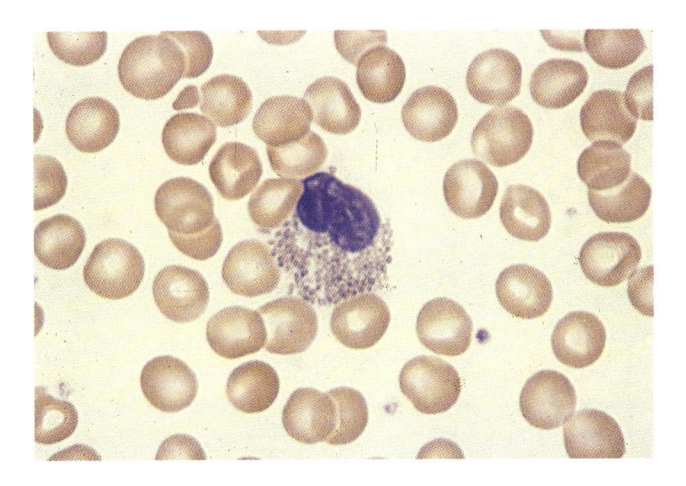

Fig. 6-9. LM of eosinophil with a bilobed nucleus in peripheral blood. Specific granules are large and acidophilic. (Wright's stain; ×1,100.)

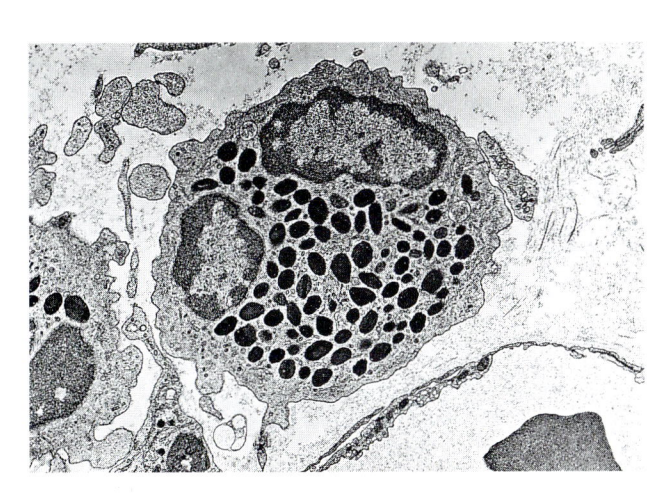

Fig. 6-10. TEM of eosinophil adjacent to capillary in connective tissue. Specific granules are large and electron-dense and usually contain angular crystalloid. Nucleus is bilobed. (×5,100.)

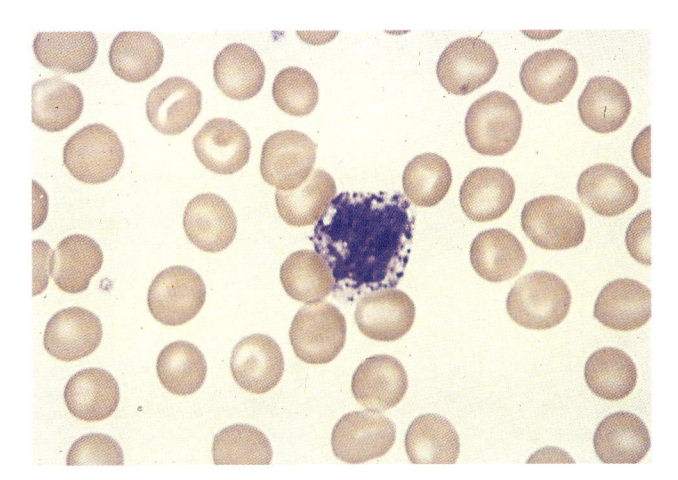

Fig. 6-11. LM of basophil in peripheral blood. Cytoplasm of mature basophil is clear and contains numerous large, basophilic specific granules, which usually overlie and obscure bilobed nucleus. (Wright's stain; ×1,100.)

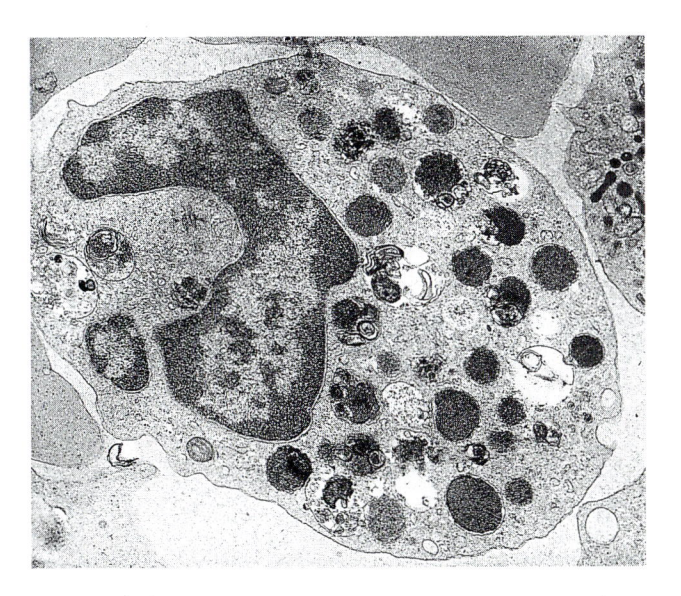

Fig. 6-12. TEM of human basophil. Specific granules are large and regular in size and shape and contain histamine, heparin, SRS (slow reacting substance), and serotonin, which are powerful vasoactive mediators. Granules are often disrupted owing to difficulty in fixing tissue. (×10,500.)

CHAPTER 7

BONE MARROW & HEMOPOIESIS

BONE MARROW, LOCATED within the medullary cavities of long bones and the intratrabecular spaces of cancellous bone, is composed of a **vascular compartment** and a **hemopoietic compartment.** The vascular compartment derives its blood supply from the nutrient artery, which eventually divides into thin-walled sinusoids having a discontinuous endothelial lining. These in turn are surrounded by a poorly developed and incomplete basement membrane and by both **adventitial cells** (fibroblast-like) and **macrophages** belonging to the mononuclear phagocytic system. The hemopoietic compartment is almost entirely extravascular and is composed of a reticular fiber stroma together with a variety of cells, many of hemopoietic origin. Connective tissue cells such as plasma cells, osteoblasts, osteoclasts, adipocytes, macrophages, and mast cells can also be present.

The principal functions of bone marrow are (1) the production of blood cells and their release into peripheral blood; (2) hematoclasis, that is, the detection and phagocytosis of defective blood cells; (3) functions of the mononuclear phagocytic system: the phagocytosis of cells and cellular debris together with the production of monocytes; (4) the production of precursors to T and B lymphocytes; and (5) an osteogenic function by cells lining the endosteum, and (6) the distribution of blood vessels to bone.

The production of blood cells to replace those leaving the peripheral blood compartment is called **hemopoiesis.** This process is essential since the life span of many cells in the peripheral blood compartment is relatively short. Leukocytes survive for only hours to days and must be constantly replenished. Red blood cells are long lived (120 days), but because of their large numbers in the peripheral blood compartment turnover of red blood cells requires that 25×10^{10} cells be replaced daily.

Erythropoiesis deals with the differentiation of red blood cells from a **totipotent stem cell.** Division of the stem cell results in the formation of **committed stem cells** (colony forming unit–erythron and burst forming unit–erythron) that are not recognizable morphologically but are responsive to hemopoietic regulators such as erythropoietin and the interleukins. Division of these committed stem cells produces **pronormoblasts** (proerythroblasts), which are the first cells recognized in the developing erythroid series. (The term "normoblast" or "erythroblast" is applied to nucleated precursor cells in the differentiation of red blood cells.) Pronormoblasts are large cells (15 to 20 μm) containing a large spherical nucleus with a delicate chromatin pattern. Nucleoli are visible and the cytoplasm is lightly basophilic as a result of the presence of free polyribosomes involved in the production of hemoglobin.

Mitosis and continued differentiation of pronormoblasts result in the formation of **basophilic normoblasts** (basophilic erythroblast). These cells are slightly smaller than pronormoblasts, being 12 to 16 μm in diameter, but because of increased RNA synthesis they have more intensely basophilic cytoplasm. Their nuclei have a condensed chromatin pattern that makes it difficult to discern nucleoli.

Upon the intracellular accumulation of hemoglobin (acidophilic), the cell is called a **polychromatic normoblast** (polychromatic erythroblast). The cytoplasm of this cell ranges from almost complete basophilia early in development to a mixed bluish-red later, making this stage in cellular differentiation highly variable in terms of cell size and cytoplasmic staining characteristics. Polychromatic normoblasts are the last stage in erythropoiesis in which cell division can occur.

The next stage is the **orthochromatic normoblast,** in which the shrunken nucleus has a highly condensed chromatin pattern and the acidophilia of the cytoplasm is almost identical to that of the mature red blood cell. Expulsion of the nucleus from the polychromatic normoblast results in the formation of a **polychromato-**

philic red blood cell (macrocyte), whereas expulsion at the orthochromatic stage forms a **reticulocyte** (RNA within the cell is recognizable by staining with vital dyes). Reticulocytes remain in the marrow for approximately 1 to 2 days and then enter the peripheral blood compartment (where 1% of RBCs are reticulocytes) to complete the maturation process into mature red blood cells.

The first recognizable cell in granulopoiesis is the **myeloblast,** a cell that can give rise to all three types of granulocytes: neutrophil, eosinophil, and basophil. The myeloblast has a large spherical nucleus with a delicate chromatin pattern and scanty but lightly basophilic cytoplasm. Continued differentiation results in the formation of a **promyelocyte** that is recognized by the presence of distinct azurophilic granules and a larger amount of basophilic cytoplasm. As the promyelocyte undergoes mitosis, cells become smaller (10 to 12 μm) and upon the appearance of characteristic specific granules are referred to as either **neutrophilic myelocytes, eosinophilic myelocytes,** or **basophilic myelocytes.**

Production of specific granules is completed in the myelocyte, which is the last stage in granulopoiesis capable of cell division. Subsequent stages in the development of each type of granulocyte involve the sharp indentation of the nucleus **(metamyelocyte stage)** and the formation of nuclei resembling a curved ribbon **(band form).** Only in these later stages of differentiation do the granulocytes acquire the properties of ameboid movement, chemotaxis, and phagocytosis.

The differentiation of lymphocytes and monocytes is called **lymphopoiesis,** but it is difficult to study with typical histologic staining methods since these cells do not possess characteristic cytoplasmic or nuclear markers that will permit one to distinguish between early and later stages in differentiation.

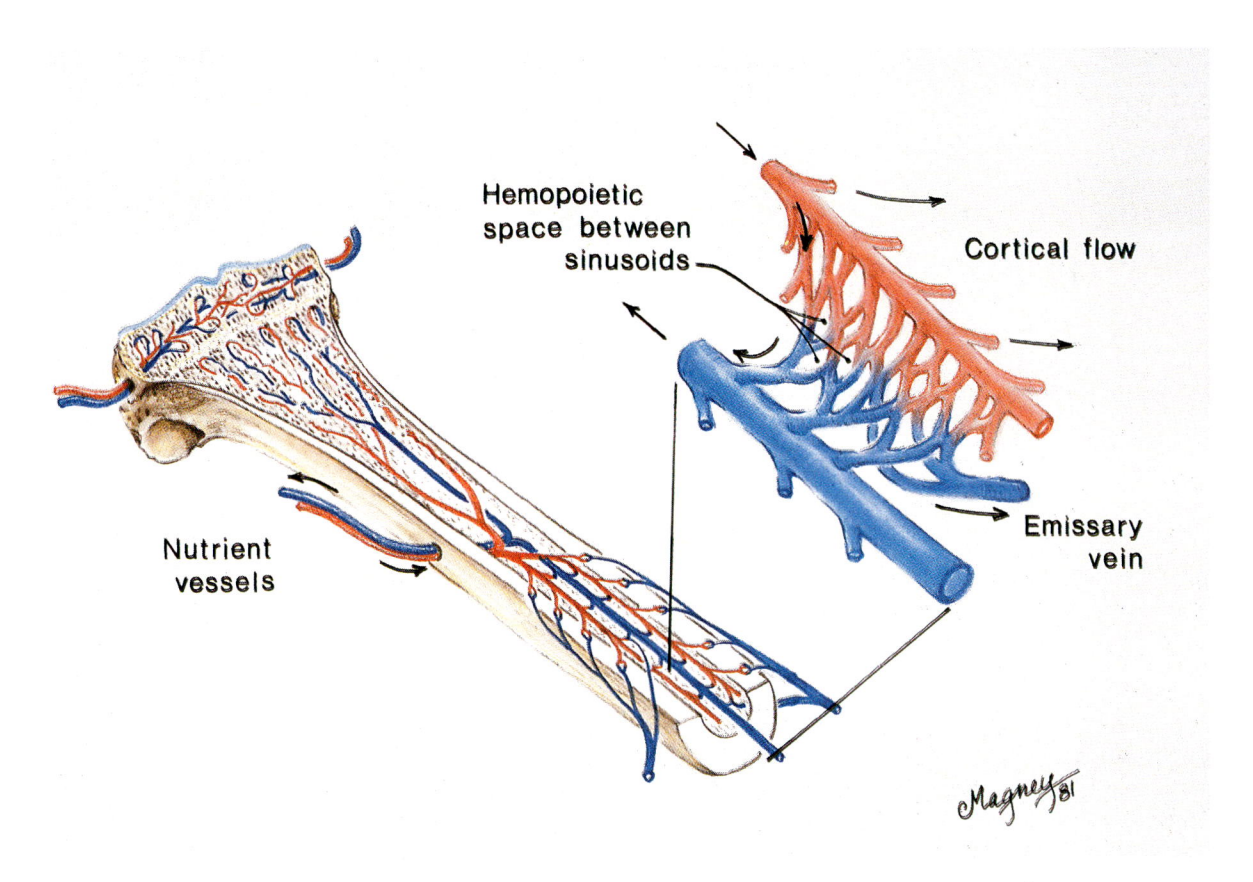

Fig. 7-1. Bone marrow vasculature and circulation. Nutrient vessels penetrate compact bone and form ascending and descending branches. Periosteal vessels also penetrate cortical osseous tissue. Both types of vessels eventually communicate with medullary sinusoids.

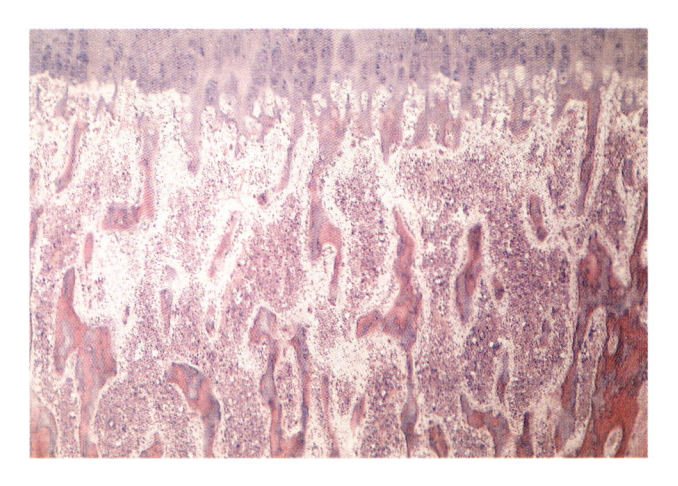

Fig. 7-2. LM of epiphyseal plate showing spicules of cancellous bone and surrounding marrow. (H&E; ×100.)

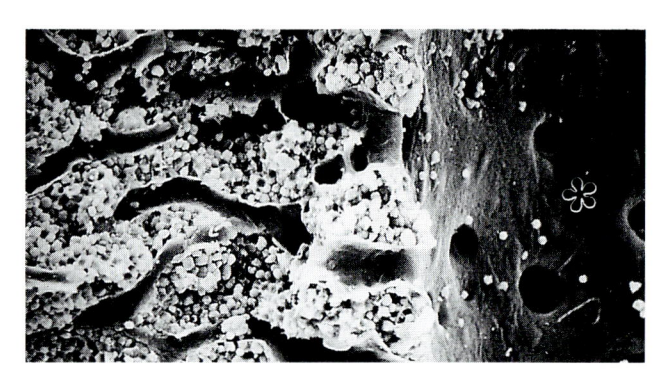

Fig. 7-3. SEM of bone marrow. Sinusoids open into lumen of vessel *(asterisk)*. Cells of the hemopoietic compartment can be seen between sinusoids. (×250.)

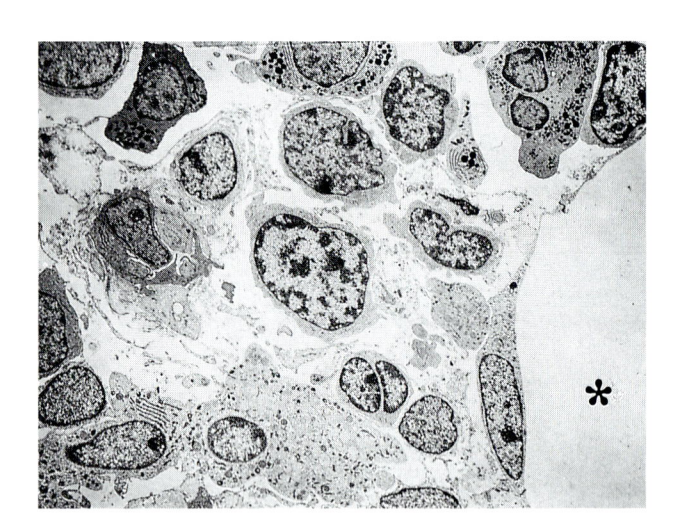

Fig. 7-4. TEM of hemopoietic cells of bone marrow adjoining sinusoid *(asterisk)* lined by endothelial cells. (×2,000.)

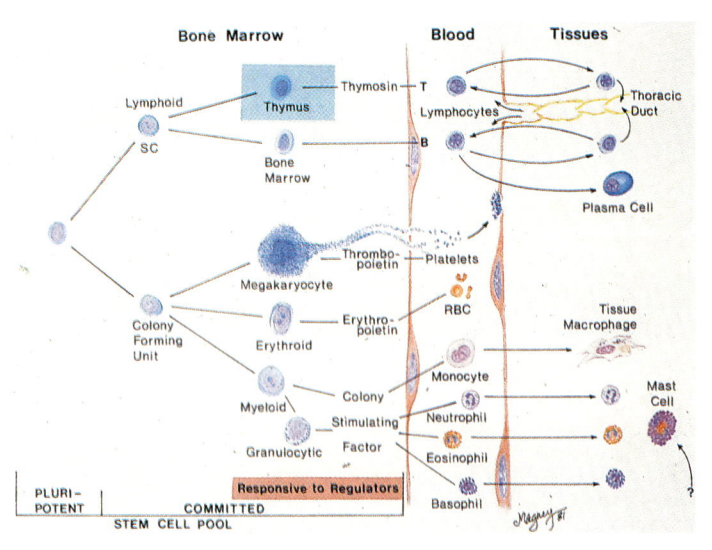

Fig. 7-5. Pluripotent stem cell in bone marrow and its differentiation into committed hemopoietic stem cell lines. Pluripotent stem cells constitute about 0.01% of nucleated marrow cells and proliferate slowly compared to more rapidly proliferating committed stem cells which are more responsive to a variety of growth factors, often referred to as colony stimulating factors because of their ability to stimulate growth in tissue culture. All cells move by diapedesis from hematopoietic to vascular compartments except for the platelet, which apparently can be shed from long processes of megakaryocytes directly into sinusoids. Functions of red blood cells (gas transport) and platelets (repair of vascular injury) are carried out within cardiovascular system, whereas lymphoid, granulocytic, and monocytic cells usually complete their life cycle after leaving the cardiovascular system and entering tissues.

BONE MARROW & HEMOPOIESIS 45

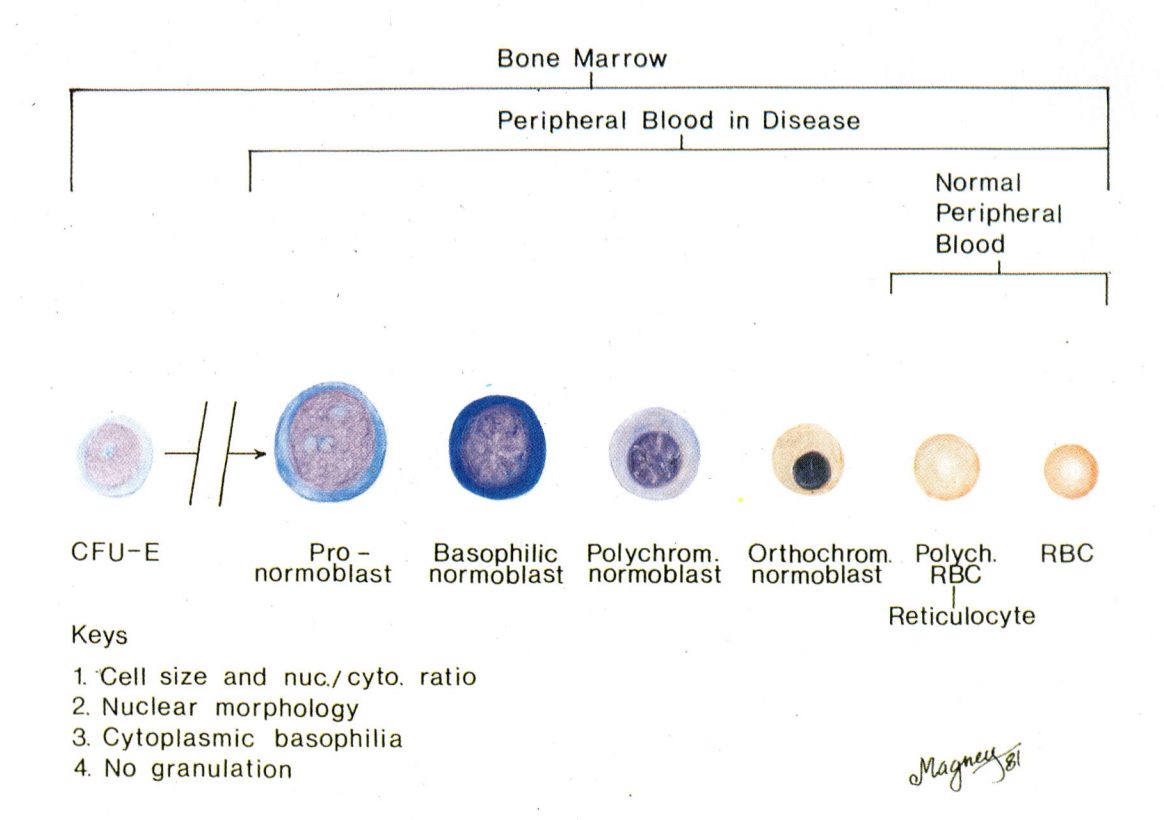

Keys
1. Cell size and nuc./cyto. ratio
2. Nuclear morphology
3. Cytoplasmic basophilia
4. No granulation

Fig. 7-6. Cytodifferentiation of erythropoietic series illustrating important morphologic keys to identification of different stages in maturation.

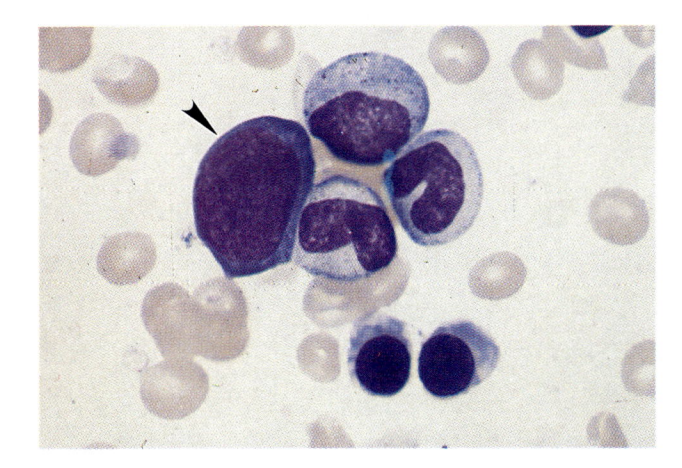

Fig. 7-7. LM of pronormoblast *(arrowhead)* with a large smooth nucleus and nucleoli. Nuclear membrane is distinct and cytoplasm relatively basophilic. Seen on right are three granulocytes, and below them two late polychromatic normoblasts, and numerous mature red blood cells. (Wright's stain; ×1,100.)

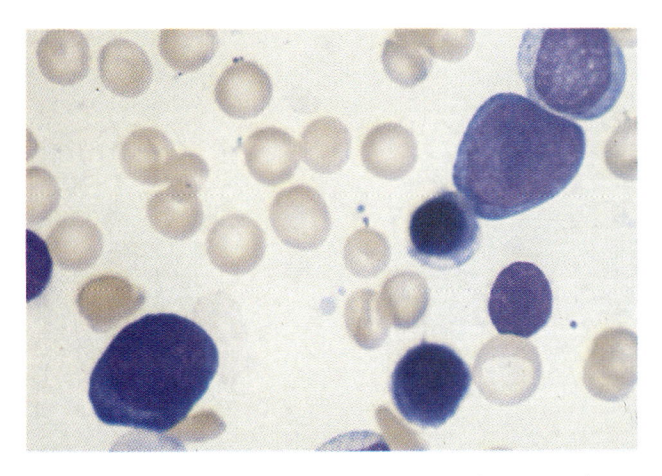

Fig. 7-8. Comparison (by LM) of pronormoblast *(upper right)* and basophilic normoblast *(lower left)*. In latter cell, nuclear chromatin is more condensed and cytoplasm is navy blue, making this the most basophilic cell in bone marrow. (Wright's stain; ×1,100.)

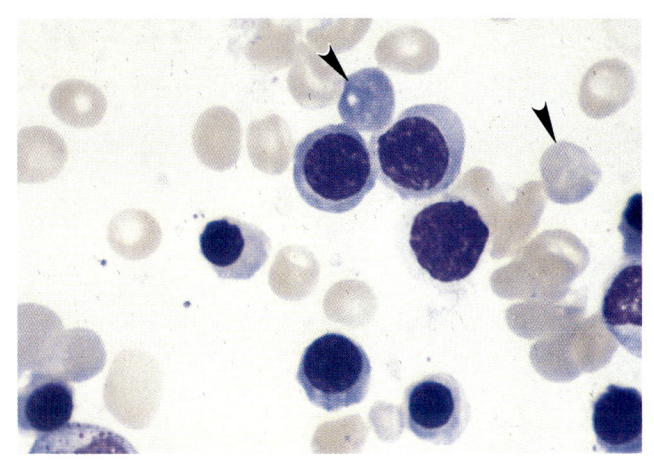

Fig. 7-9. LM of group of polychromatic normoblasts, showing variation in size and in cytoplasmic staining. Larger polychromatic normoblasts are less mature than smaller ones, which exhibit very dense pyknotic nuclei. Several polychromatophilic red blood cells *(arrowheads)* with bluish-staining cytoplasm of various shades can be seen. Just left of center is a normoblast that is about to extrude its nucleus. (Wright's stain; ×1,100.)

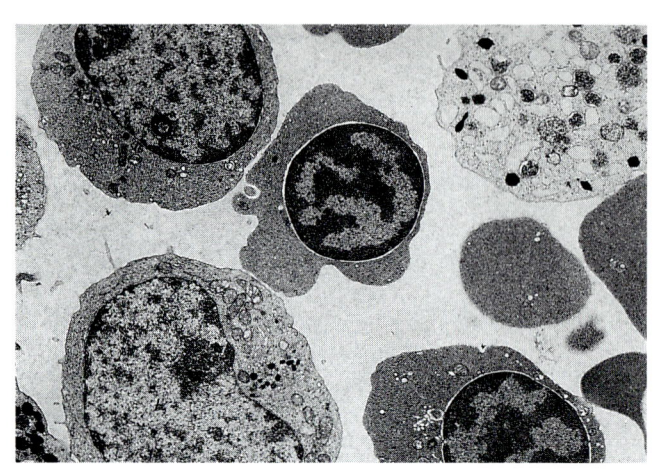

Fig. 7-10. TEM of basophilic normoblast *(upper left)* with numerous ribosomes, and two polychromatic normoblasts which are smaller, with more condensed nuclear chromatin. Parts of granular leukocytes are also visible *(lower left, upper right)*. (×4,000.)

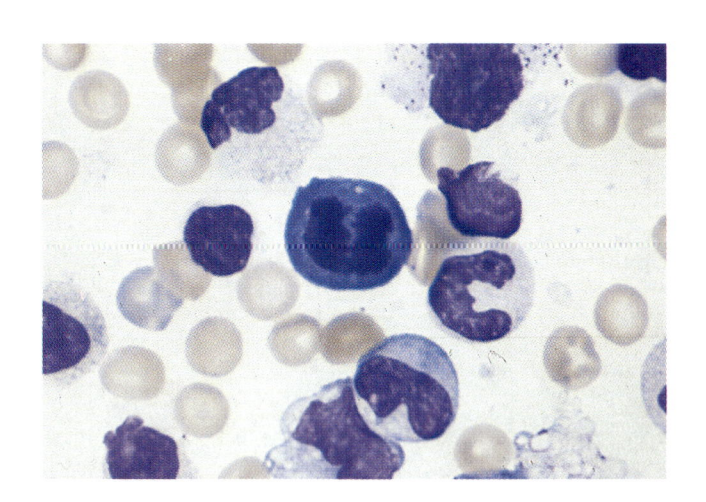

Fig. 7-11. LM of polychromatic normoblast in mitosis *(center)* surrounded by developing neutrophils. (Wright's stain; ×1,100.)

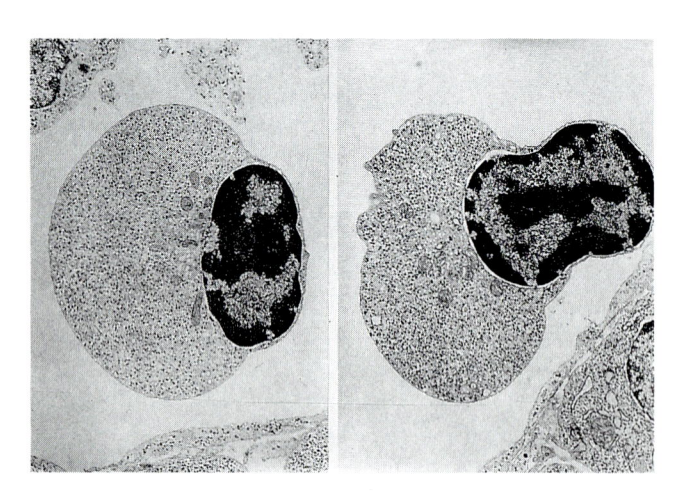

Fig. 7-12. Normoblasts as seen by TEM in two stages of nuclear extrusion. Note that a thin rim of cytoplasm is carried away with the extruded nucleus. (×1,900.)

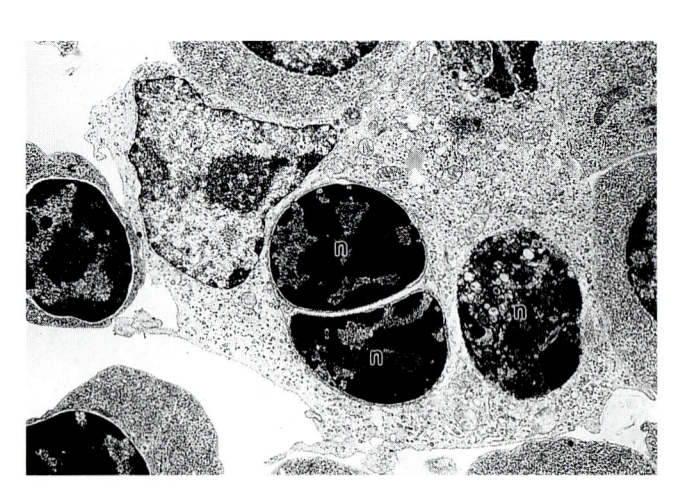

Fig. 7-13. TEM of macrophage that has ingested extruded normoblast nuclei *(center)*. Parts of two polychromatic normoblasts are visible *(left)*. (×1,800.)

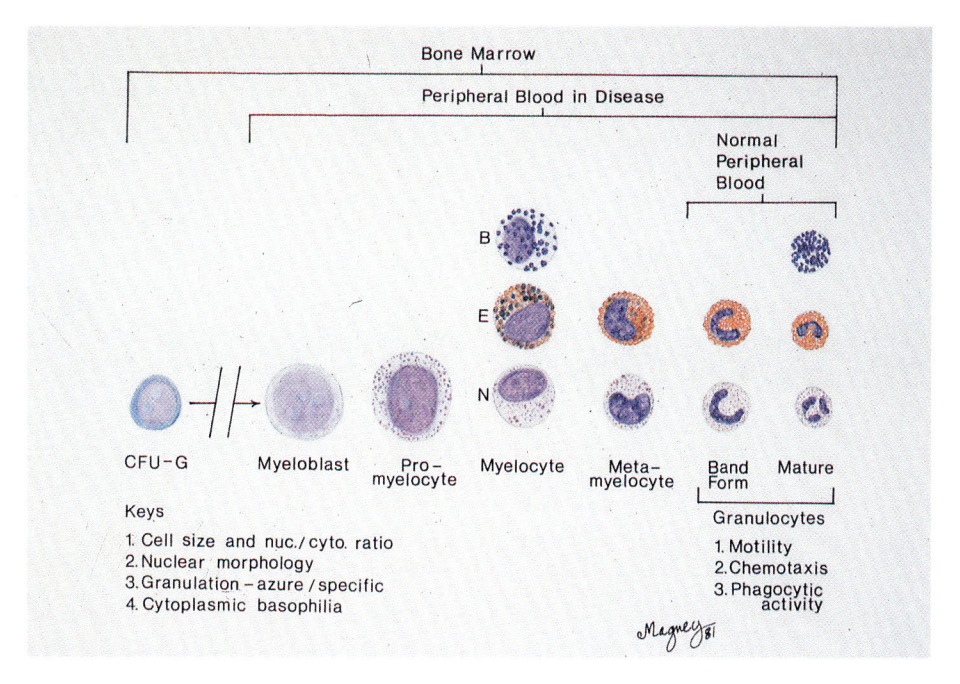

Fig. 7-14. Cytodifferentiation of granulocytic series illustrating important morphologic keys for identification of different stages in maturation.

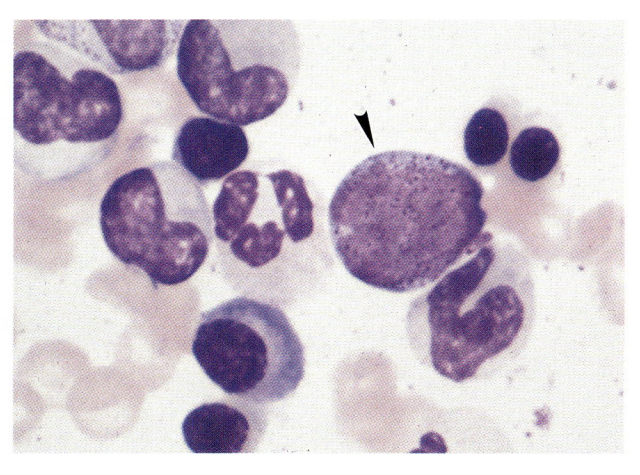

Fig. 7-15. LM of myeloblast *(arrowhead)*. This cell has a very large vesicular nucleus, an indistinct nuclear membrane, and scattered cytoplasmic azure granulation. (Wright's stain; ×1,100.)

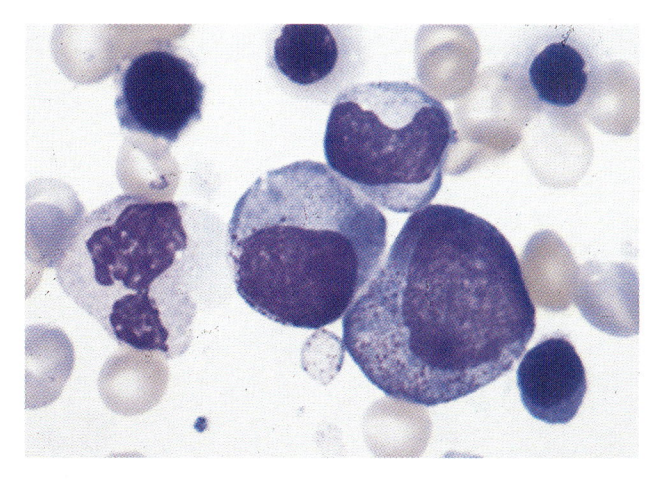

Fig. 7-16. Promyelocyte *(lower right)* showing larger proportion of cytoplasm as compared with myeloblast or with later stages in development. Many large azurophilic granules are present in cytoplasm. Nuclear membrane is distinct. Compare to myeloblast in Fig. 7-15. Observe neutrophilic myelocyte *(left)* and neutrophilic metamyelocyte *(top)*. (Wright's stain; ×1,100.)

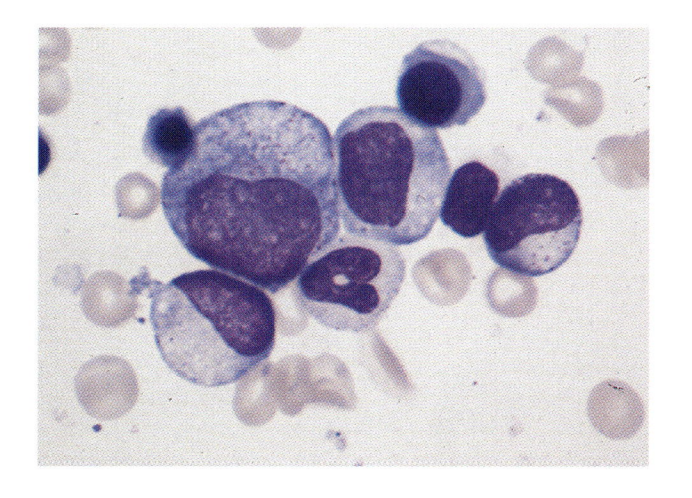

Fig. 7-17. LM comparison of large promyelocyte *(upper left)* with succeeding stages of neutrophilic maturation. Observe neutrophilic myelocyte next to it on either side *(upper center, lower left)*, neutrophilic metamyelocyte with slightly indented nucleus *(far right)*, and band form neutrophil *(below and to the right of promyelocyte)*. (Wright's stain; ×1,100.)

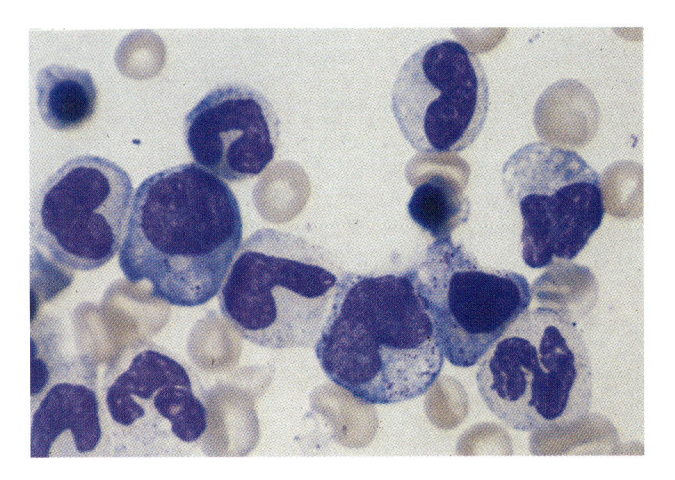

Fig. 7-18. LM of neutrophilic series. Neutrophilic myelocyte (round nucleus) is seen at left center adjacent to several neutrophilic metamyelocytes (indented nuclei), two band forms, and two almost mature neutrophils. (Wright's stain; ×1,100.)

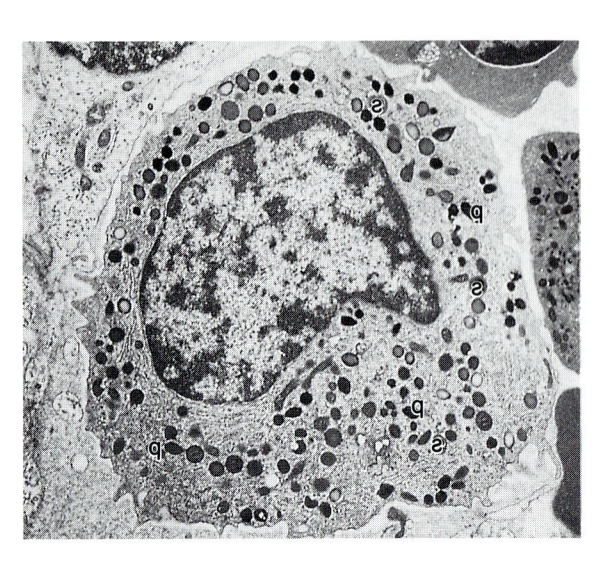

Fig. 7-19. TEM of neutrophilic myelocyte. Note that specific granules (s) present in cell are variable in size, shape, and density. Some azurophilic, or primary (P), granules are also seen. (×5,500.)

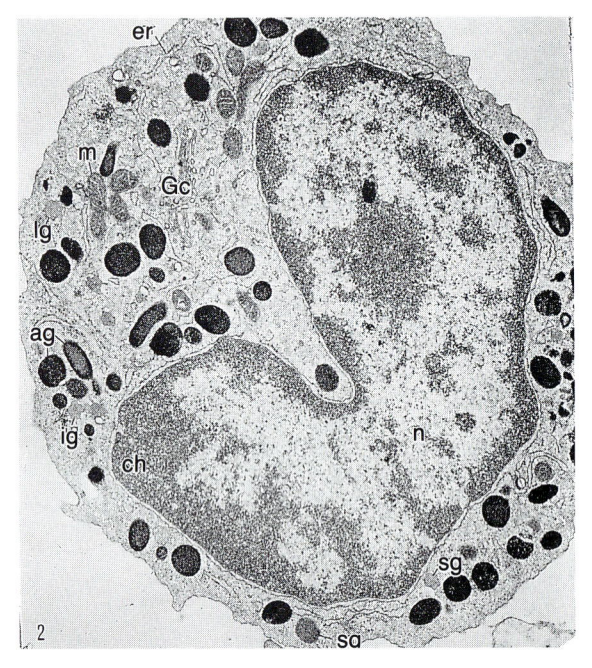

Fig. 7-20. TEM of neutrophilic metamyelocyte with a deeply indented nucleus. n, Nucleus; ch, chromatin; Gc, Golgi complex; er, rough endoplasmic reticulum; m, mitochondria; ag, azure granule; ig, immature granule; sg, specific granule. (×6,400.)

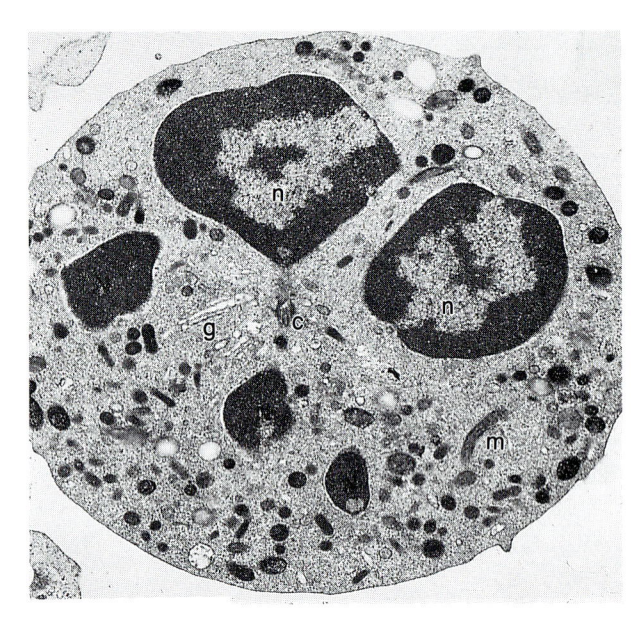

Fig. 7-21. Mature neutrophil (TEM) exhibiting lobulated nucleus (N). Lobules are connected by strands of nucleoplasm, which are out of the plane of section. Organelles and secretory granules are clearly visible. g, Golgi; c, centriole; m, mitochondrion. (×7,000.)

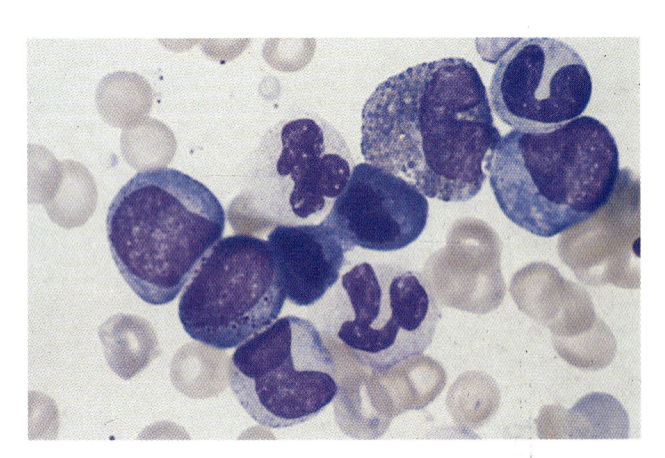

Fig. 7-22. LM showing a number of different bone marrow cells, including several developing granulocytes, a polychromatic normoblast in mitosis, and two mature neutrophils. Identify early-stage granulocytes. (Wright's stain; ×1,100.)

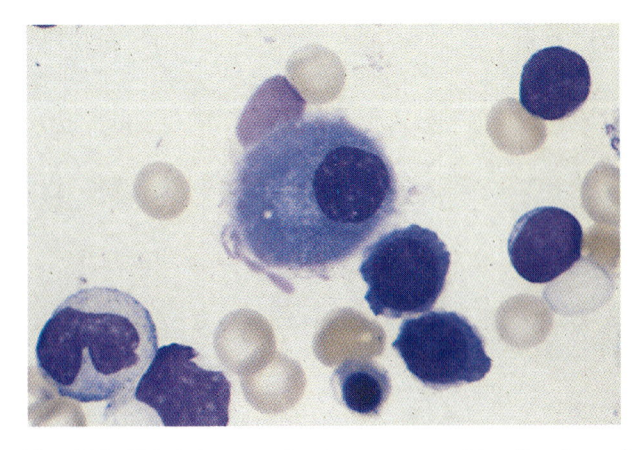

Fig. 7-23. LM of plasma cell in bone marrow. Identify other cell types. (Wright's stain; ×1,100.)

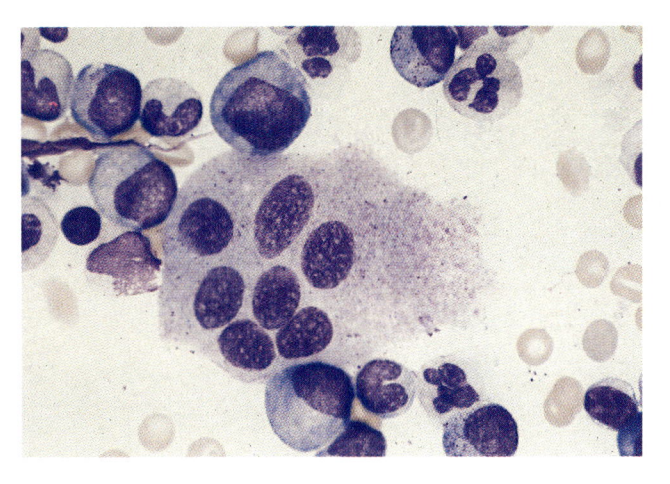

Fig. 7-24. LM of a multinucleated osteoclast in bone marrow surrounded by differentiating granulocytes. Identify them by using cytoplasmic/nuclear keys listed in Fig. 7-14. (Wright's stain; ×500.)

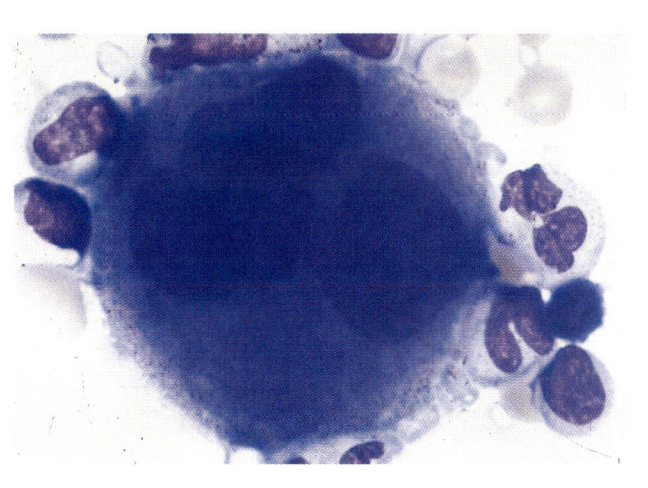

Fig. 7-25. LM of megakaryocyte in bone marrow displaying large, lobulated nucleus. These polyploid cells form long filopodia-like cytoplasmic processes that extend into sinusoids. Platelets appear to form by budding from distal ends of processes. (Wright's stain; ×750.)

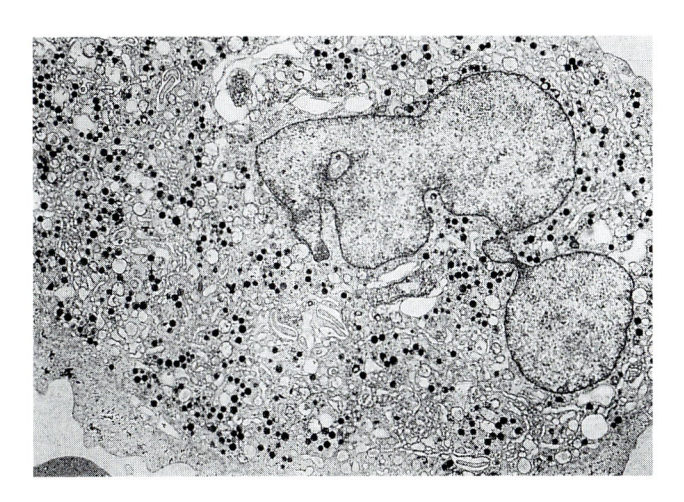

Fig. 7-26. TEM of megakaryocyte with large polymorphic nucleus. Cytoplasm contains granules of various density. Extensive SER, called platelet demarcation membrane, divides cytoplasm into developing platelets, which contain microfilaments and cytoplasm, but are largely devoid of other organelles. (×4,000.)

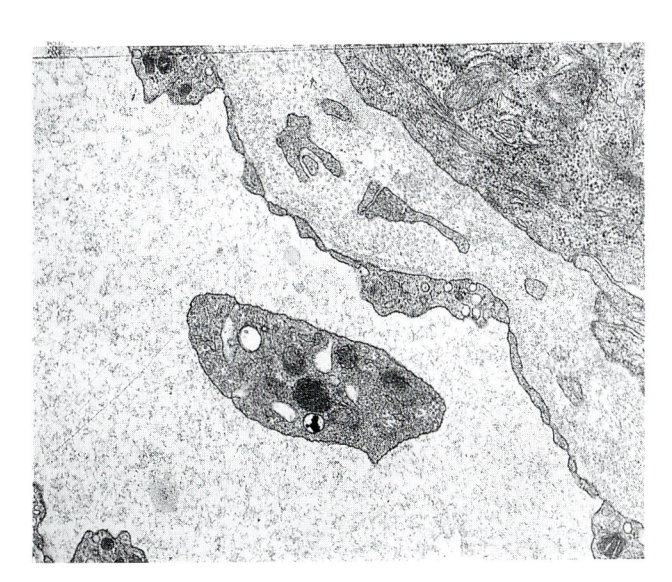

Fig. 7-27. TEM of circulating platelet in capillary of lamina propria of small intestine. (×12,000.)

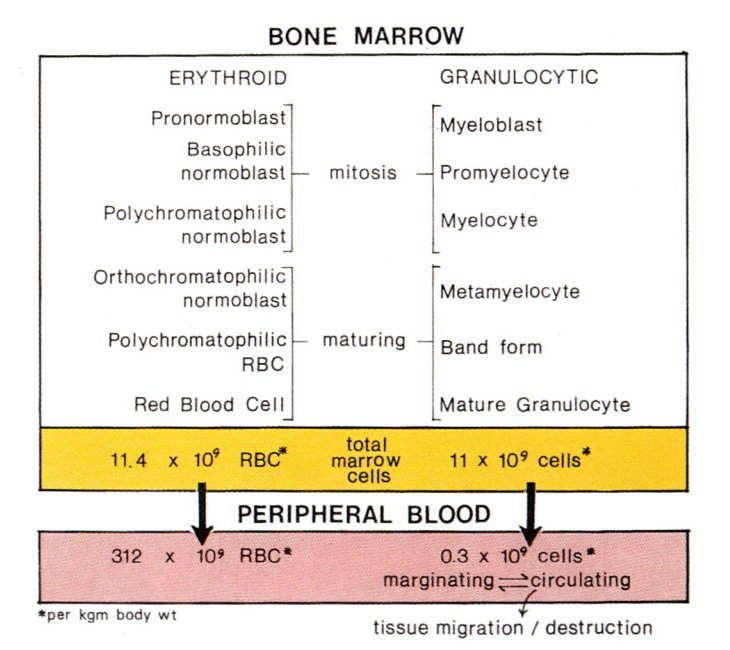

Fig. 7-28. Comparison of maturation of red and white blood cell lines together with total number of cells (per kilogram body weight) found in bone marrow and in peripheral blood compartments. Lifespan of RBCs is about 120 days. Approximately 1% of all RBCs are produced/destroyed daily, which is comparable to the reserve of maturing RBC in bone marrow. On the other hand, WBCs have a lifespan of hours to days, and there is a 40-fold excess or reserve of developing WBCs in marrow compared to WBCs circulating in peripheral blood compartment.

CHAPTER 8

MUSCLE

MUSCLE TISSUE CONSISTS of cells that have been modified to respond to external or internal stimuli by contracting. Such tissue is responsible for most kinds of body movement. There are three types of muscle: **smooth, cardiac,** and **skeletal.** An abundance of the contractile proteins **actin** and **myosin** and the specialized attachment of these microfilaments (myofilaments) to the muscle cell membrane characterize all muscle cells (myofibers). However, the arrangement of organelles within the cells and the attachment of the myofilaments to the cell membrane are different in each of the muscle types. Connective tissues are associated with force transmission in each, although variations exist here also.

Smooth muscle, found in the walls of internal organs, is responsible for activities such as peristalsis, vasoconstriction, or micturition. Smooth muscle cells are fusiform, 15 to 100 μm in length by 3 to 8 μm in diameter, and surrounded by a basal lamina (external lamina) and a fine network of reticular fibers **(endomysium)** that acts in force transmission. Nuclei are oval and centrally placed, and most organelles are located in the cytoplasm near the nuclear poles. Bundles of thick (myosin) and thin (actin) myofilaments are anchored to the cell membrane **(sarcolemma)** at electron-dense regions called **dense bodies.** It is believed that during contraction the myofilaments slide past each other and through their attachment to the sarcolemma, cause shortening of the cell. Contracted smooth muscle cells observed by light microscopy appear coiled or pleated and exhibit folded nuclei. **Gap junctions** between adjacent cells allow the transmission of excitation signals from cell to cell. Contraction of smooth muscle is involuntary and may be inherently myogenic (i.e., in response to stretch); however, signals from the autonomic nervous system, hormones, or local chemical mediators may also stimulate contraction.

Skeletal muscle is attached to bone and provides for movement of the body as a whole or of its parts. Cells are much larger (1 to 40 mm in length by 10 to 100 μm in diameter) than smooth muscle cells and have a cylindrical shape. Multiple nuclei are located peripherally just beneath the sarcolemma. Within the cytoplasm **(sarcoplasm),** long, tightly packed cylindrical myofibrils lie parallel with each other and with the long axis of the cell and are associated with numerous mitochondria. **Myofibrils** are composed of subunits called **sarcomeres,** which contain bundles of actin and myosin myofilaments arranged in register so that the myofibrils and the cell as a whole appear cross-striated. Sarcomeres are connected end to end at **Z lines.** One end of an actin (thin) filament attaches to a Z line and the other end interdigitates with myosin (thick) filaments, which are located in the center of the sarcomere and form an electron-dense region called the **A band.** A lighter **H band,** consisting only of myosin filaments with no overlapping actin, is centered in the A band and is itself bisected by the M line, a region where myosin filaments form lateral interconnections. The I band (formed of the parts of actin filaments of adjacent sarcomeres that do not overlap myosin filaments) is bisected by the Z line to which the actin filaments attach.

Sliding of actin filaments past myosin filaments results in shortening (contraction) of each sarcomere and of the muscle as a whole. This is called excitation-contraction coupling. In skeletal muscle, stimulus for contraction is received from lower motor neurons by way of neuromuscular junctions called **motor end plates** (MEP). The neurotransmitter acetylcholine is released from an axon terminal into the synaptic cleft and then is bound by receptors on the muscle cell membrane, where it initiates a wave of membrane depolarization. Regular invaginations of the sarcolemma called **T tubules** pass deeply into the muscle cell, where they form **triads** (at the junction of the A and I bands) with a highly organized sarcoplasmic reticulum (SER). Depolarization passing down T tubules causes the release of calcium from the sarcoplasmic reticulum and initiates the complex series of events leading to muscle contraction.

Skeletal muscle cells transmit their contractile forces to bone by means of a harness of connective tissues. **Endomysium** (reticular fibers) covers each muscle cell, linking cells into bundles called fascicles that are surrounded by a connective tissue layer called **peri-**

mysium. Fascicles are bound together into a muscle by **epimysium,** an outermost dense connective tissue sheath. All of these connective tissue layers blend together and with the fibers of tendons that attach the muscle to bone.

Cardiac muscle makes up the myocardium, or muscular wall of the heart, and is responsible for pumping blood throughout the body. Cardiac muscle cells are elongated and branched, and have cental nuclei. They are 50 to 100 μm in length and 15 to 20 μm in diameter. Like skeletal muscle, cardiac muscle cells are striated and have subunits called **myofibrils** composed of sarcomeres attached end to end. An abundance of mitochondria, residual bodies, and a modified sarcoplasmic reticulum (which is associated with T tubules to form diads at the Z line of sarcomeres) are typical of cardiac muscle. The cells and their branches are joined end to end at specialized membrane junctions called **intercalated disks,** which include fascia adherens that anchors actin filaments of terminal sarcomeres, macula adherens for mechanical attachment of cells to each other, and gap junctions for communication between cells. Cardiac muscle cells are also surrounded with a delicate endomysium, which attaches them to each other and to a rigid connective tissue **cardiac skeleton** against which the contracting muscle pulls to force blood from the chambers of the heart. Specialized nodal cells initiate the impulse for contraction, which passes through the heart by way of modified cardiac muscle cells called **Purkinje fibers.** These cells, specialized for conduction, are deficient in myofilaments but possess more glycogen in their cytoplasm and are rich in gap junctions. The rate and force of contraction are modulated by the autonomic nervous system.

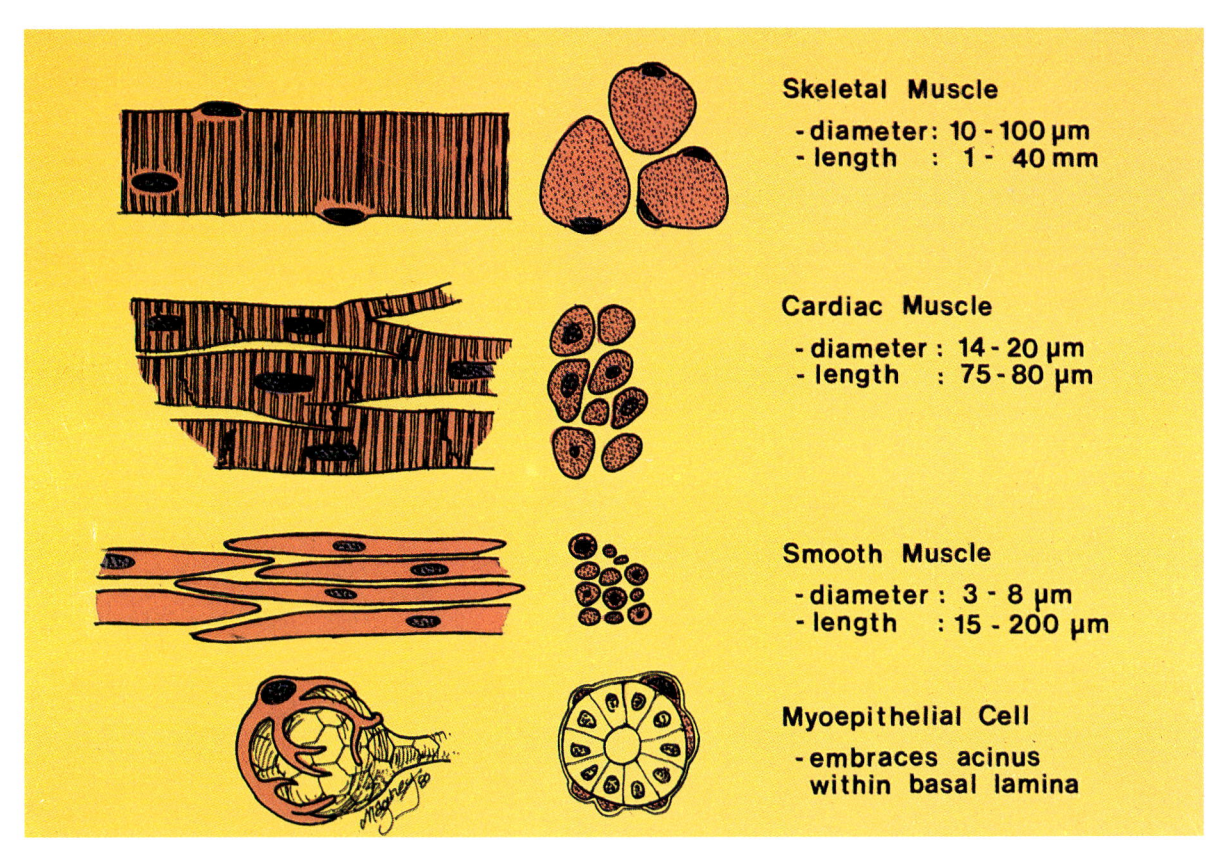

Fig. 8-1. Cells of three classifications of muscle in longitudinal and cross section, with approximate size comparisons. Myoepithelial cells are contractile cells that compress walls of secretory acini/alveoli or ducts so that luminal contents are ejected into or along a duct system.

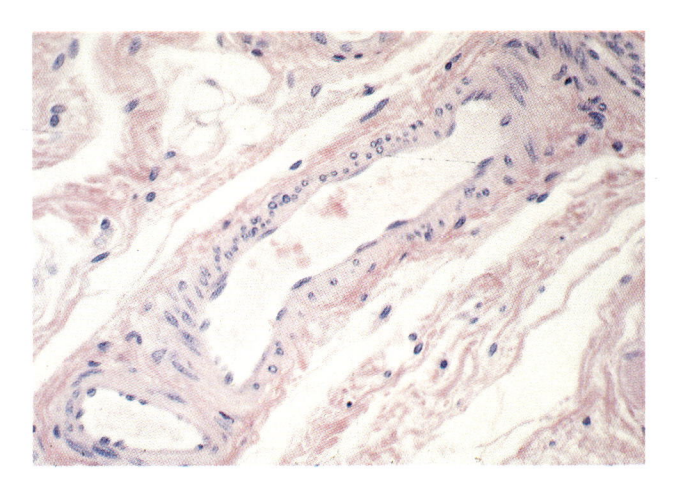

Fig. 8-2. LM of a small muscular artery providing examples of both longitudinal and cross sections of smooth muscle. (H&E; ×200.)

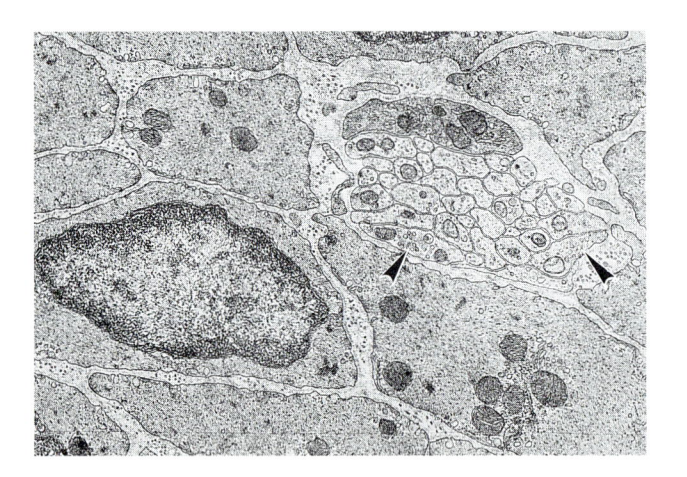

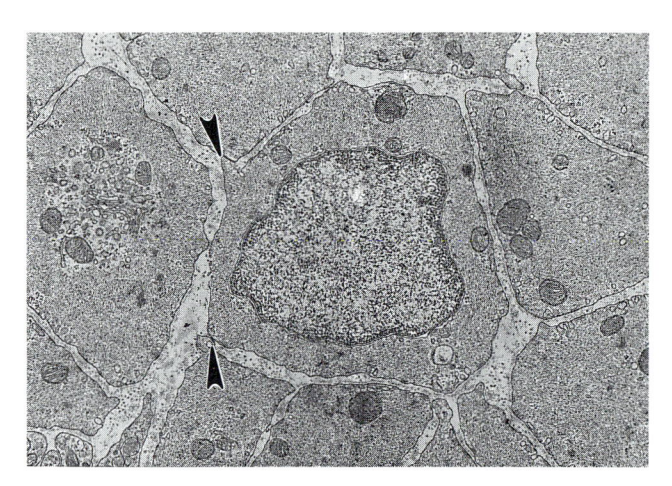

Fig. 8-3. Cross section of smooth muscle by TEM. Because of elongate, fusiform shape of smooth muscle cells, plane of section may not include nucleus of all cells. Golgi apparatus and other organelles are located between nucleus and poles of cell. Communication between adjacent smooth muscle cells occurs by gap junctions *(arrowheads)*. See Fig. 8-1. (×10,800.)

Fig. 8-4. TEM of smooth muscle. Part of an unmyelinated nerve lies within a bundle of smooth muscle. Accumulations of synaptic vesicles in dilatations of axons *(arrowheads)* suggest sites of neurotransmitter release. Note presence of external lamina, myofilaments, and dense bodies on sarcolemma which serve as sites of myofilament attachment. (×4,400.)

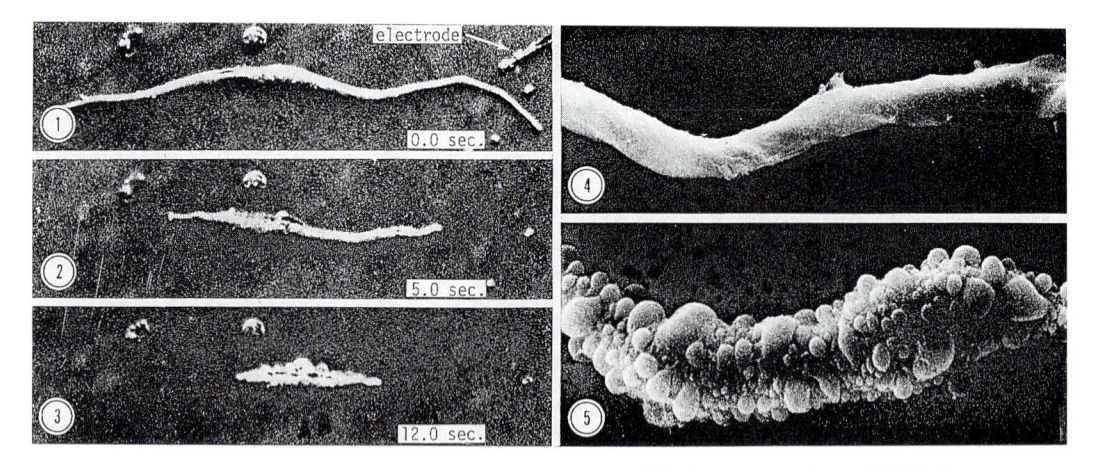

Fig. 8-5. In vitro contraction of smooth muscle as seen by LM cinematography and SEM. Frames 1 to 3 illustrate an isolated smooth muscle cell before electrical stimulation (0.0 seconds in *frame 1*) and 5 and 12 seconds after initiation of synchronous contraction *(frames 2 and 3)*. Note changes in cell length during contraction. By SEM, surface of smooth muscle cell before electrical stimulation appears smooth and cellular diameter is narrow *(frame 4)* (compare to LM in frame 1). After synchronous contraction, cell diameter is increased due to shortening of cell, and surface membrane exhibits massive blebbing *(frame 5)* (compare to LM in frame 3). (*1-3*, ×375; *4*, ×1,900; *5*, 1,800.)

Fig. 8-6. Arrangement of cells (fibers) in skeletal muscle and their relationship to connective tissue coverings. Cross striations apparent by light microscopy are caused by registration of myofibrils within muscle cell. Individual cell or fiber is enclosed in connective tissue sheath called endomysium, bundles (fascicles) of cells in perimysium, and entire muscle in epimysium.

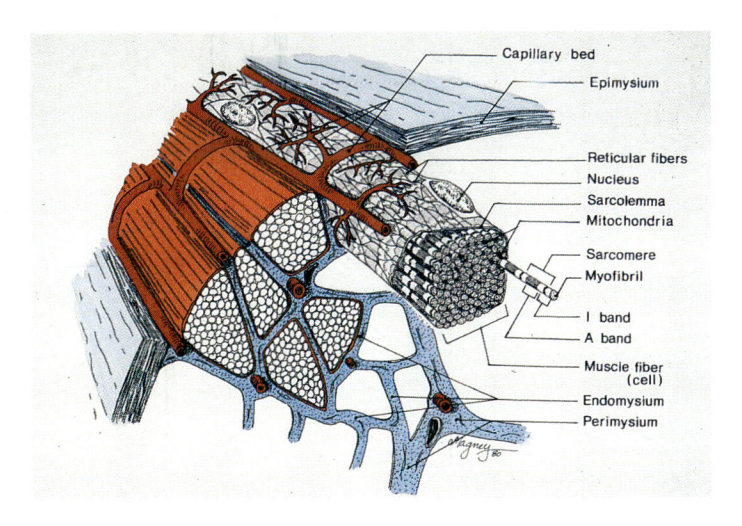

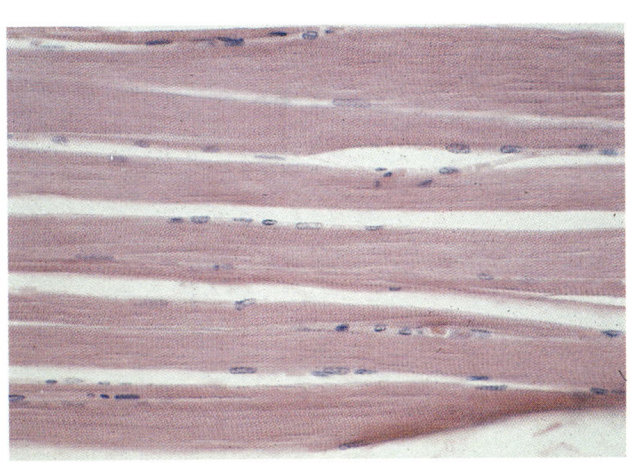

Fig. 8-7. Skeletal muscle cells in longitudinal section (LM) exhibiting cross striation. Notice peripherally placed nuclei within each cell and delicate endomysium surrounding cell. (H&E; ×450.)

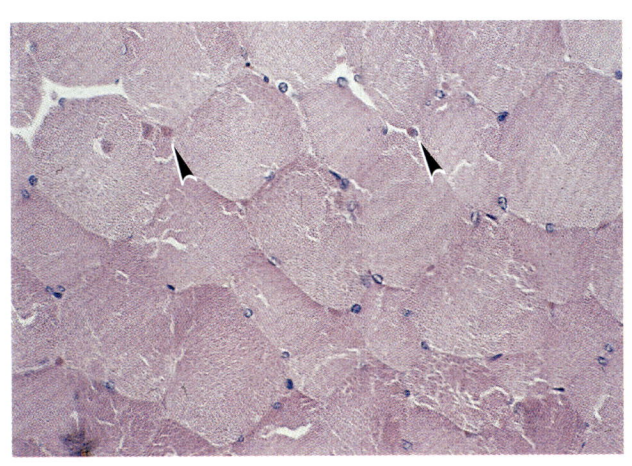

Fig. 8-8. Fascicle of skeletal muscle seen in cross section by LM. Individual cells (fibers) have peripherally placed, multiple nuclei. At this magnification only a few fibers of endomysium are evident; however, occasional red blood cell indicates presence of capillaries *(arrowheads)* within interstitium. (H&E; ×500.)

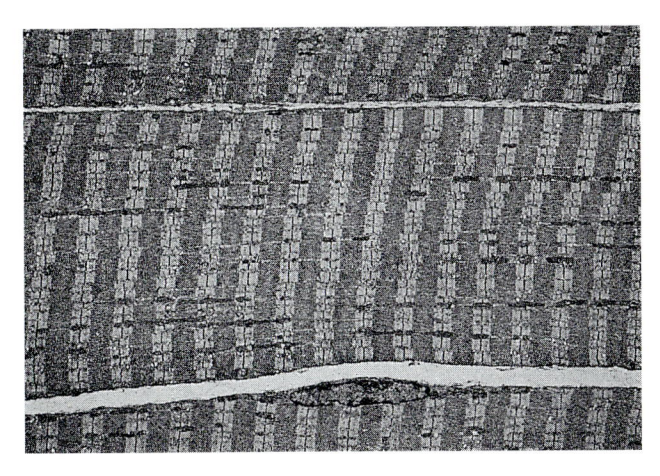

Fig. 8-9. TEM illustrating longitudinal section of skeletal muscle fiber. Portions of two other muscle cells are seen at the top and bottom of micrograph. Bottom cell exhibits peripheral nucleus. Details of cross striations that were visible by LM are apparent and should be compared to Fig. 8-6. Cells are subdivided into long myofibrils within which myofilaments are arranged in subunits called sarcomeres. (×2,400.)

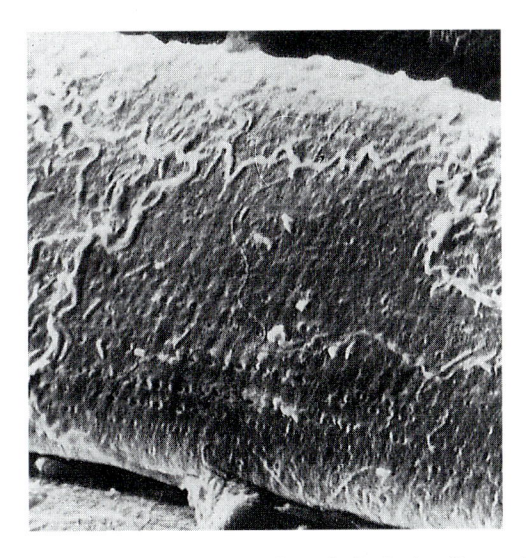

Fig. 8-10. SEM of skeletal muscle cell. Reticular fibers of endomysium form loose network on the sarcolemma. Invaginations of sarcolemma form T tubules, which penetrate deep into cell to carry membrane depolarization to every myofibril. See Fig. 8-11. (×2,500.)

Fig. 8-11. Ultrastructure of individual muscle cell. Study arrangement of actin and myosin myofilaments into myofibrils, which are aligned parallel with long axis of cell. T tubules, invaginations of plasma membrane, transmit membrane depolarization signals deep into cell interior. T tubules together with expansions of sarcoplasmic reticulum (smooth endoplasmic reticulum) called terminal cisternae form triads. Release of Ca^{++} from proteins in sarcoplasmic reticulum results in excitation-contraction coupling. Myofilaments slide past each other to cause muscle contraction, and energy (ATP) for process is provided by mitochondria that lie between myofibrils.

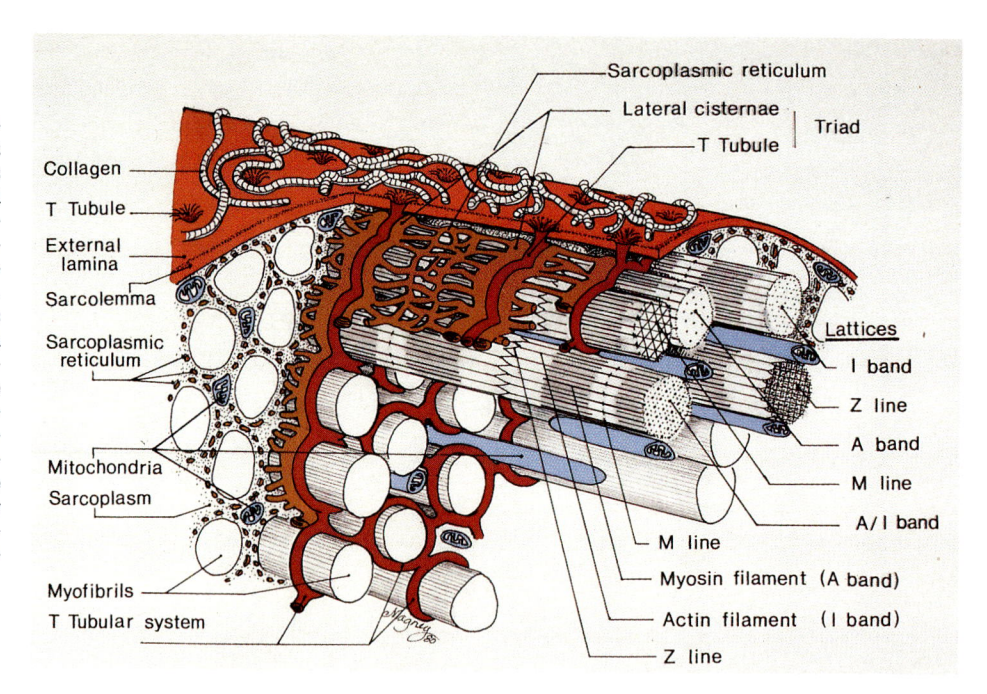

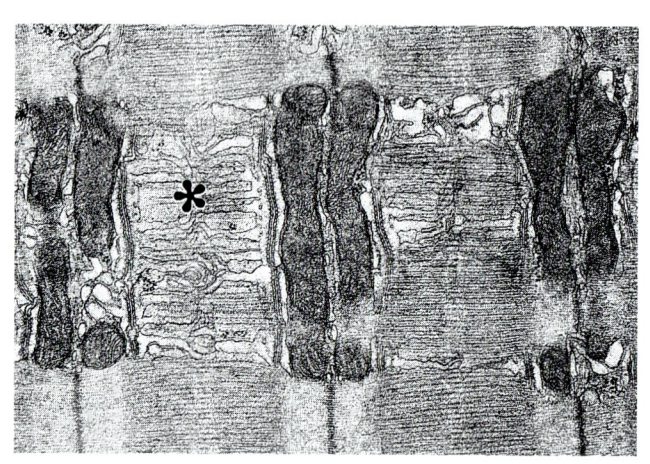

Fig. 8-12. High-magnification TEM revealing sarcomeres in mouse skeletal muscle. Because of tangential plane of section, the tubular network (*) of sarcoplasmic reticulum surrounding myofilaments (of sarcomere) can be seen. ($\times 14,000$.)

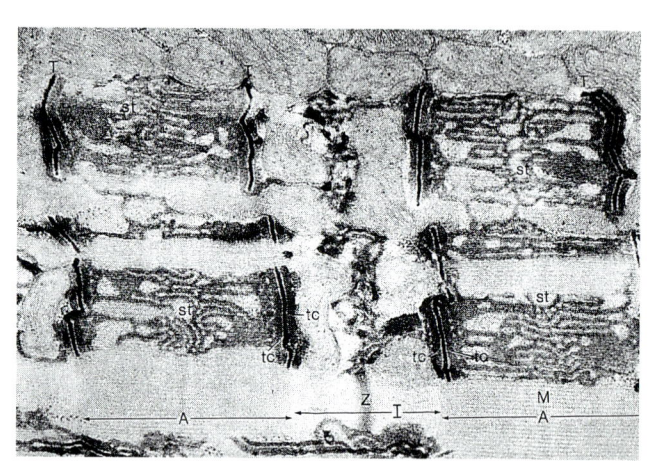

Fig. 8-13. Sarcoplasmic reticulum of two adjacent sarcomeres, which appears electron dense by TEM because of staining with heavy metal. Subdivisions of sarcoplasmic reticulum include sarcotubules *(st)* surrounding sarcomere and terminal cisternae *(tc)* seen at junction of A and I bands in mammalian skeletal muscle. Association of two terminal cisternae with T tubule *(t)*, an invagination of plasmalemma, forms triad. *A*, A-band; *I*, I-band; *M*, M-line; *Z*, Z-line. ($\times 15,500$.)

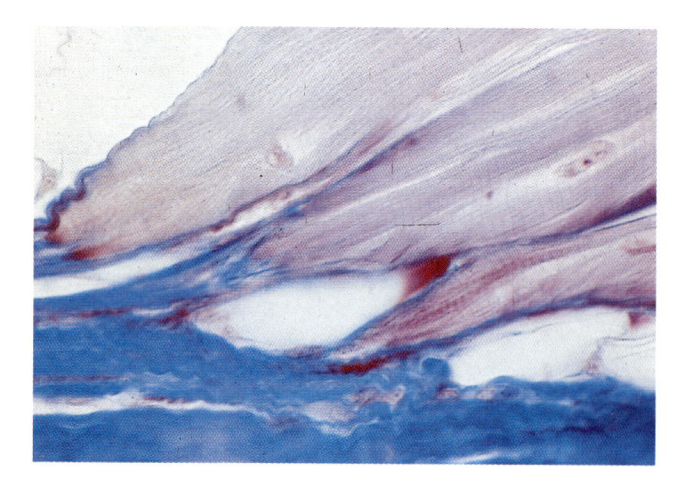

Fig. 8-14. LM of myotendinous junction showing interface between striated skeletal muscle and tendon. Collagen (stained blue) of endomysium and perimysium blends with collagen bundles of tendon. (Azan stain; $\times 600$.)

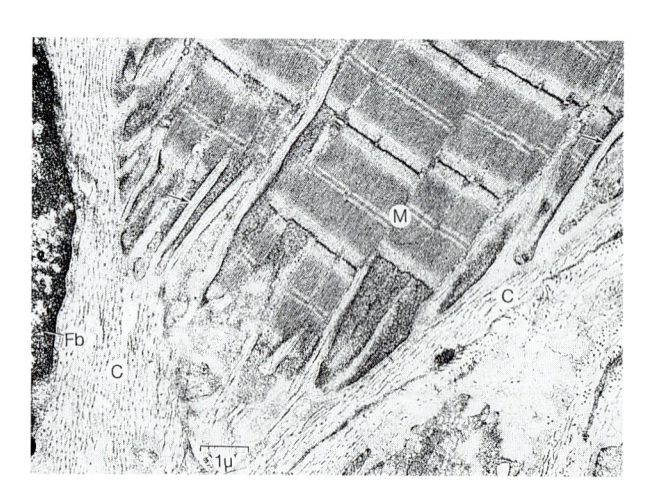

Fig. 8-15. Myotendinous junction by TEM. Note that indentation of cell membrane increases surface area for attachment of endomysium to cell surface. Sarcomeres terminate in modified Z lines on sarcolemma. *Fb*, Fibroblasts; *C*, collagen; *M*, muscle. ($\times 6,900$.)

MUSCLE 55

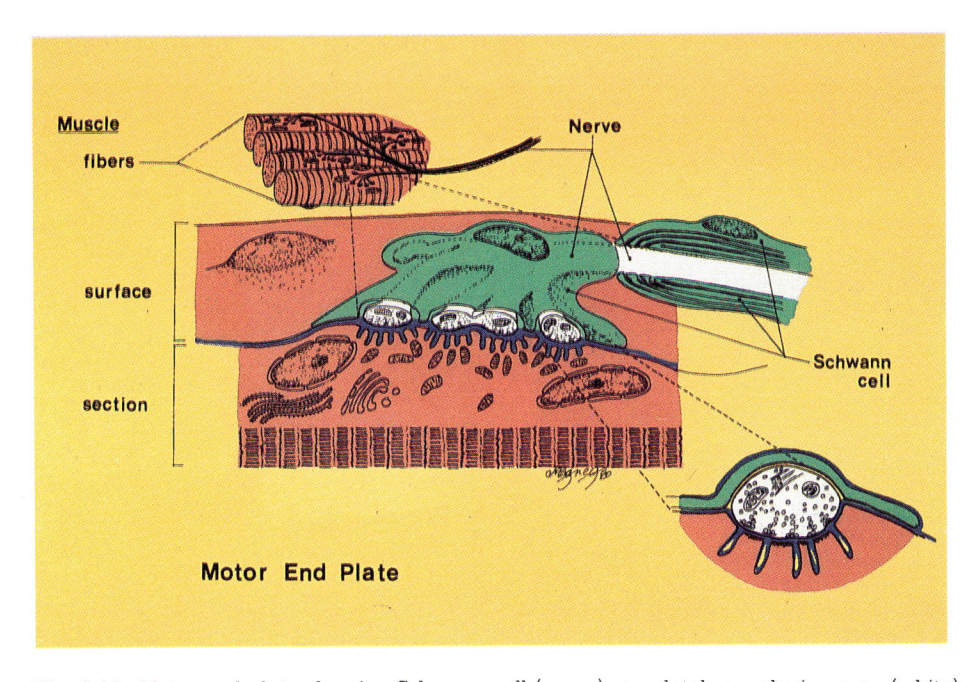

Fig. 8-16. Motor end plate showing Schwann cell (green) completely enveloping axon (white) and exposed surface of axon terminals, which are in direct apposition to primary synaptic cleft. Infoldings of muscle cell membrane, called junctional folds, produce secondary synaptic clefts (subneural clefts).

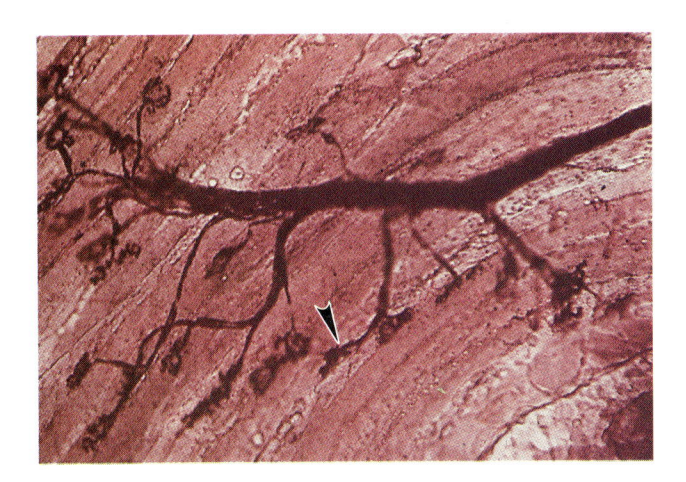

Fig. 8-17. LM of whole mount of skeletal muscle showing nerve fiber dividing into terminal branches. Each branch ends in motor end plate characterized by multiple synaptic terminals *(arrowhead).* (Silver stain; ×400.)

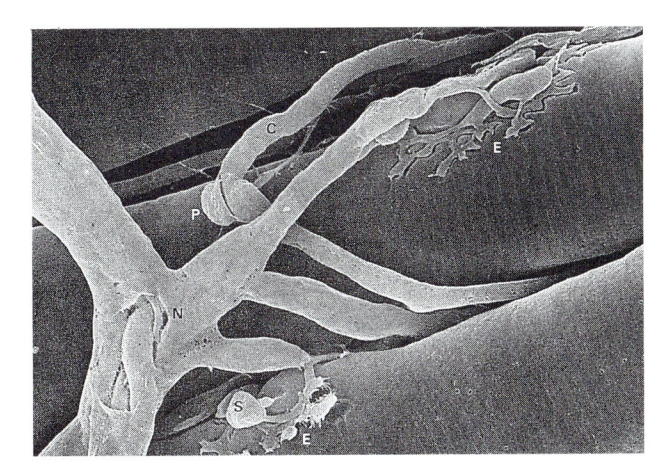

Fig. 8-18. SEM of motor end plate. Collagen and external lamina of muscle and nerve cells have been removed. Bundle of nerves *(N)* can be seen to end in two motor end plates *(E)*. Observe branching of terminal portion of nerve fiber in motor end plate, where it is in apposition to muscle cell. Schwann cell *(S)* covers axon and terminals. Small blood capillary *(C)* and pericyte *(P)* are also visible. (×750.)

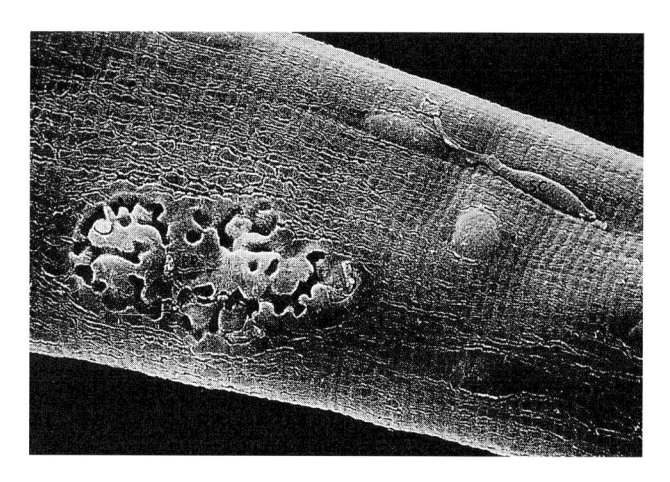

Fig. 8-19. SEM of mouse skeletal muscle cell revealing site *(left)* where motor end plate occupies deep furrows (synaptic cleft) in cell surface. Identify also striations of sarcomeres in myofibrils, nuclei of muscle cell, and satellite cell. (×1,000.)

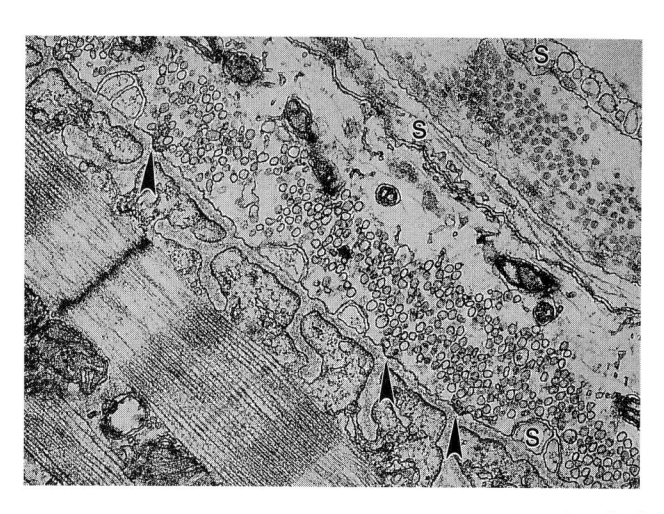

Fig. 8-20. Motor end plate seen by TEM. Terminal is sheathed by a Schwann cell process *(s, top)*, which intrudes fingers *(s, lower right)* between terminal and muscle cell. Synaptic vesicles cluster around specialized regions of presynaptic membrane *(arrowheads)*, which are subtended by dense cytoplasmic material forming bands that face junctional folds. Postsynaptic muscle membrane at top of folds is also underlaid by electron-dense material that may represent its active or receptive zone. Compare with Fig. 8-19 and 8-21. (×18,400.)

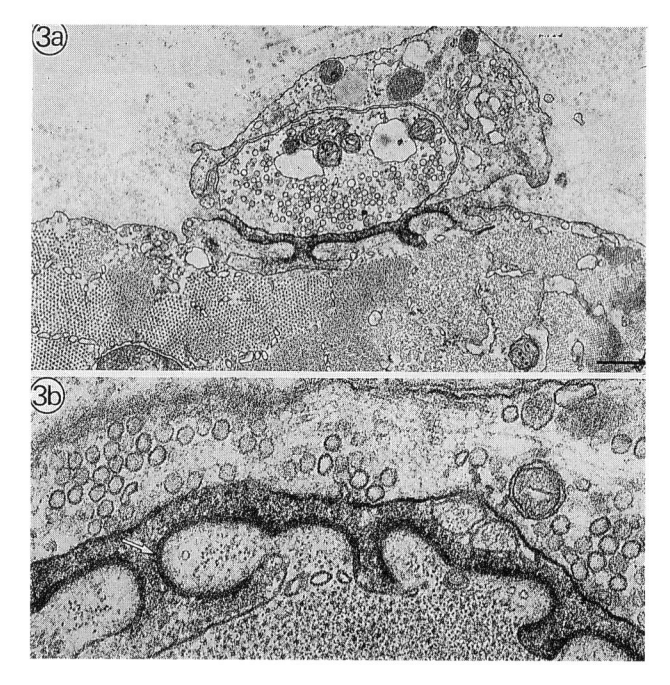

Fig. 8-21. TEM of motor end plates in which cholinergic receptors have been localized using HRP-labeled alpha-bungarotoxin. Compare normal morphology *(frame 3A)* with localization of cholinergic receptors *(frame 3B)*. In latter, dense staining, which represents presence of cholinergic receptors, is seen on postsynaptic membrane at top of, and partly down sides of, junctional folds of muscle cell. (3A, ×7000; 3B, ×24,800.)

MUSCLE 57

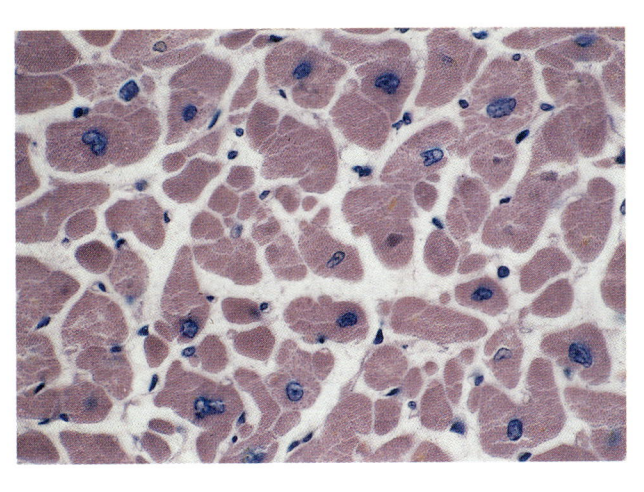

Fig. 8-22. Cross section of cardiac muscle cells by LM. Nuclei of muscle cells (fibers), when in plane of section, are centrally located in cell. (H&E; ×400.)

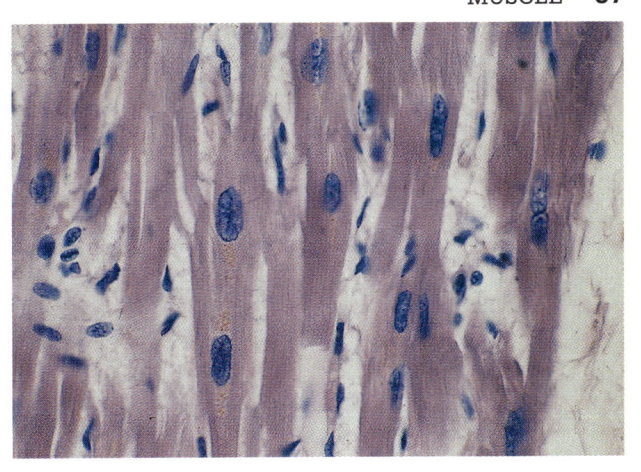

Fig. 8-23. Cardiac muscle seen (LM) in longitudinal section. Many capillaries lie between muscle fibers. Muscle cell nuclei are central, with lipofuscin pigment (gold-brown granules) concentrated at nuclear poles. (H&E; ×400.)

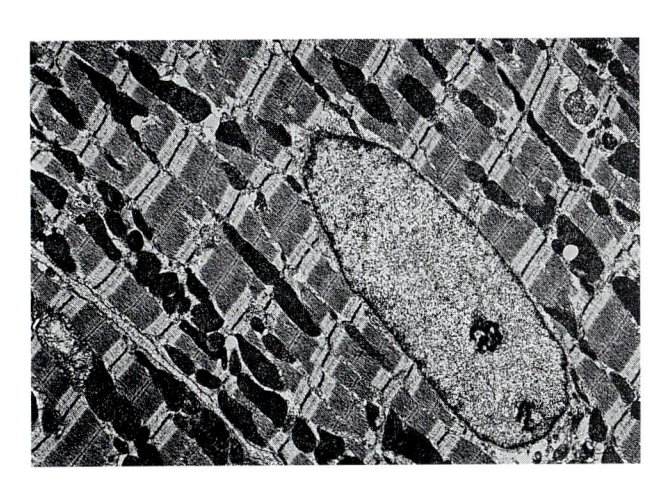

Fig. 8-24. Cardiac muscle in longitudinal section (TEM). Sarcomere registration is less precise than in skeletal muscle. Mitochondria are prominent. (×3,600.)

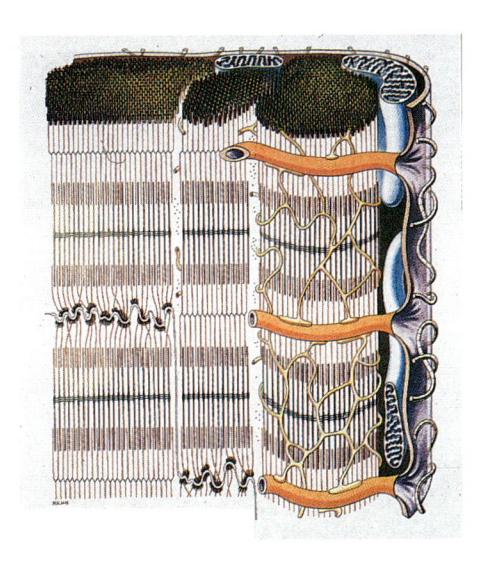

Fig. 8-25. Cardiac muscle showing differences in location of T tubules (at Z lines) and in arrangement of sarcoplasmic reticulum (in diads) as compared to skeletal muscle. Seen at left is intercalated disk composed of actin filaments attached to sarcolemma (fascia adherens), desmosome, and gap junction.

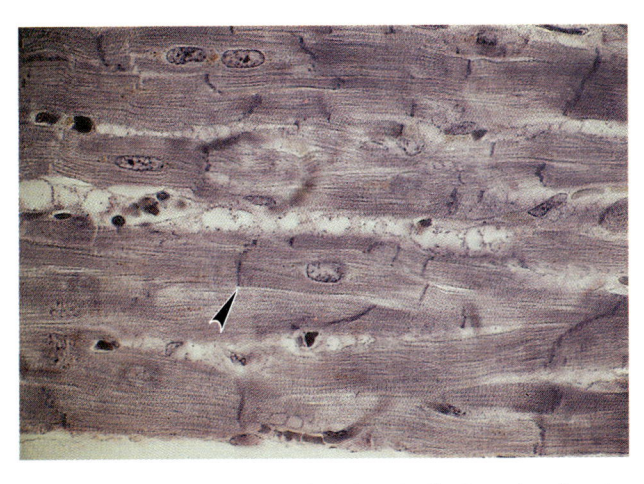

Fig. 8-26. LM of cardiac muscle in longitudinal section showing branching of fibers and intercalated disks (arrowhead), which are junctional complexes that join cardiac muscle cells and their branches end to end. (H&E; ×400.)

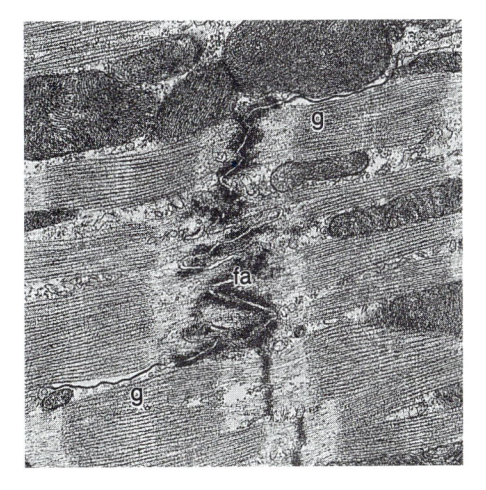

Fig. 8-27. High-magnification TEM of intercalated disk in cardiac muscle showing regions of cell membrane that correspond to gap junctions (g) and fascia adherens (fa). Intercalated disks are modified Z lines, since actin filaments in terminal sarcomeres are anchored in fascia adherens. (×12,500.)

58 COLOR ATLAS OF HISTOLOGY

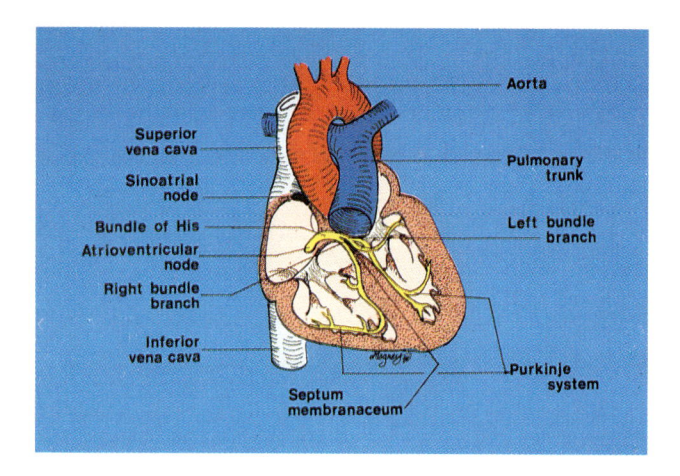

Fig. 8-28. Conducting system of heart identifying sinoatrial node, atrioventricular node, atrioventricular bundle of His, and bundle branches.

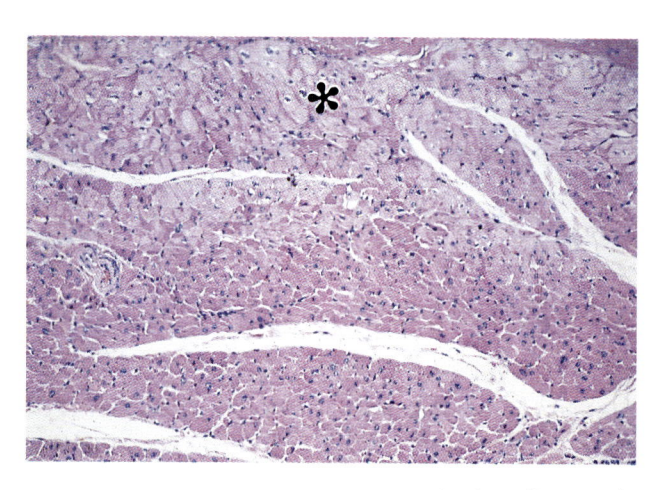

Fig. 8-29. LM of myocardium. Lightly stained cardiac muscle cells (*) seen in upper half are called Purkinje fibers. They are modified for conduction. Their staining is less intense because of reduced numbers of myofibrils within cell. (H&E; ×100.)

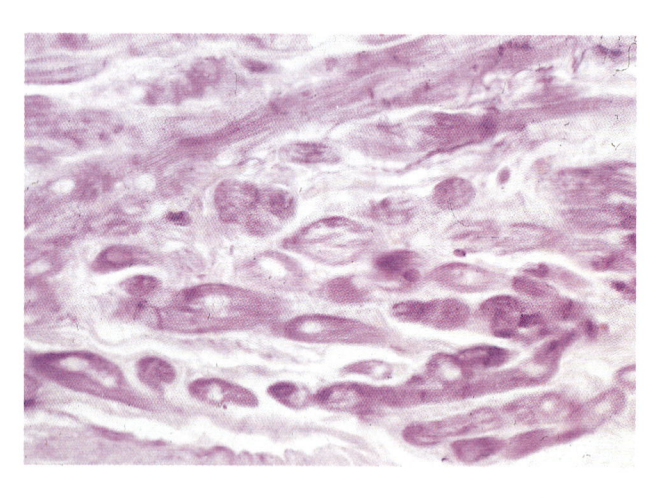

Fig. 8-30. Purkinje system consisting of modified cardiac muscle cells. Cells are stained magenta color by periodic acid–Schiff because of their high content of glycogen. Nuclei appear as negative images. (PAS stain; ×400.)

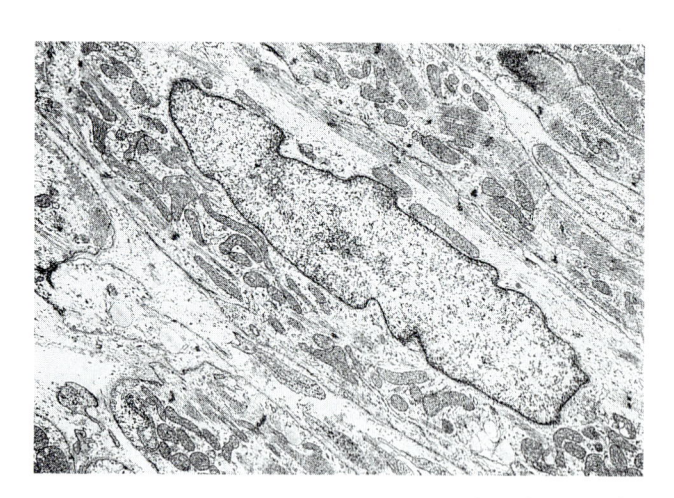

Fig. 8-31. Longitudinal section of Purkinje fiber from monkey heart seen by TEM. Note paucity of myofibrils within cytoplasm and their irregular distribution. (×5,000.)

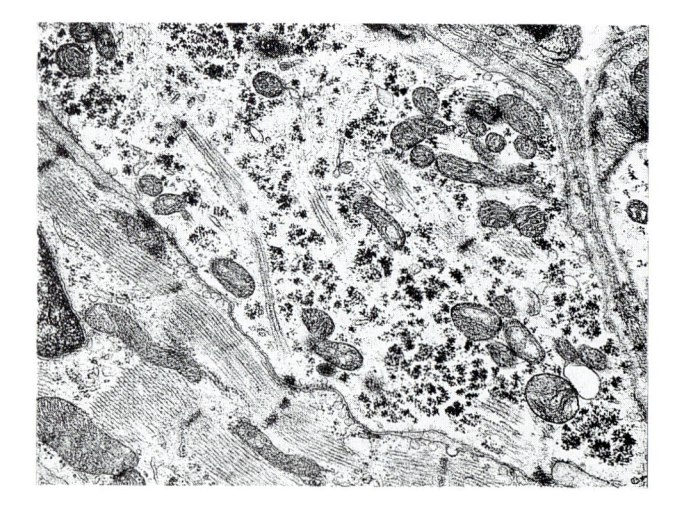

Fig. 8-32. High-magnification TEM of Purkinje fiber. Compare this specialized fiber with normal cardiac muscle cell at bottom of field. Large amounts of glycogen and few myofibrils are seen in Purkinje fiber. (×10,200.)

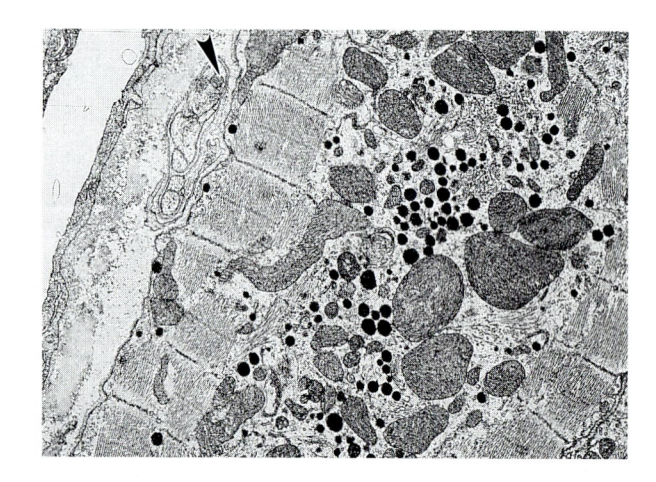

Fig. 8-33. TEM of atrial cardiac muscle cell. Unmyelinated nerve containing synaptic vesicles *(arrowhead)* is seen in endomysium between muscle cell and endothelial cell at left. Small dense granules are characteristic of atrial muscle cells and are presumed to contain atrial natriuretic peptide. (×6,400.)

CHAPTER 9

NERVE

THE FUNCTION OF the nervous system is to sense change in the external or internal environment of the body and to respond by causing the body to react appropriately to change. The nervous system can be subdivided into the **central nervous system,** including the brain and spinal cord, and the **peripheral nervous system,** which constitutes all nerve fibers and aggregates of neurons outside the central nervous system. On the basis of function, the nervous system can be classified into **somatic** or voluntary components (motor and sensory) and **visceral** or **autonomic nervous system** regulating involuntary functions of the body.

Nerve tissue consists of cells called **neurons** that have the capacity to respond (**irritability**) to a wide variety of stimuli and to transmit (**conductivity**) excitation to other nerve cells or effector organs such as muscle and glands. A neuron cell body, or **soma,** has multiple cytoplasmic processes called **dendrites** that receive information and a single process, the **axon,** used to carry information to other cells. Neurons may be classified according to the numbers and distribution of their processes (i.e., multipolar, bipolar, pseudounipolar) or process length (Golgi I, Golgi II); according to function (i.e., sensory, motor, excitatory, inhibitory); or by the chemical nature of the neurotransmitter (i.e., adrenergic, cholinergic).

The euchromatic nucleus with its prominent nucleolus is indicative of a cell active in protein synthesis. Polysomes and rough endoplasmic reticulum (RER), essential for protein synthesis, are so prominent in the neuronal cytoplasm that they were called **Nissl bodies** by early light microscopists. Other cellular organelles are present, including numerous mitochondria and bundles of microfilaments called **neurofibrils.** End-stage lysosomes (lipofuscin granules by LM) may be numerous in aged nerve cells.

Dendrites are usually short and contain cytoplasmic organelles. Small evaginations of the membrane, called **dendritic spines,** are receptive areas for synapse with other neurons. Dendrites always carry a wave of depolarization toward the cell soma; however, in the case of sensory bipolar or pseudounipolar neurons, the long peripheral process has all the characteristics of an axon with a small receptive (dendritic) region at some distance from the cell body.

Axons vary in length from less than a millimeter to approximately a meter. At the soma, an **axon hillock,** largely devoid of Nissl bodies, gives rise to a short, unmyelinated initial segment of the axon where synapses may occur. Microtubules, microfilaments, smooth endoplasmic reticulum (SER), and mitochondria are present in the cytoplasm (**axoplasm**) of axons and are implicated in axonal transport. There is a single axon per cell, but it may produce collaterals along its length, all of which end in terminal branches called **telodendria** that form synaptic terminals. Axons are classified according to diameter (A, B, C) and the presence or absence of a myelin sheath. In myelinated axons **nodes of Ranvier** indicate an unmyelinated region between adjacent myelin segments. An internodal (myelinated) segment is approximately 1 mm in length.

Chemical synapses, which comprise most synapses in the nervous system, are regions where telodendria come into proximity with other neurons or skeletal muscle. A synapse has two compartments: the **presynaptic** axon terminal and the **postsynaptic** region, which may be on a nerve cell body (**axosomatic**), a dendrite (**axodendritic**), the initial segment of an axon (**axo-initial segment**), a presynaptic knob near the axon terminal (**axoaxonic**), or a **motor end plate** of skeletal muscle. A **synaptic cleft** (20 to 30 nm wide) separates the pre- and postsynaptic membranes. Within the presynaptic terminal are vesicles containing **neurotransmitters,** which may be excitatory (round vesicles) or inhibitory (flat vesicles). A number of neurotransmitters are known (noradrenaline, dopamine, serotonin, peptides, acetylcholine, glutamic acid, gamma-aminobutyric acid), and more than one may be found in a terminal. Also present in the terminal are mitochondria, microtubules, and neurofilaments. Vesicles fuse with the presynaptic membrane to release neurotransmitter by exocytosis into the synaptic cleft. The neurotransmitter diffuses across the cleft and binds with postsynaptic membrane receptors to cause depolarization or hyperpolarization of the postsynaptic cell membrane. Excess neurotransmitter is destroyed by enzymes present in the postsynaptic region (i.e., acetylcholinesterase). A variation of synaptic structure is demonstrated by the innervation of smooth or cardiac muscle, which differs from the motor end plates of skeletal muscle in that no specialized contacts are formed with the muscle cells but, instead, the axons terminate as swellings within the endomysium where their neurotransmitter is released into the extracellular space.

Peripheral sensory receptors assume a variety of forms (i.e., **Meissner's corpuscle, Pacinian corpuscle, end bulb of Krause, naked nerve endings**) and transmit over peripheral processes toward pseudounipolar cell bodies that lie within the dorsal root or sensory ganglia near the central nervous system (CNS). Without passing through the cell soma, the impulse is carried into the spinal cord or brainstem by a central process (axon).

Associated with neurons in nerve tissue are a variety of supporting cells. In the CNS are neural crest–derived neuroglial cells including **protoplasmic astrocytes** and **fibrous astrocytes,** which provide mechanical and nutritional support and protection (blood-brain barrier) to the neurons, and **oligodendrocytes,** which myelinate axons in the CNS. **Microglial cells** are macrophages of the CNS that arise from blood-borne monocytes rather than the neural crest and are not true glial cells. In the peripheral nervous system (PNS), the cells surrounding and supporting ganglionic neurons are called **satellite** or **capsule cells. Schwann cells** form an investment called the neurilemma around all nerve fibers in the peripheral nervous system. Nerve fibers covered only with Schwann cell cytoplasm are referred to as **unmyelinated fibers,** while those surrounded by multiple wrappings of Schwann cell membranes and cytoplasm (myelin) are known as **myelinated fibers.** In axons the rate of propagation of the action potential along the fiber is proportional to the thickness of the myelin sheath.

In the PNS sensory and motor axons are wrapped together in layers of connective tissue to form nerves. Individual nerve fibers and their Schwann cell coverings are surrounded by an incomplete layer of reticular fibers called **endoneurium;** a number of fibers are bundled into fascicles by **perineurium;** and groups of fascicles bound together by **epineurium** form a nerve. There is little or no connective tissue in the CNS, where bundles of axons called **tracts** (instead of nerves) are supported by neuroglia.

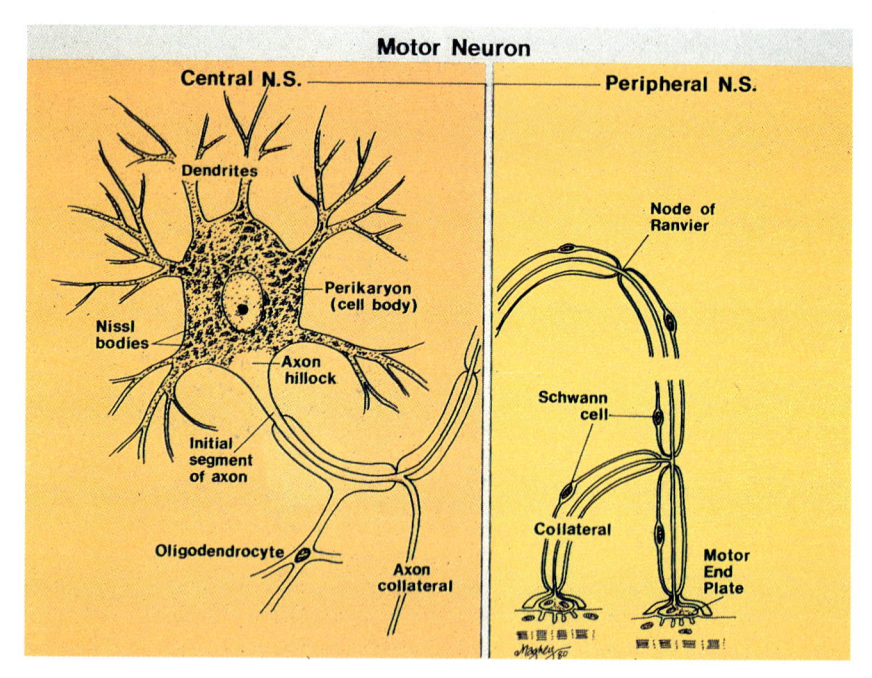

Fig. 9-1. Motor neuron in ventral horn of spinal cord. Neuronal perikaryon or cell body is located in gray matter of ventral horn. Axonal process begins at axon hillock (devoid of Nissl bodies [RER] and ribosomes). Motor axon extends from central nervous system into peripheral nervous system, where it terminates in motor end plates on skeletal muscle. In the central nervous system oligodendrocytes form myelin sheath around axons, whereas in the peripheral nervous system this is accomplished by Schwann cells.

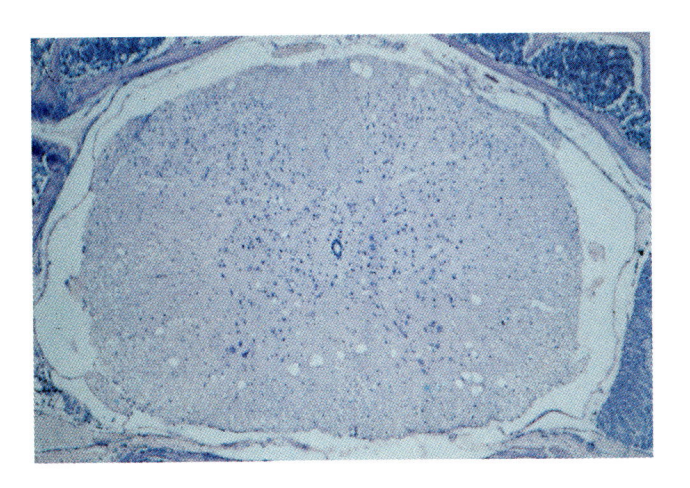

Fig. 9-2. LM of mouse spinal cord showing both white matter (myelinated axons) and gray matter (cell bodies of neurons in dorsal and ventral horns). Large basophilic cells (lower motor neurons) are seen in ventral horns. (H&E; ×30).

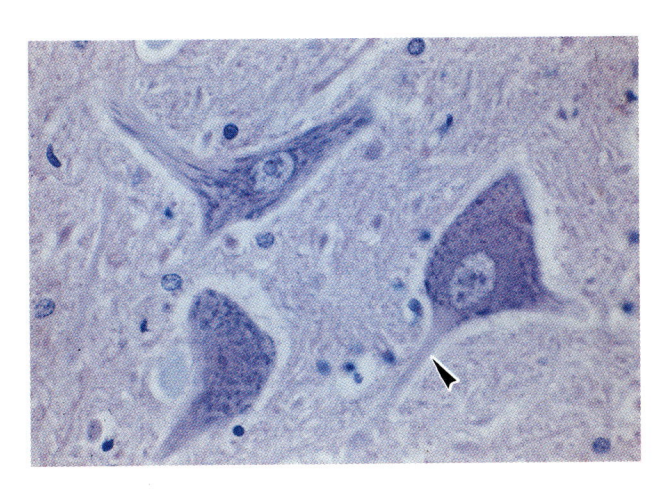

Fig. 9-3. High-magnification LM reveals three lower motor neurons within human spinal cord. Two of these neurons exhibit large euchromatic nuclei with prominent nucleoli and basophilic rough endoplasmic reticulum called Nissl substance. Axon hillock *(arrowhead)* is recognized by absence of Nissl substance. Nuclei of neuroglial cells are seen in surrounding neuropil (see Fig. 9-4). (H&E; ×400.)

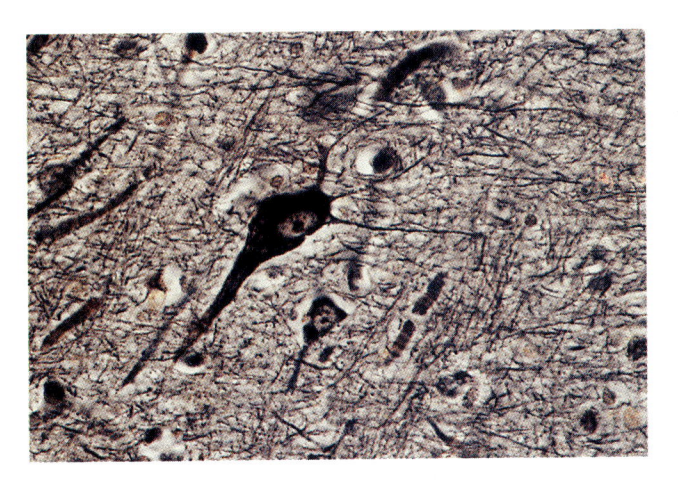

Fig. 9-4. LM of neuron in cerebral cortex. Use of silver impregnation reveals neuronal processes extending from perikaryon, and numerous processes from other cells. These processes and neuroglia are referred to as neuropil. (Silver stain; ×400.)

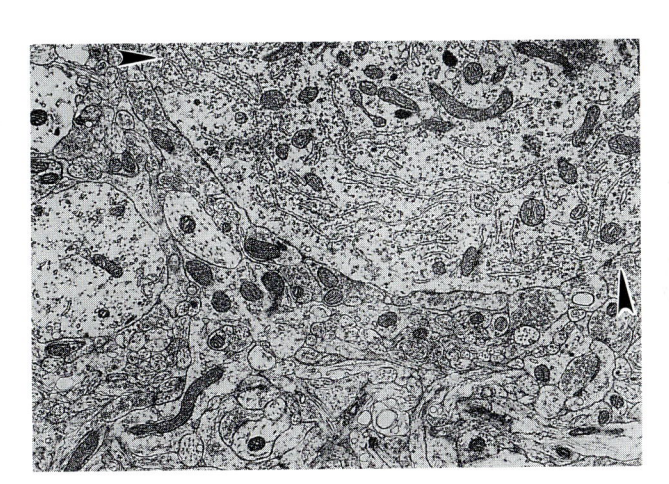

Fig. 9-5. TEM of neuronal cytoplasm *(upper right)* in central nervous system showing numerous profiles of rough endoplasmic reticulum, called Nissl substance at LM levels, and many mitochondria. Plasmalemma of cell runs from midright to upper left *(arrowheads)* and separates neuronal cytosol from surrounding neuropil and synaptic endings. (×7,200.)

Fig. 9-6. Peripheral nervous system (PNS). Cell bodies of lower motor neurons are located in gray matter of spinal cord and brainstem; those of sensory neurons are found within dorsal root or sensory ganglia. Sensory and motor processes/axons in PNS have myelin sheaths of variable thickness produced from wrapping of Schwann cell membrane and cytoplasm. Unmyelinated fibers lack this wrapping of membranes but are still individually covered by Schwann cell cytoplasm. Layers of connective tissue formed by fibroblasts surround nerves in the PNS. Each nerve fiber is surrounded by a layer called endoneurium, while groups of fibers (fascicles) are enveloped by perineurium. Bundles of fascicles surrounded by an external connective tissue layer called epineurium form the spinal nerve.

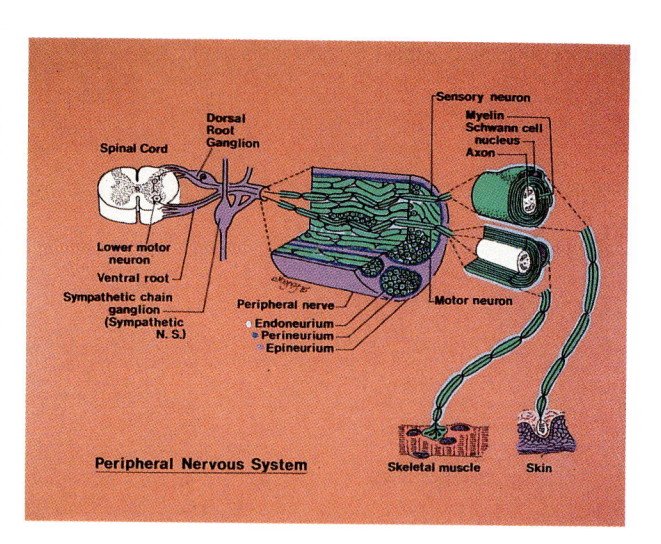

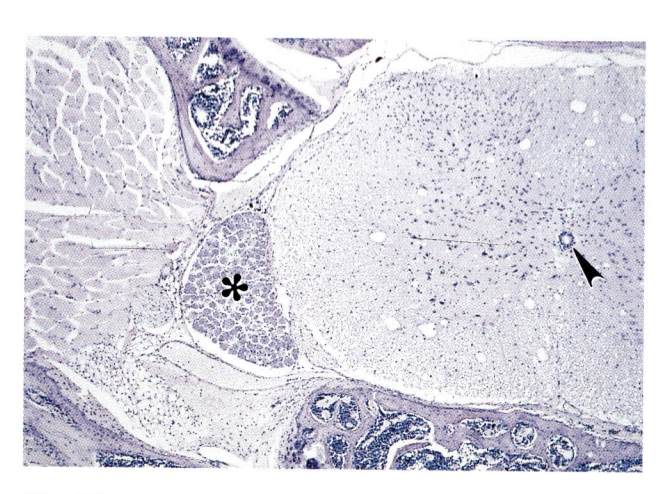

Fig. 9-7. Cross section of mouse spinal cord by LM showing central canal *(arrowhead)*, white and gray matter, and a dorsal root ganglion *(asterisk)*. Note vertebrae, their medullary cavities, and dorsal body wall musculature. (H&E; ×40.)

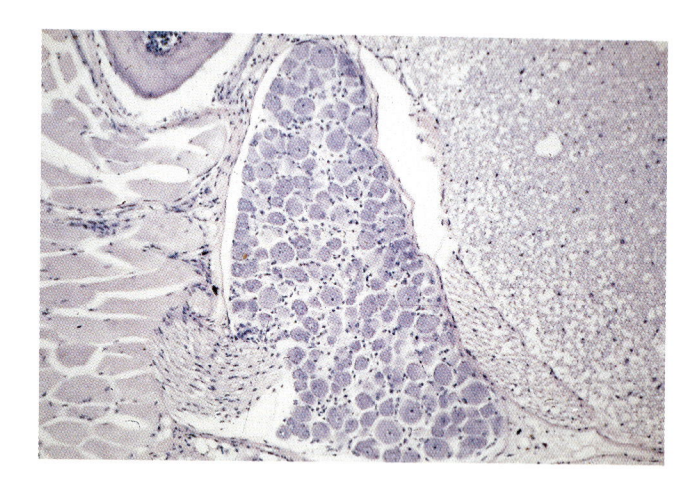

Fig. 9-8. Dorsal root ganglion of mouse spinal cord at higher magnification (LM). Satellite cells surround perikarya of neurons. (H&E; ×100.)

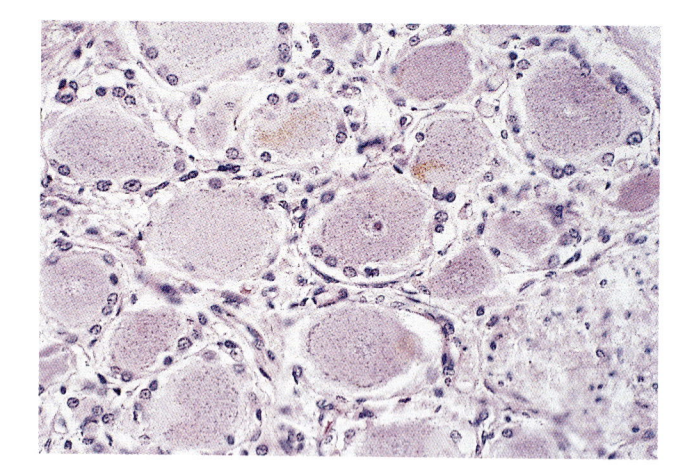

Fig. 9-9. Higher magnification LM of dorsal root ganglion cells containing lipofuscin pigment. Observe perineuronal satellite cells. All neurons in a dorsal root ganglion are sensory neurons. (H&E; ×500.)

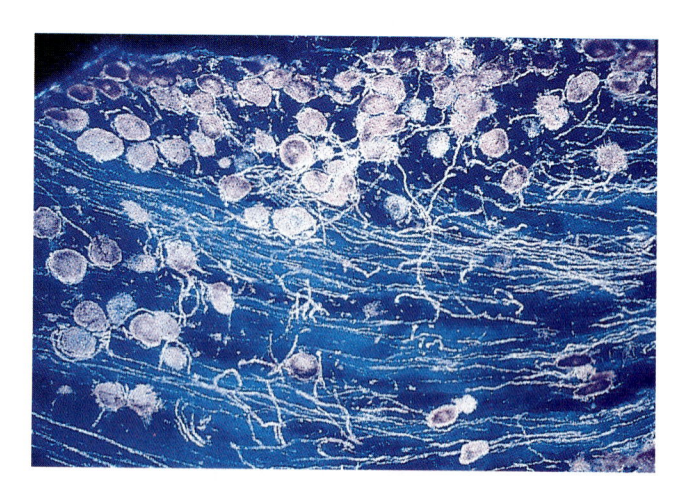

Fig. 9-10. Dorsal root ganglion as viewed by dark field microscopy (LM) after neuronal uptake of horseradish peroxidase. Note abundant nerve processes, which appear white while cell bodies are pink. (×150.)

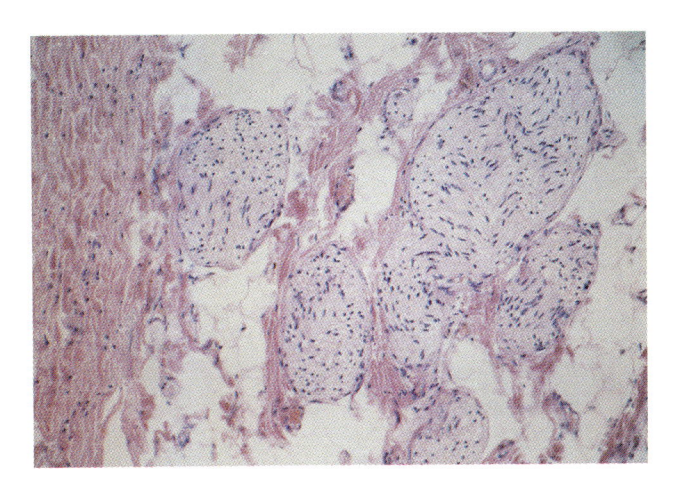

Fig. 9-11. LM of peripheral nerve surrounded by connective tissue epineurium and divided by perineurium into fascicles. Individual fibers (axons) within nerve are ensheathed by endoneurium and are seen in both cross and longitudinal sections. (H&E; ×60.)

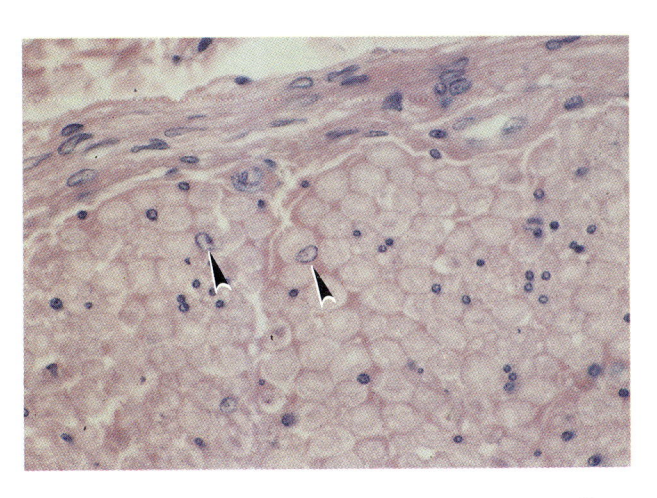

Fig. 9-12. LM of axons surrounded by myelin. Schwann cell nuclei *(arrowheads)* are large and vesicular and found within endoneurial sheaths that surround individual axons. (H&E; ×400.)

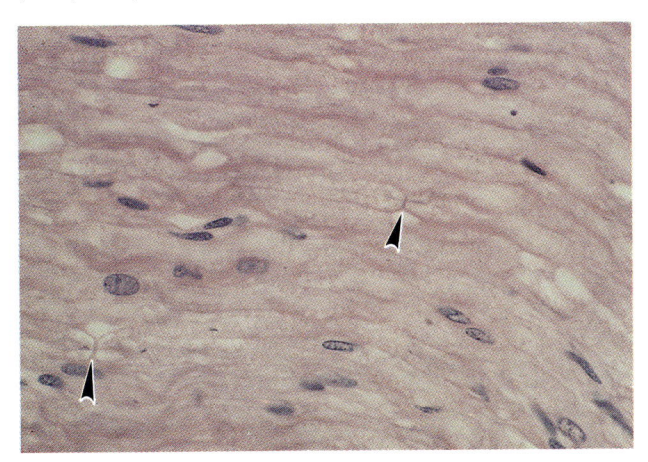

Fig. 9-13. LM of nerve in longitudinal section. Clear nodal cytoplasm of Schwann cells helps distinguish two nodes of Ranvier *(arrowheads)*. Small flattened nuclei of fibroblasts and endothelial cells and large vesicular nuclei of Schwann cells may be seen. (H&E; ×400.)

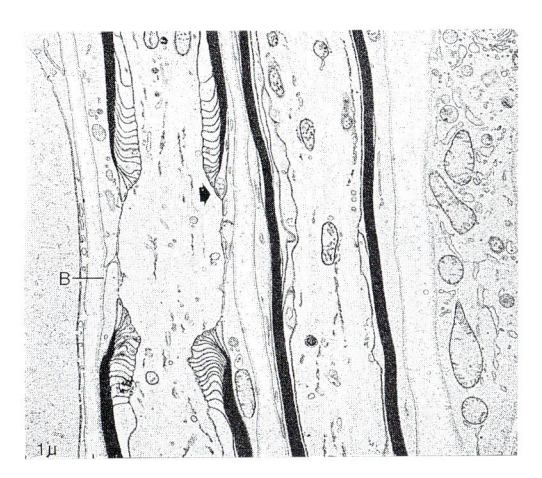

Fig. 9-14. TEM showing longitudinal section through node of Ranvier. Myelin sheaths of adjoining Schwann cells show distended individual lamellae *(arrowhead)*, each of which is closely apposed to axon membrane. Node of Ranvier is covered by cytoplasmic processes of Schwann cell. These processes are separated from connective tissue interstitium by an external lamina *(b)*, which is type IV collagen resembling basal lamina of epithelium. (×9,600.)

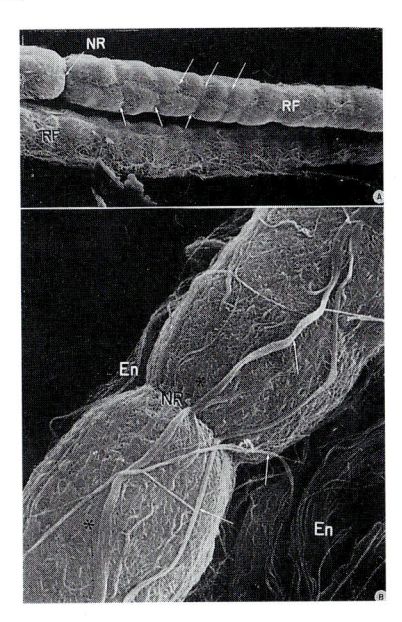

Fig. 9-15. SEM of isolated myelinated fibers of sciatic nerve. In **A**, endoneurial sheath *(En)* and node of Ranvier *(NR)* are clearly evident. Segmented appearance of nerve fiber *(arrows)* is due to a number of incisures (clefts of Schmidt-Lantermann) in myelin sheath. **B** is an SEM at higher magnification of node of Ranvier *(NR)* showing terminal portions of two Schwann cells (*). Delicate reticular fibers, together with some collagen fibers *(arrows)*, form endoneurial sheath *(En)*. (Upper ×600; lower ×4,800.)

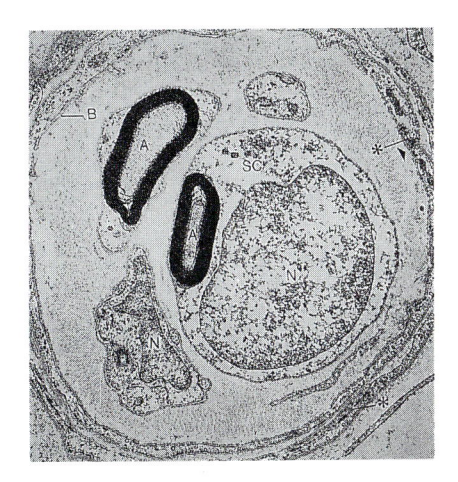

Fig. 9-16. Cross section through branch of facial nerve seen by TEM. In center of this endoneurial sheath are four Schwann cells, two of which contain myelinated **(A)** axons and two, unmyelinated axons. All are surrounded by collagenous sheath and two layers of flattened connective tissue cells. These fibroblasts are unique in that they are covered with external lamina **(B)**. This cellular perineural sheath may function as barrier to nutrients diffusing from capillaries to Schwann cells and nerve fibers within sheath. *SC*, Schwann cell; *N*, nucleus; *, junctional area. (×3,800.)

64 COLOR ATLAS OF HISTOLOGY

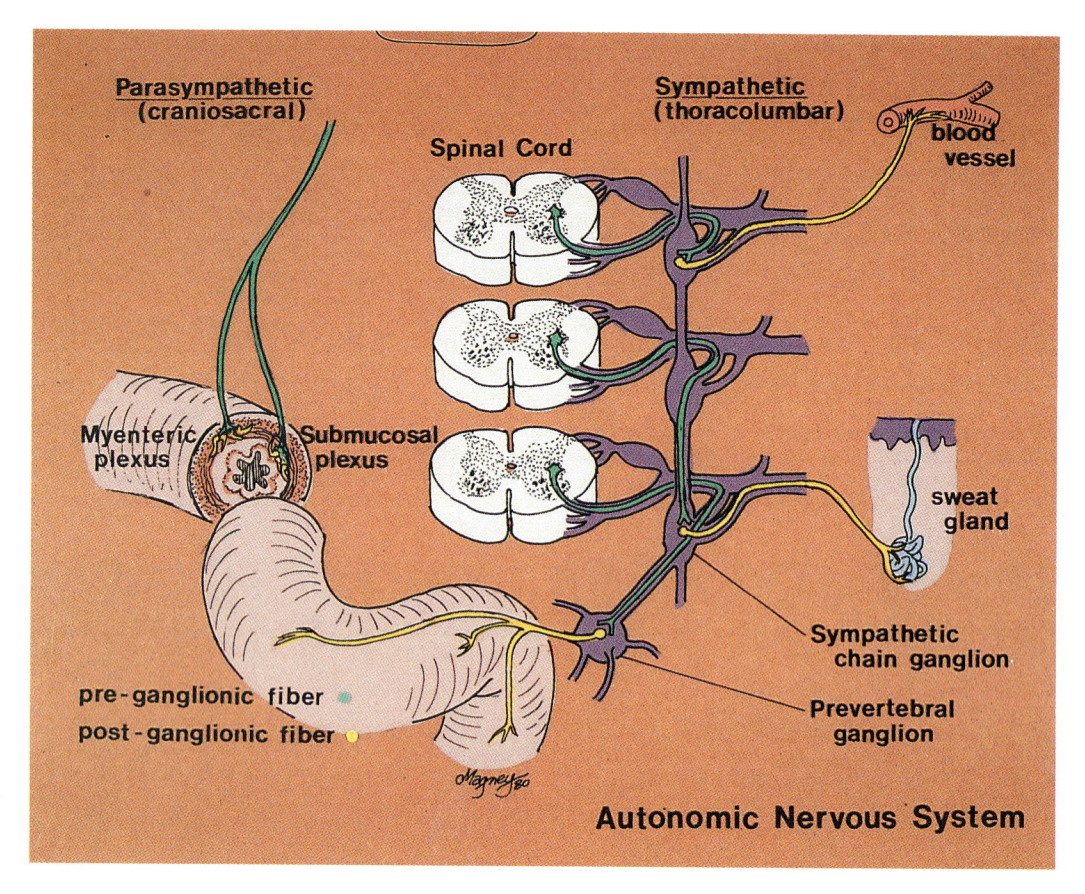

Fig. 9-17. Autonomic nervous system with sympathetic and parasympathetic divisions.

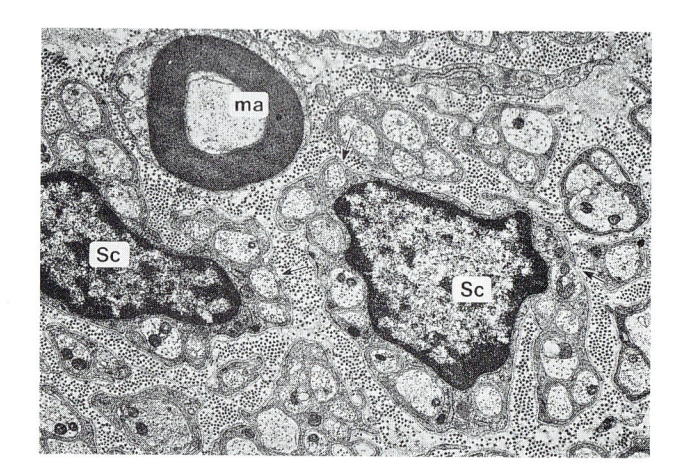

Fig. 9-18. TEM of unmyelinated nerve in connective tissue. Axons are enfolded in Schwann cell cytoplasm, and some contain synaptic vesicles. Schwann cell has external lamina. (×1,600.)

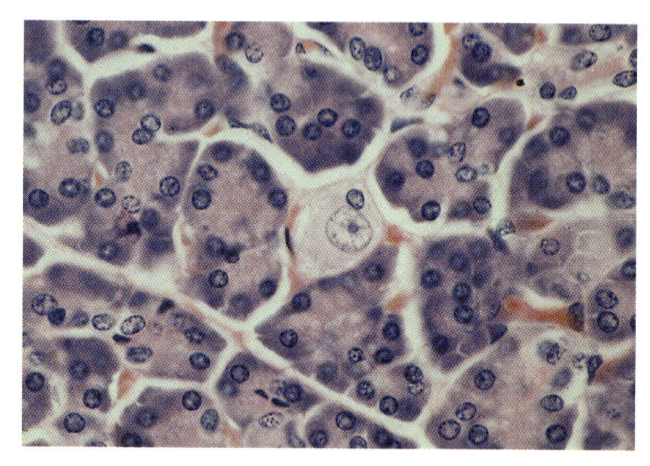

Fig. 9-19. Parasympathetic postganglionic neuron and its adjacent satellite cell seen amid pancreatic acinar cells. (H&E; ×800.)

NERVE 65

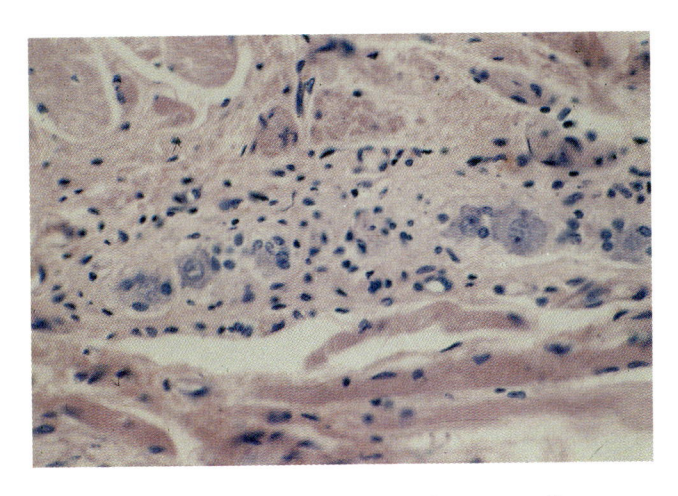

Fig. 9-20. High-magnification LM of esophagus revealing myenteric plexus of Auerbach. Large basophilic cell bodies are postganglionic parasympathetic neurons and are surrounded by satellite cells. (H&E; ×350.)

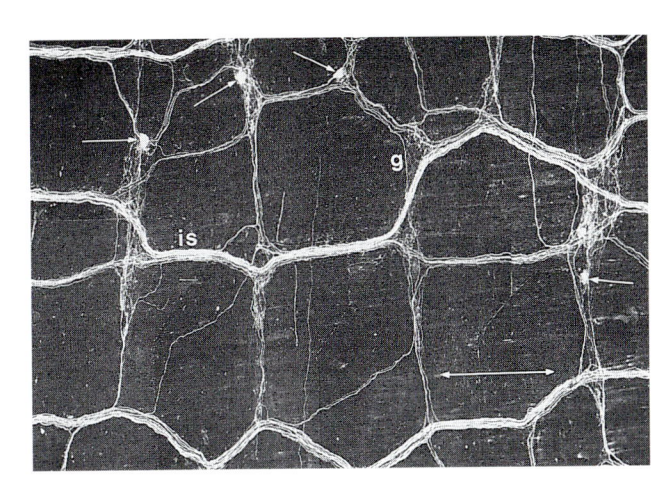

Fig. 9-21. Low-power LM of myenteric plexus in whole mount of small intestine showing distribution of fibers stained for 5-hydroxytryptamine immunoreactivity. Double arrows indicate orientation of longitudinal muscle. Immunoreactivity is seen in fibers of internodal strands *(is)*. Nerve cell bodies can be seen *(single arrows)* within ganglia of plexus *(g)*. (×80.)

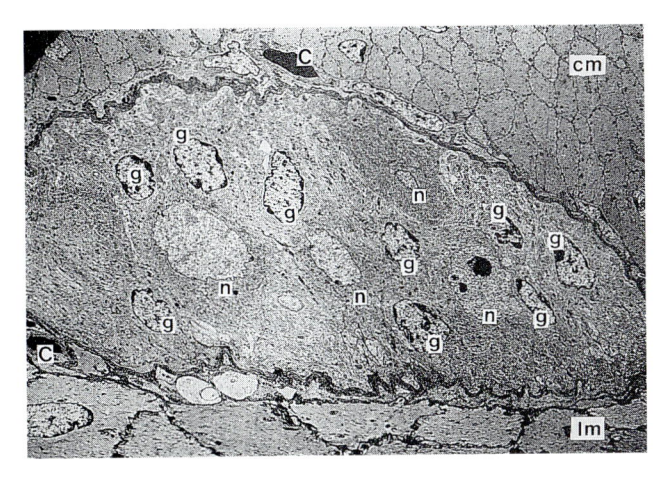

Fig. 9-22. TEM of parasympathetic neuronal cell bodies in the myenteric plexus. Observe "glial-like" satellite or capsule cells surrounding neuronal cell bodies. *cm*, Circular muscle; *lm*, longitudinal muscle; *n*, neuron; *g*, capsule or satellite cells; *c*, connective tissue. (×1,300.)

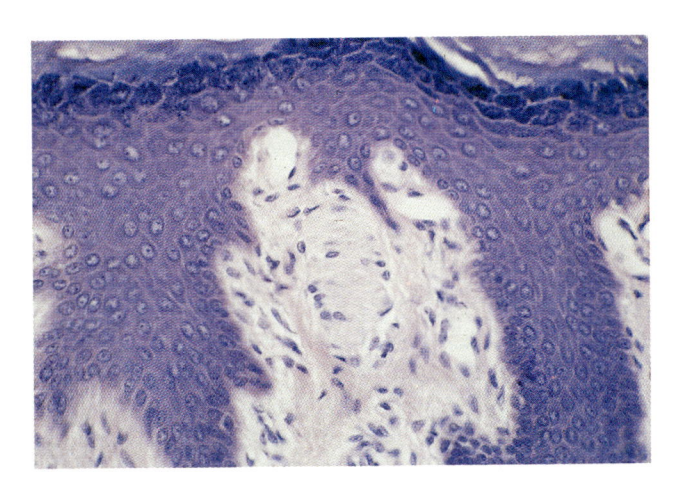

Fig. 9-23. LM of Meissner's corpuscle *(center)* in skin. It is a touch receptor in papillary layer of dermis. (H&E; ×350.)

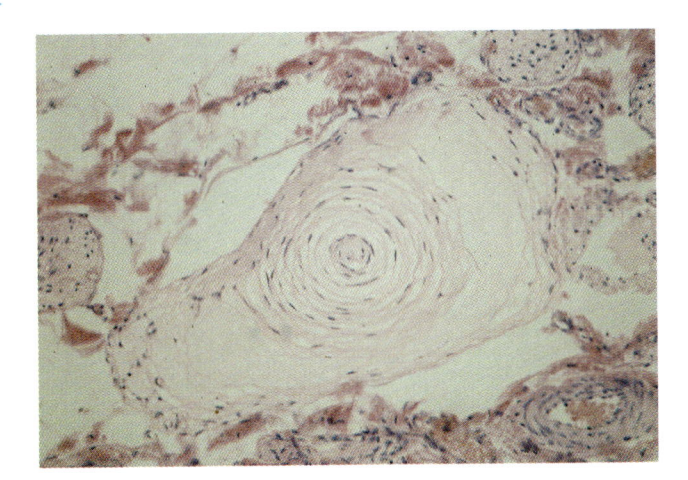

Fig. 9-24. Pacinian corpuscle. This corpuscle is a pressure receptor distributed throughout dermis and subcutaneous connective tissue (as shown here) and also in joint capsules, mesenteries, urinary bladder, and other tissues that may be deformed by pressure. (H&E; ×100.)

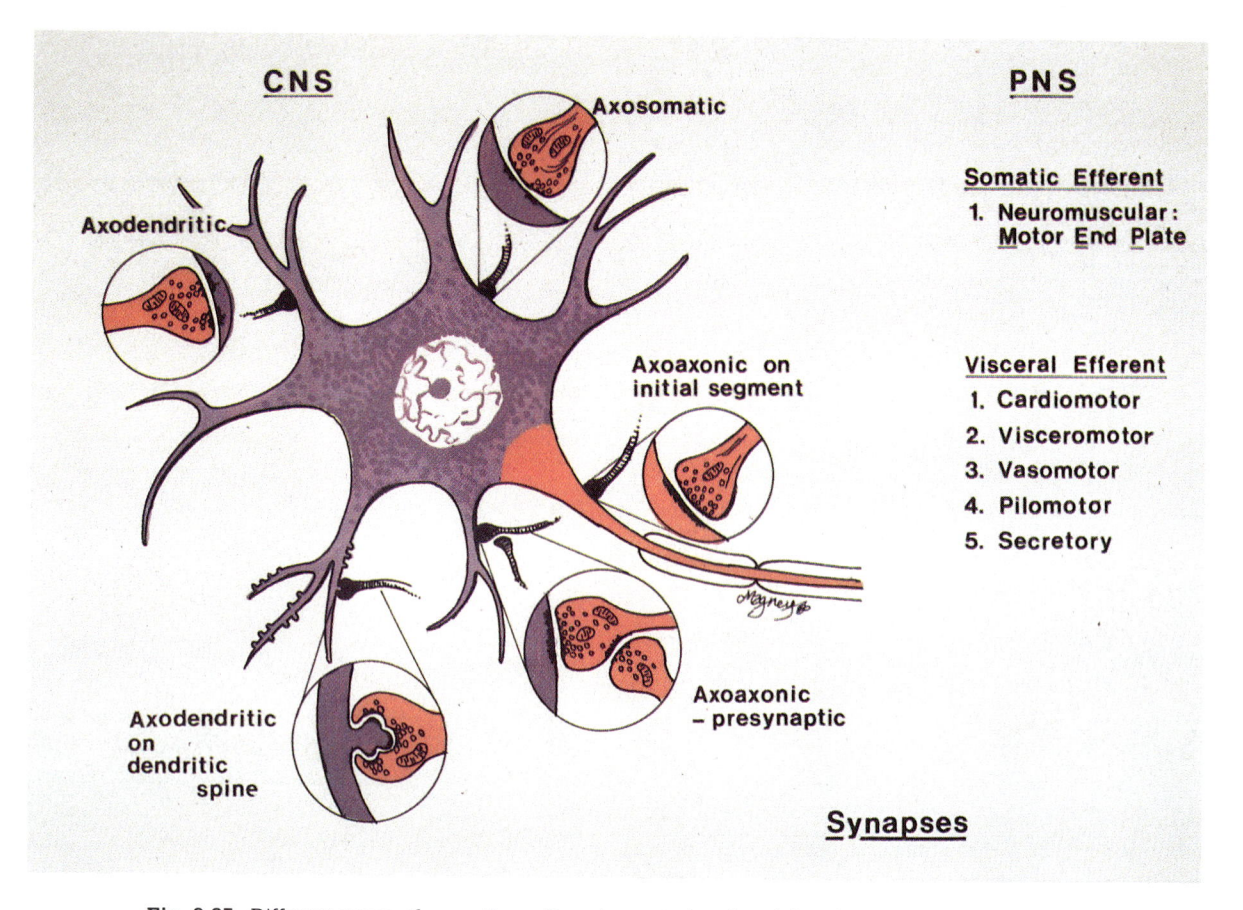

Fig. 9-25. Different types of synaptic endings in central and peripheral nervous systems. Synapses may occur on cell body (soma), on dendrites or dendritic spines, or on axons (initial segments or terminal boutons). In PNS synaptic endings of somatic efferent fibers terminate on skeletal muscle, while those of visceral efferent fibers innervate smooth muscle, cardiac muscle, and glands.

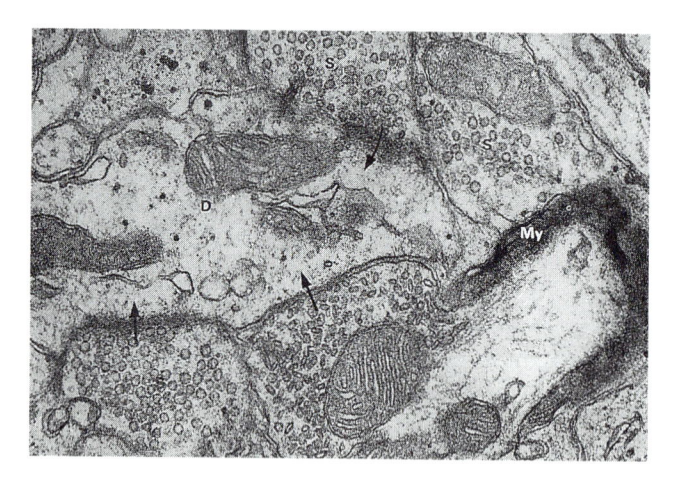

Fig. 9-26. TEM of synapses between terminal boutons and dendrite (D). Arrows indicate direction of tranmission. Vesicles exhibit different shapes: round vesicles are thought to contain excitatory neurotransmitters; flattened vesicles, inhibitory neurotransmitters. *M*y, Myelin. (×35,000.)

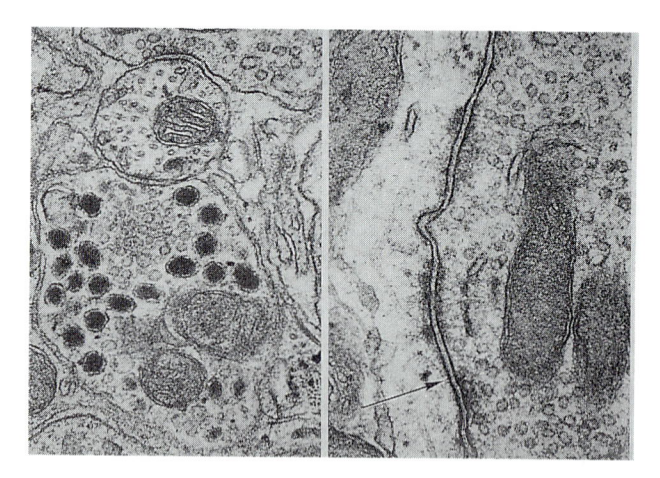

Fig. 9-27. TEM of synaptic terminals revealing pre- and postsynaptic thickening of plasmalemma. Note mitochondria and synaptic vesicles. Presynaptic terminal *(left)* contains round vesicles with excitatory neurotransmitters and dense-cored vesicles that contain adrenergic-peptidergic neurotransmitters. Arrow in right portion points to postsynaptic membrane thickening in opposing cell. (Right ×37,000; left ×38,500.)

CHAPTER 10

CARDIOVASCULAR SYSTEM

THE CARDIOVASCULAR SYSTEM moves blood throughout the body by virtue of a muscular pump, the heart, which is connected to vessels that carry blood from the heart to the tissues and back again to the heart. This closed tubular system transports oxygen and nutrients to cells and removes the byproducts of cellular metabolism, carbon dioxide and wastes by transporting them to organs responsible for their elimination from the body. Moreover, blood carries hormones from endocrine glands to target organs, provides for the recirculation of immune system cells, and regulates body temperature.

The organs of the cardiovascular system are the four-chambered heart and blood vessels, which assume a variety of configurations based on function. Blood vessels are hollow organs with layered walls. In all cases the wall adjacent to the lumen has an endothelial lining that is attached to underlying muscle by connective tissue. This forms a layer called the **endocardium** in the heart or the **tunica intima** in blood vessels. The middle layer of the heart is called **myocardium** and is composed of cardiac muscle; a **tunica media** consisting of smooth muscle is found in blood vessels. A connective tissue **epicardium** covers the heart, while a **tunica adventitia** surrounds blood vessels.

HEART

The cardiac muscle of the heart forms irregularly concentric layers that attach to a fibrous **skeleton** in such a way as to form a double pump. The right side of the heart receives deoxygenated blood and pumps it through a **pulmonary circuit** to the lungs where it exchanges carbon dioxide for oxygen. The blood returns to the left side of the heart and from there is distributed through the **systemic circuit** to all tissues of the body. Two thin-walled **atria** receive venous blood—the right atrium from the systemic circulation and the heart itself, the left atrium from the pulmonary circulation. Because venous blood is at low pressure, the walls of the atria are relatively thin. Right and left **ventricles,** responsible for pumping blood from the heart through the pulmonary and systemic circuits against higher peripheral resistance, have correspondingly thicker walls. Within the walls of the right atrium are two nodal regions. The **sinoatrial** (SA) node, at the base of the superior vena cava, and the **atrioventricular** (AV) node, in the atrial interventricular septum, are both composed of modified cardiac muscle. Their activity may be modulated by the autonomic nervous system. The sinoatrial node initiates a wave of depolarization that passes throughout the atrial muscle, causing atrial contraction, and also activates the atrioventricular node. Modified cardiac muscle cells called **Purkinje fibers,** characterized by a paucity of myofibrils and much glycogen, carry the wave of depolarization from the AV node along the **bundle of His** and bundle branches to both ventricles, which then contract. Purkinje fibers can be seen just beneath the endocardium on each side of the interventricular septum. Certain atrial (cardiac) muscle cells produce secretion granules known to contain **atrial natriuretic peptide,** a hormone that acts in the kidney to produce diuresis and natriuresis.

ARTERIES

Arteries are classified into three major groups: **elastic arteries, muscular arteries,** and **arterioles.** The major arteries leaving the heart—the pulmonary trunk and the aorta—together with their principal branches are classified as **elastic arteries.** These vessels are designed to expand when blood is ejected from the heart (systole) and to recoil during relaxation of the ventricles (diastole). Therefore the thick tunica media consists of layers of smooth muscle in a network of elastic fibers. Nutritional support to the tunica intima and the innermost portion of the tunica media is derived by diffusion from the lumen of the vessel, while small arterioles or capillaries **(vasa vasorum)** located in the outer tunica media and the tunica adventitia supply these parts of the vessel wall. **Muscular** (or **distributing**) **arteries** carry blood to specific regions of the body; the tunica media of these vessels contains a moderate amount of smooth muscle and less elastin. Regulation of blood pressure within the arterial system is accomplished by **arterioles.** These are small in diameter, contain only a few smooth muscle cells in the tunica media, and by their vasoconstriction or vasodilation regulate the flow of blood to capillary beds.

CAPILLARIES

Capillaries are thin-walled vessels formed by squamous endothelial cells; they lack the tunica media and tunica adventitia seen in arteries or veins. Based on the ultrastructure of the endothelial cell, capillaries can be divided into three types. **Continuous** capillaries are found in muscle tissue and the nervous system, while **fenestrated** capillaries lie in organs where rapid exchange of small peptides or molecules occurs (i.e., endocrine glands, intestinal villi, kidney glomeruli). Both of these capillary types possess an intact basement membrane. **Sinusoidal** capillaries are usually larger in diameter and are characterized by large gaps in the endothelial wall and an incomplete basement membrane. They appear to be designed for the movement of cells or large molecules through the vessel wall (as occurs in bone marrow, spleen, and liver). Blood usually flows from arterioles to capillaries to venules. However, in **portal systems** blood flows through two capillary beds connected by either a vein (liver, pituitary) or arteriole (kidney). Capillary beds may also be short circuited by direct **arteriovenous anastomosis.**

VEINS

Veins return blood from capillary beds to the heart. **Venules** are larger than capillaries and, like them, may be partially surrounded by pericytes, which often share the basememt membrane of the endothelial cells. Pericytes have been reported to have contractile activity and also to possess potential for transformation into other cell types. Unlike capillaries, endothelial cells in venules have "loose" tight junctions (zonula occludens), and they serve as a major site for the exchange of small molecules across the vessel wall. **Postcapillary venules (high endothelial venules [HEV])** differ from capillaries in having a tall cuboidal endothelial lining that possesses surface receptors that facilitate the recognition of circulating lymphocytes and their movement through the venule wall.

In small venules the tunica media is greatly reduced, but as the caliber of veins increases to **small** and **medium** sized veins, all three tunics (intima, media, and adventitia) can be recognized in the wall. Because of low venous pressure, the tunica media contains few smooth muscle cells and the tunica adventitia predominates as the major layer of the vessel wall. To prevent backflow, veins that return blood against gravity possess valves of connective tissue covered with endothelium. **Large veins** (superior and inferior venae cavae) entering the heart and their major tributaries are characterized by a tunica adventitia, which contains numerous bundles of smooth muscle arranged parallel to the long axis of the vessel.

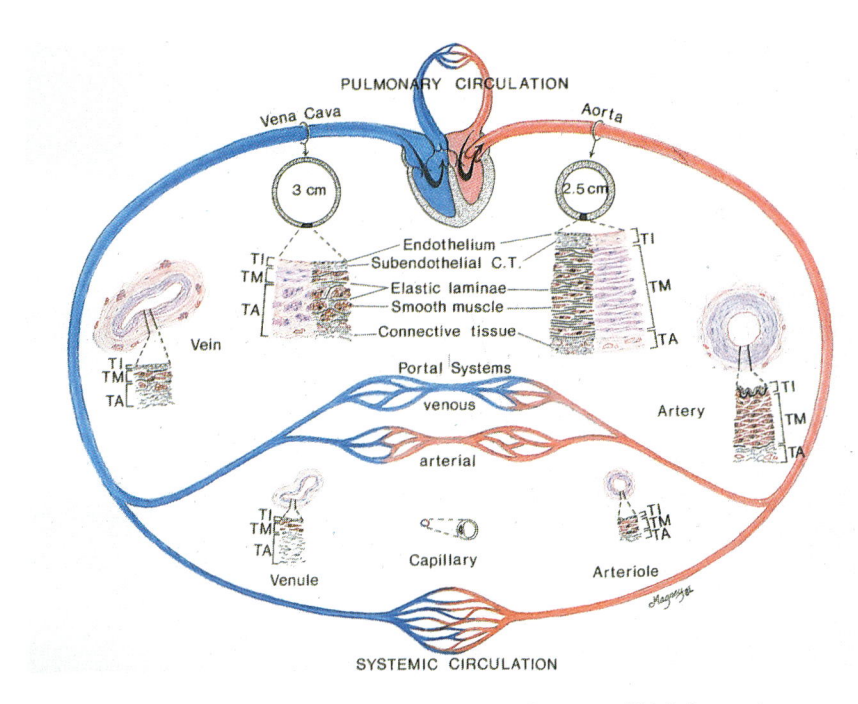

Fig. 10-1. Vessels comprising systemic circulation. Because of high internal pressure (100 mm Hg) in arterial circulation, walls of vessels exhibit multiple layers of smooth muscle and relatively little connective tissue. On the other hand, pressure within veins is low (<15 mm Hg), so walls of these vessels consist largely of connective tissue with small amounts of smooth muscle. Notice that large veins close to heart have longitudinally oriented bundles of smooth muscle in tunica adventitia. *TI*, Tunica intima; *TM*, tunica media; *TA*, tunica adventitia.

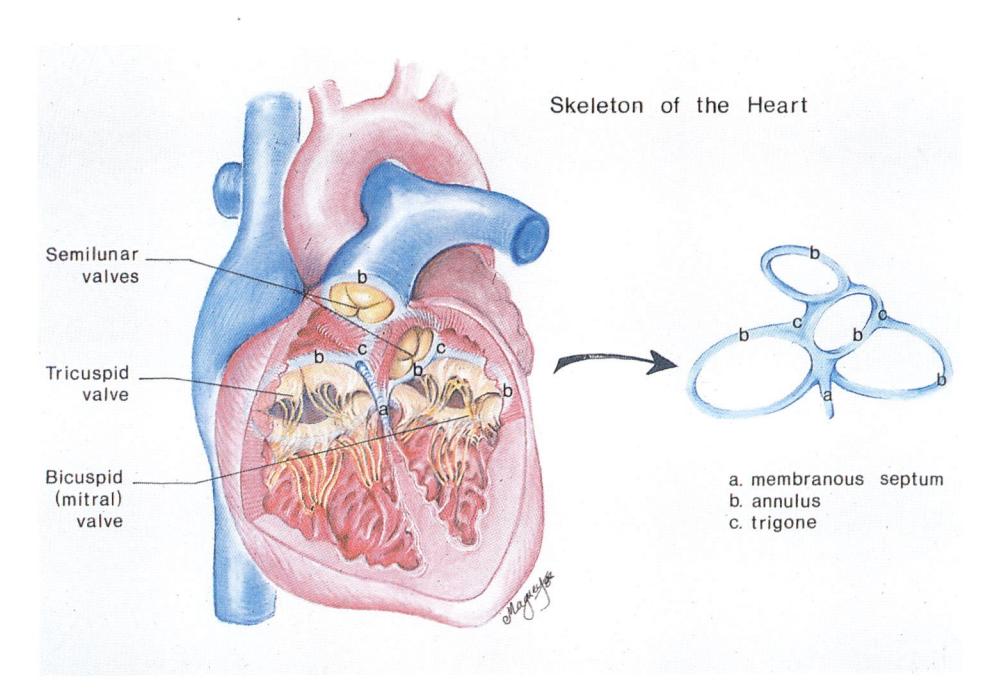

Fig. 10-2. Skeleton of heart and its relationships to both heart valves and cardiac muscle cells, which attach (origin and insertion) to this connective tissue framework. Cardiac skeleton is composed of three parts: the annuli fibrosi, trigones, and membranous interventricular septum. Annuli fibrosi are fibrous rings from which valve leaflets originate. Trigones consist of areas of dense connective tissue joining annuli fibrosi. Membranous septum is part of interventricular septum adjacent to atrial chambers. Purkinje system of heart, which coordinates contraction of chambers, pierces cardiac skeleton near membranous interventricular septum and descends in the septum.

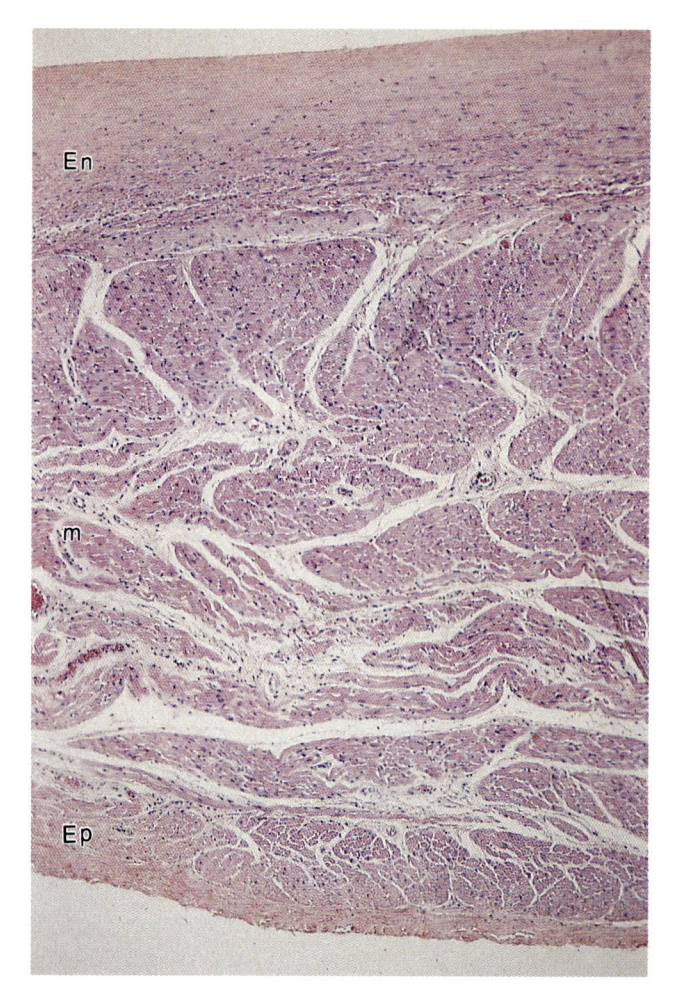

Fig. 10-3. LM showing full thickness of atrial wall. Easily distinguished are three layers of heart: endocardium *(En)*, adjacent to lumen; myocardium *(M)*, consisting mainly of cardiac muscle; and epicardium *(Ep)*, containing significant amount of fat. (H&E; ×25.)

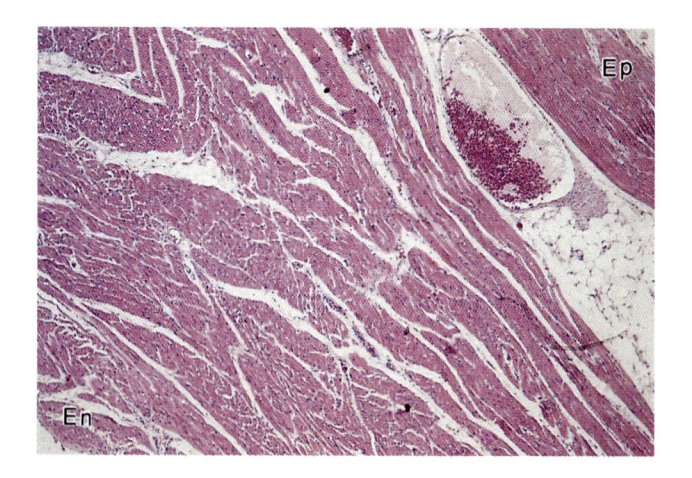

Fig. 10-4. Low-magnification LM of ventricular wall. Observe thickness of myocardium between endocardium *(En)* and epicardium *(Ep)*. (H&E; ×6.)

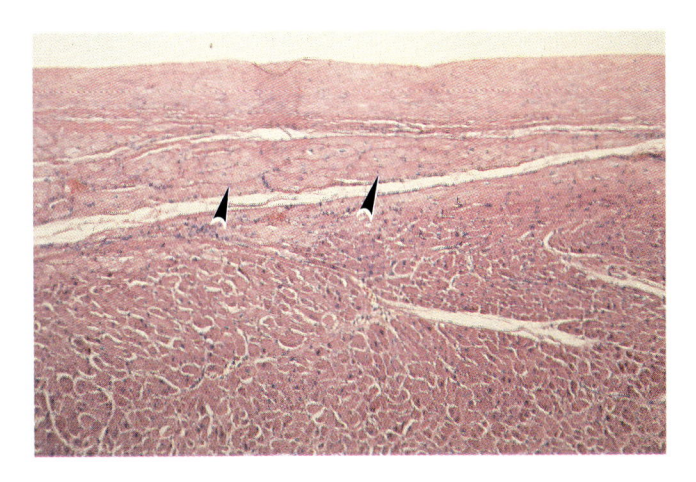

Fig. 10-5. LM of ventricular wall. Purkinje fibers *(arrowheads)* can be seen in subendocardial connective tissue. Compare their size and staining characteristics with those of underlying cardiac muscle cells in myocardium. (H&E; ×40.)

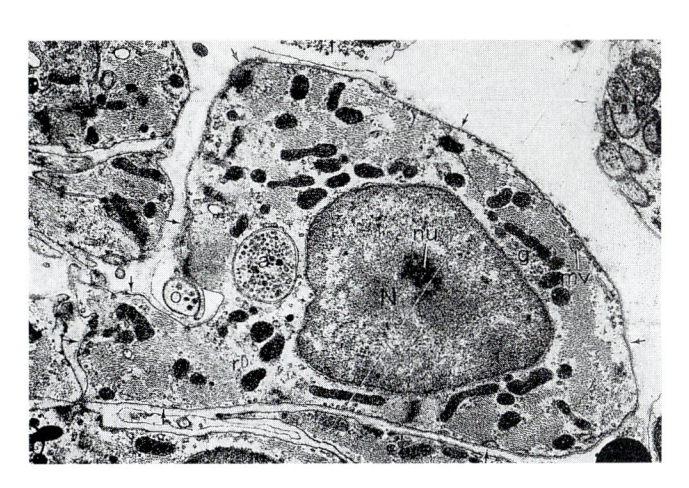

Fig. 10-6. TEM portraying cross-sectional profile of nodal cell in atrioventricular node of mouse heart. Typical intercalated disks are absent in these cell types; however, junctional specializations between contiguous nodal cells do occur. Note junction in lower left-hand corner of this cell. Profile of cell is delineated by short arrows directed toward cell surface. *N*, Nucleus; *nu*, nucleolus; *a*, nerve process with synaptic vesicles; *o*, Schwann cell invested autonomic nerve fiber; *b*, nerve bundle; *g*, Golgi complex; *mn*, multivesicular body; *r*, rough endoplasmic reticulum; *f*, fibroblast. (×4,500.)

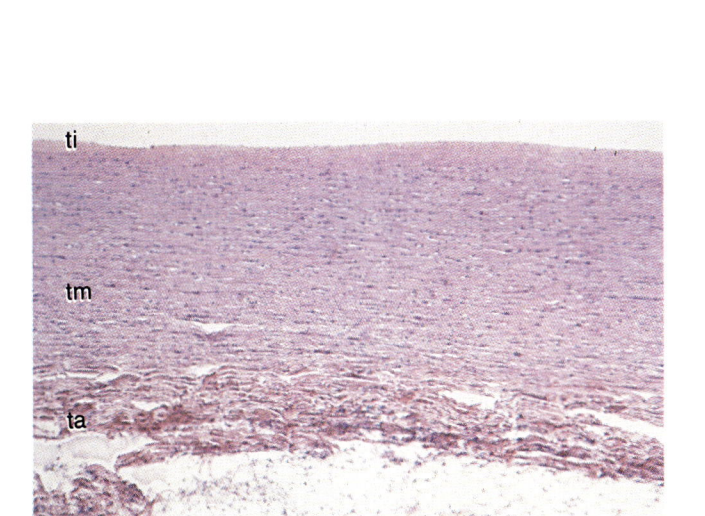

Fig. 10-7. LM of aorta illustrating tunica intima *(ti)*, tunica media *(tm)*, and tunica adventitia *(ta)*. Compare structure of wall to that in Fig. 10-1. (H&E; ×70.)

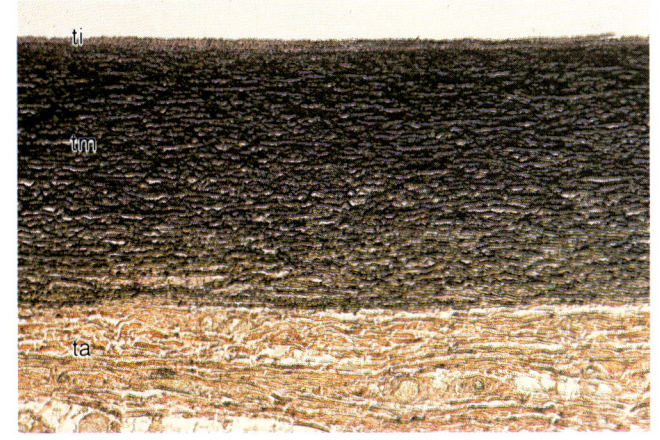

Fig. 10-8. Cross section of aorta as seen with Verhoeff stain. Note distribution of elastin (stained black) within aortic wall. *ti*, Tunica intima; *tm*, tunica media; *ta*, tunica adventitia. (×70.)

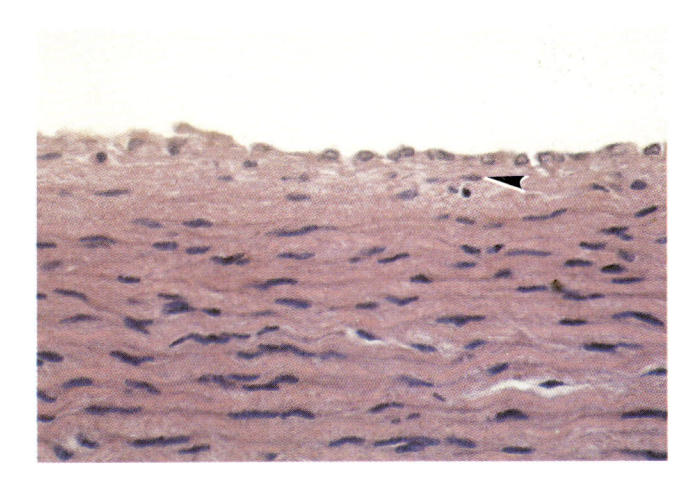

Fig. 10-9. High-magnification LM of tunica intima and part of tunica media of aorta. Subendothelial connective tissue *(arrowhead)* forms interface between endothelium and underlying tunica media. The latter consists of smooth muscle cells and a network of elastic fibers. (H&E; ×400.)

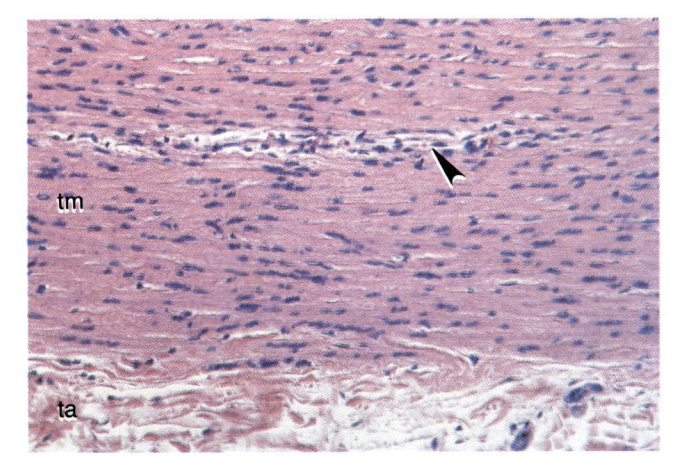

Fig. 10-10. LM of tunica media *(tm)* and tunica adventitia *(ta)* of aorta. Small vessels called vasa vasorum *(arrowhead)* can be seen within adventitia and tunica media. (H&E; ×150.)

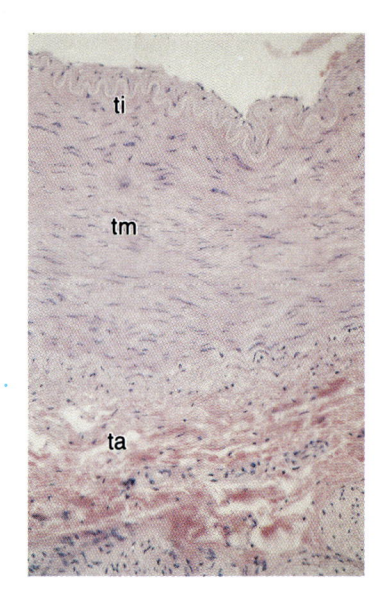

Fig. 10-11. LM of muscular artery illustrating tunica intima *(ti)*, tunica media *(tm)*, and tunica adventitia *(ta)*. (H&E; ×70.)

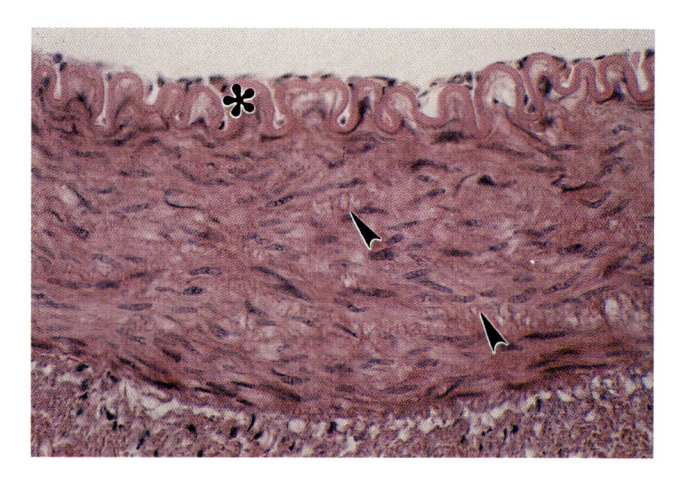

Fig. 10-12. Higher-magnification LM of wall of muscular artery. Refractile nature of elastin *(arrowheads)* permits its recognition within tunica media, internal elastic lamina (*), and tunica adventitia. (H&E; ×200.)

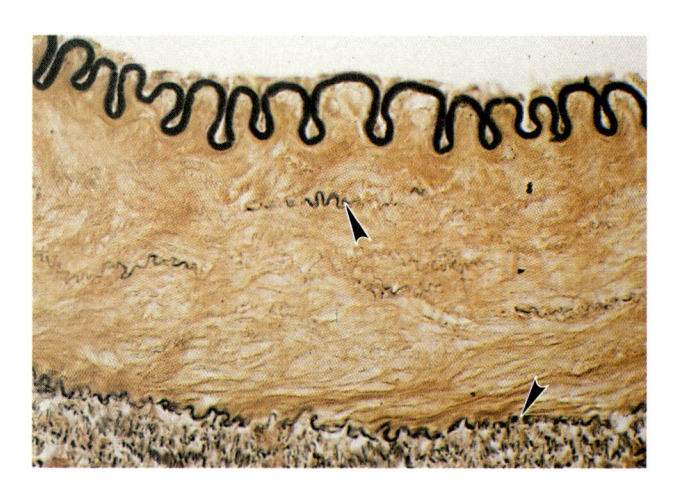

Fig. 10-13. LM of cross section of muscular artery stained with Verhoeff method. Observe distribution of elastin *(arrowheads)* within walls of vessel and compare with that seen in Fig. 10-12. (×200.)

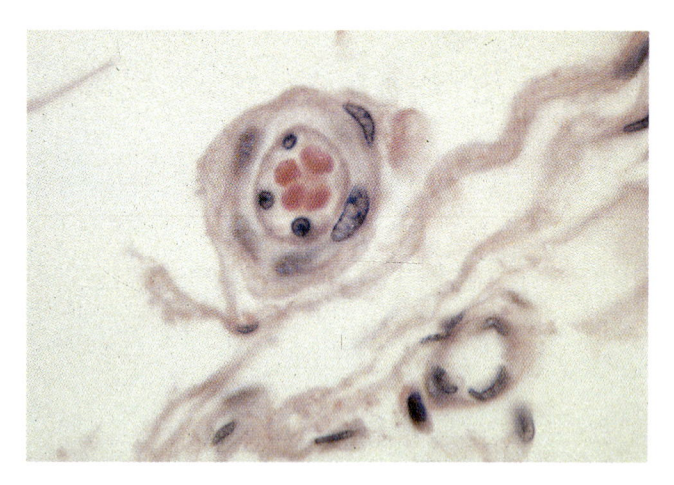

Fig. 10-14. High-magnification LM of cross section of small arteriole in connective tissue. Observe endothelial cell nuclei cut in cross section and longitudinal section of smooth muscle cells in tunica media. Compare thickness of arteriolar wall to that of aorta (see Figs. 10-1 and 10-7) and muscular artery (Fig. 10-11). (H&E; ×900.)

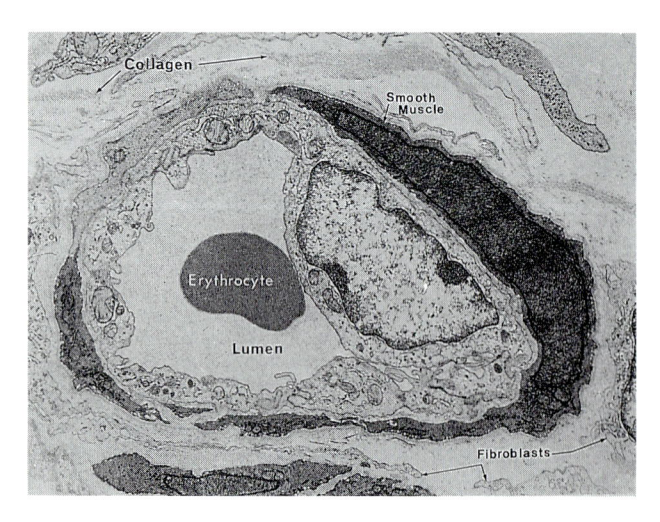

Fig. 10-15. TEM of small arteriole. Compare morphology of this arteriole at ultrastructural level with that seen by light microscopy in Fig. 10-14. (×3,000.)

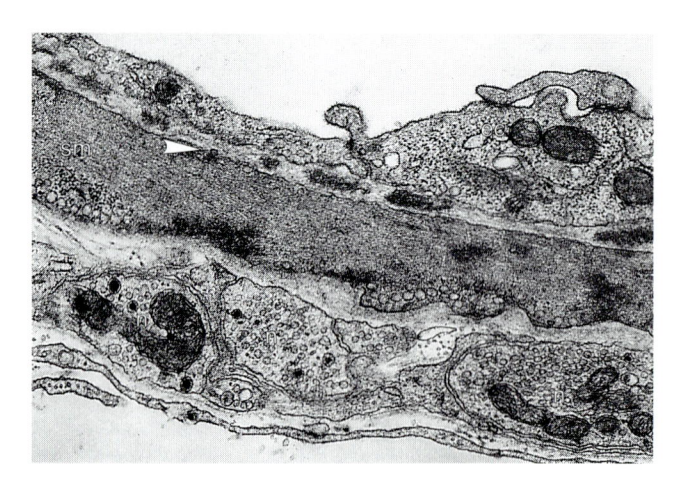

Fig. 10-16. TEM of arteriole wall revealing several portions of endothelial cells *(ec)* connected by junctions, basement membrane *(arrowhead)*, smooth muscle cell *(sm)* belonging to the tunica media, and various neuronal processes *(n)* in tunica adventitia. Neuronal vesicles of varying size, shape, and electron density can be seen within these processes. (×12,000.)

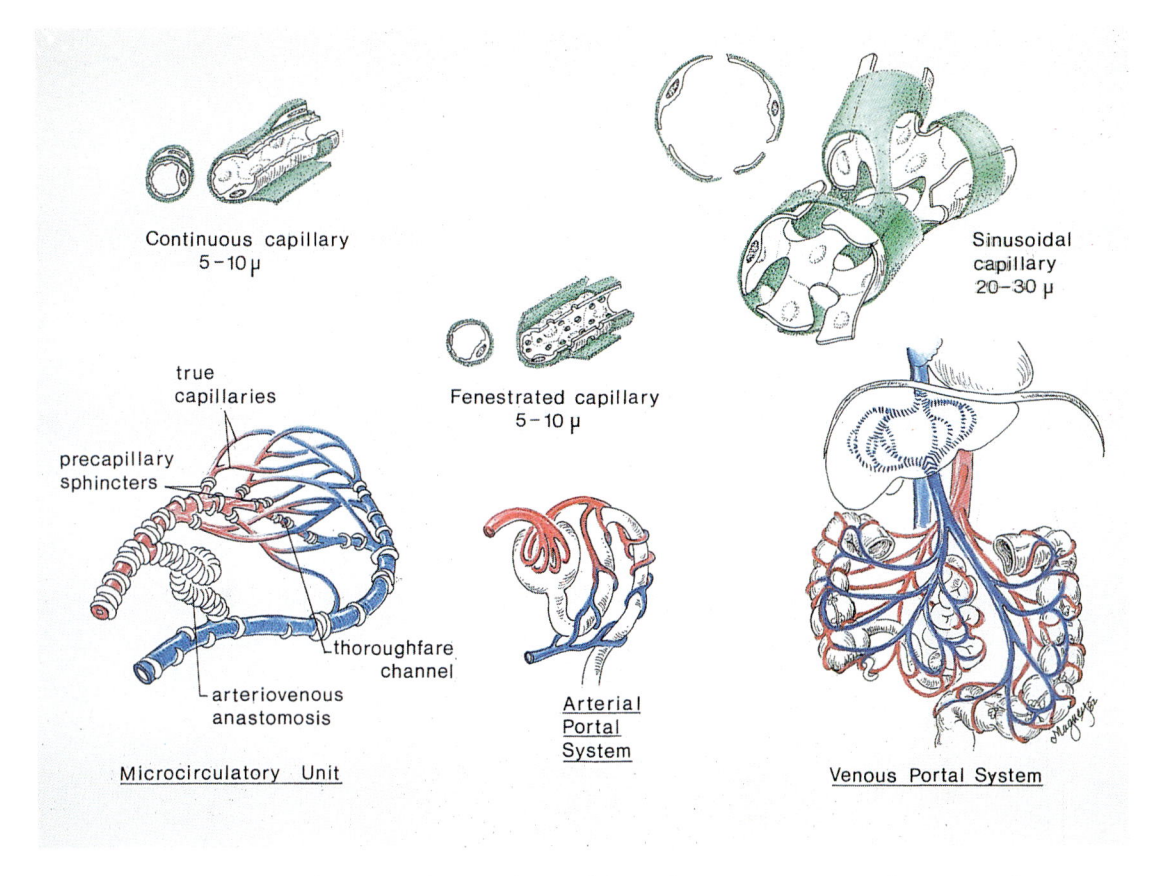

Fig. 10-17. Diagram of microcirculatory unit, arterial portal system, venous portal system, and three types of capillaries found within body. Fenestrated capillaries are located in tissues where rapid exchange takes place, such as kidney, endocrine glands, and intestine. Sinusoids facilitate exchange of macromolecules and cells; examples are found in liver and hemopoietic organs. Continuous capillaries are found in brain and muscle. In microcirculatory unit note that smooth muscle sphincters are used to control flow of blood through these vessels.

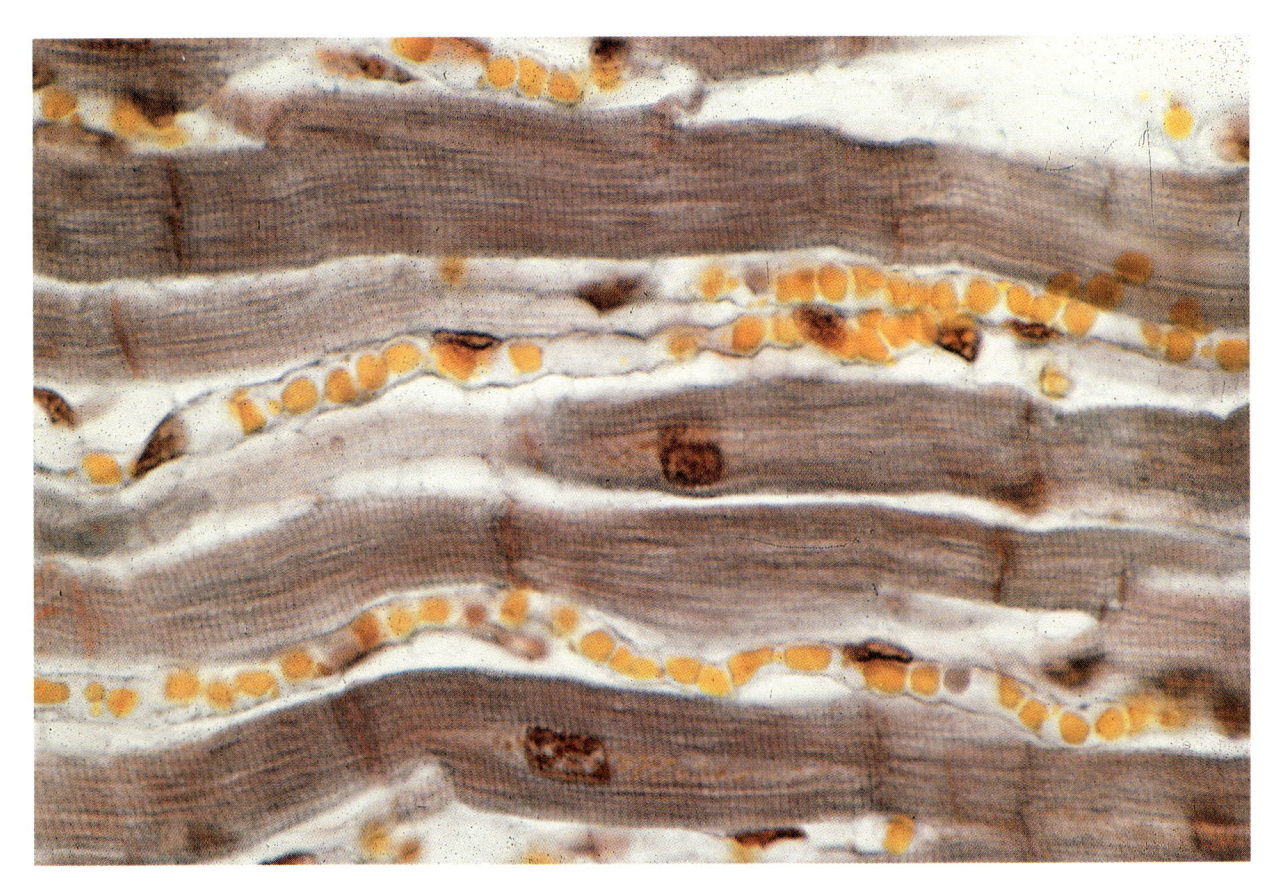

Fig. 10-18. High-magnification LM of cardiac muscle richly supplied with capillaries (note red blood cells stained orange) seen here in longitudinal section. Nuclei of endothelial cells are arranged with their long axes parallel to flow of blood. (Masson's trichrome stain; ×1,000.)

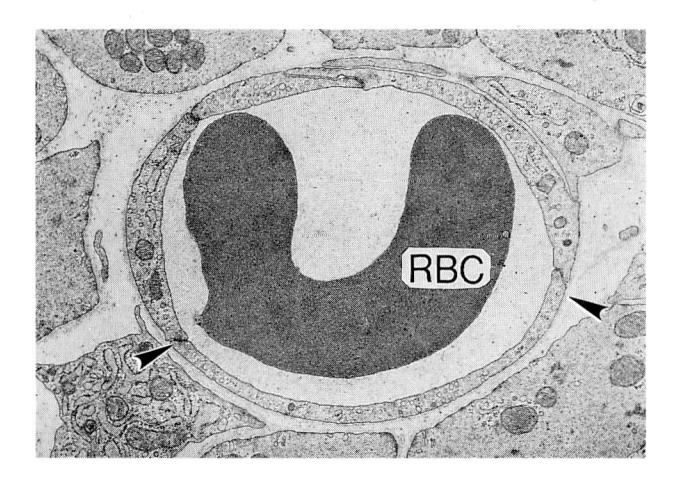

Fig. 10-19. TEM of continuous capillary in smooth muscle. Note thickness of endothelial cell wall and presence of junctions *(arrows)* between portion of adjacent endothelial cells. (×7,000.)

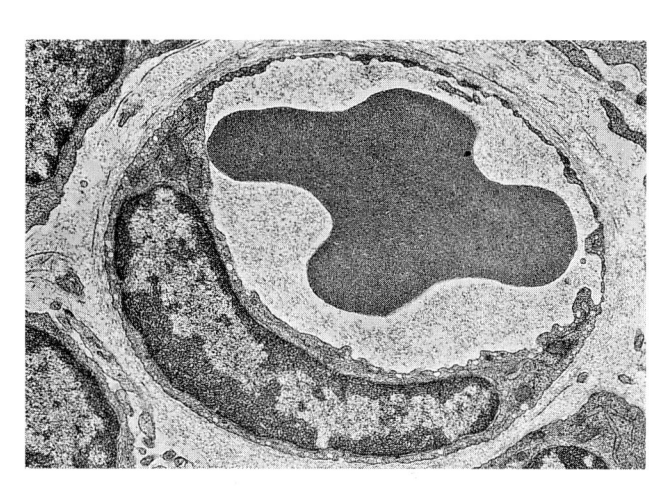

Fig. 10-20. TEM cross section of fenestrated capillary. Numerous fenestrae can be seen in endothelial cell wall. Compare this morphology with that of continuous capillary in Fig. 10-19. (×8,200.)

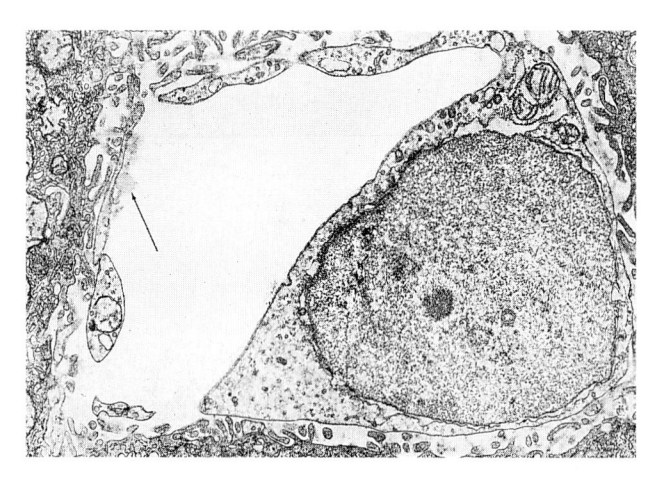

Fig. 10-21. TEM of sinusoidal capillary in liver. Note gaps within endothelial cell wall and lack of continuous basement membrane around endothelial cell. Arrow points to small chylomicron within lumen of capillary. (×7,500.)

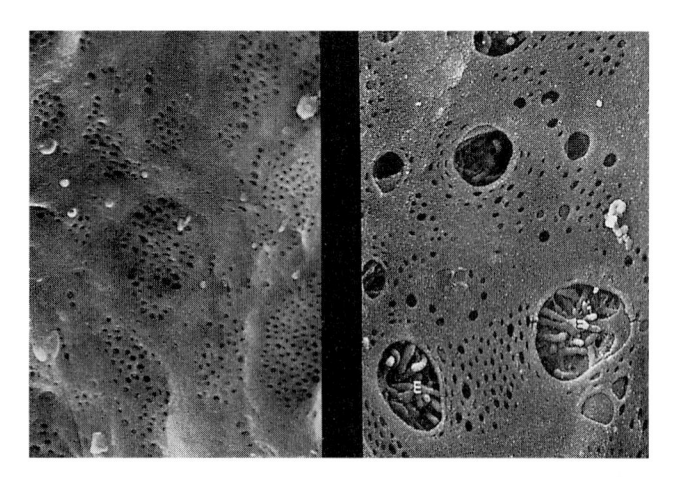

Fig. 10-22. SEM of fenestrated capillary *(left)* and sinusoidal capillary *(right)*. Observe that fenestrae are present within both types of vessels and that sinusoidal capillary has large discontinuities in the wall through which microvillous-like processes of a liver cell can be seen. (×12,000.)

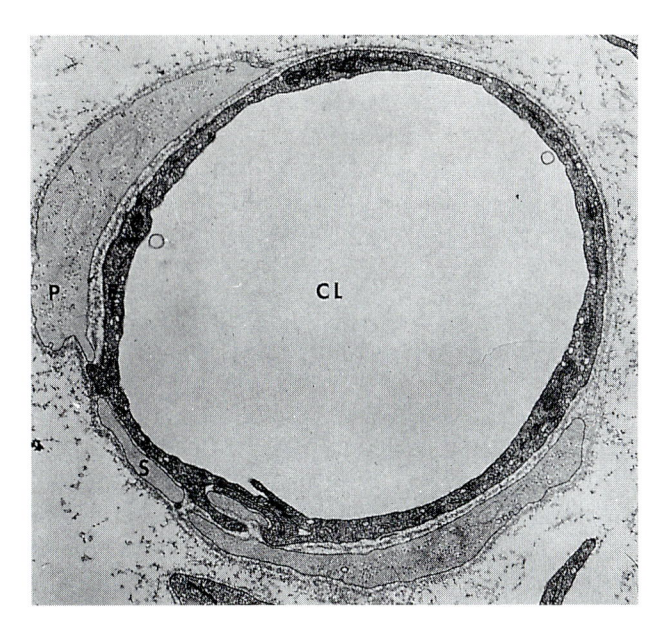

Fig. 10-23. TEM of capillary within muscle showing relationships of pericyte to capillary wall and to basal lamina. *CL,* Capillary lumen; *S,* process of pericyte; *P,* pericyte. (×8,600.)

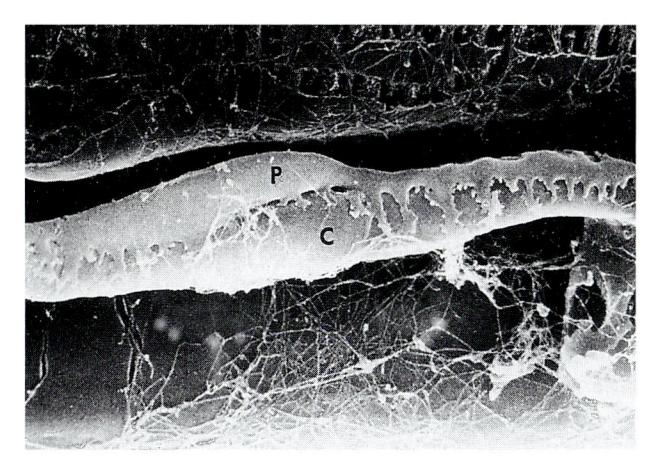

Fig. 10-24. High-magnification SEM of pericyte on capillary in muscle. Intimate contact can be seen between (1) cytoplasmic processes arising from body and branches of pericyte and (2) surface of capillary. *C,* Capillary; *P,* pericytes. (×1,100.)

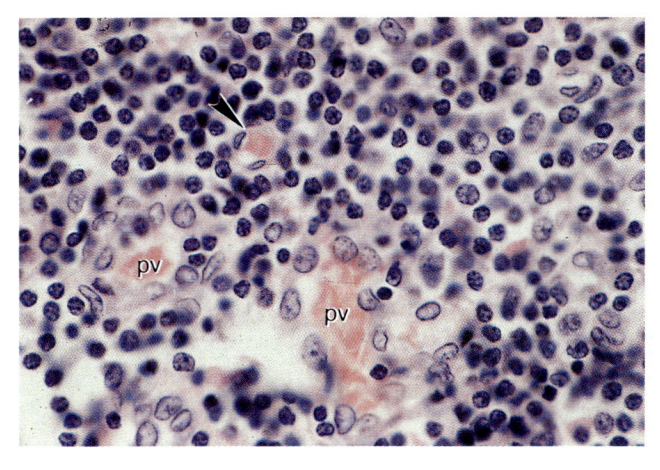

Fig. 10-25. LM of postcapillary venule in lymph node. Compare shape of endothelial cells in postcapillary venule *(pv)* with that of capillary *(arrowhead)* within the same field. (H&E; ×500.)

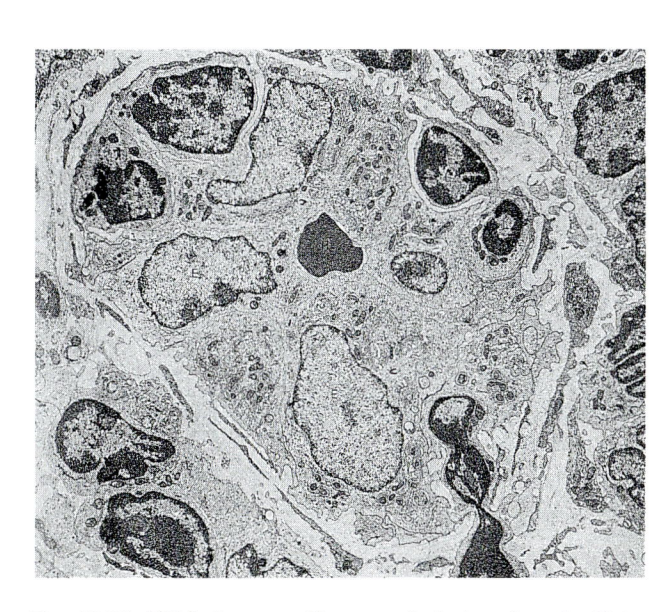

Fig. 10-26. TEM of postcapillary venule in lymph node. Note presence of lymphocytes within endothelial cell wall, and at lower right of venule, single lymphocyte in process of diapedesis. Its nucleus (beaded appearance) is deformed as a result of cell's passage through venule wall. (×1,500.)

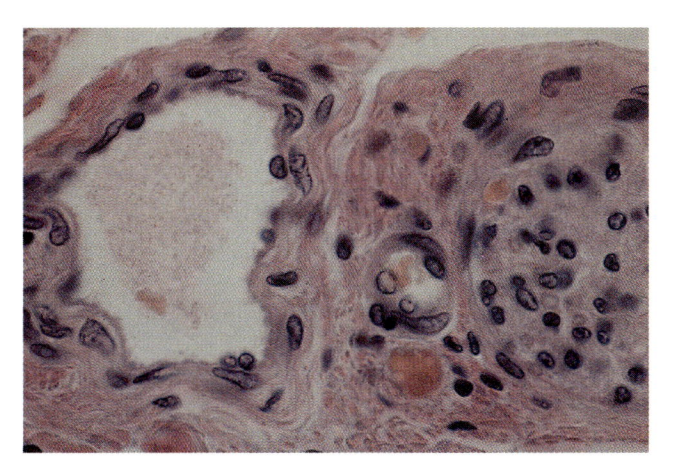

Fig. 10-27. LM of small neurovascular unit with peripheral nerve *(right),* small arteriole *(center),* and small venule *(left).* Note thickness of walls of venule and its irregular shape. Compare to arterial and other venous vessels shown in Fig. 10-1. (H&E; ×500.)

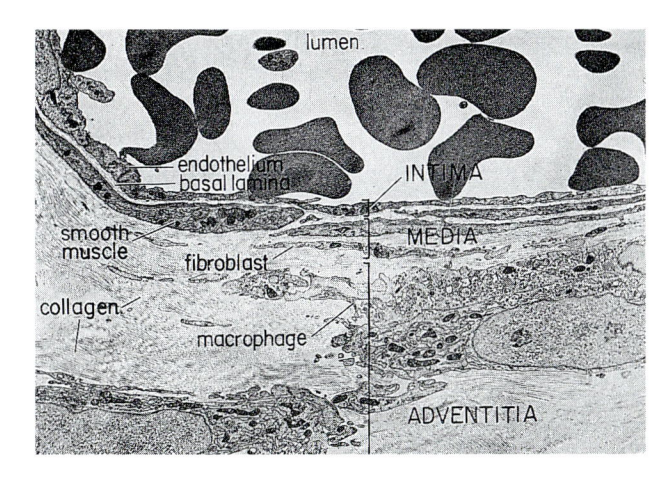

Fig. 10-28. TEM of small venule. Observe relative thickness of tunica intima, tunica media, and tunica adventitia. (×2,100.)

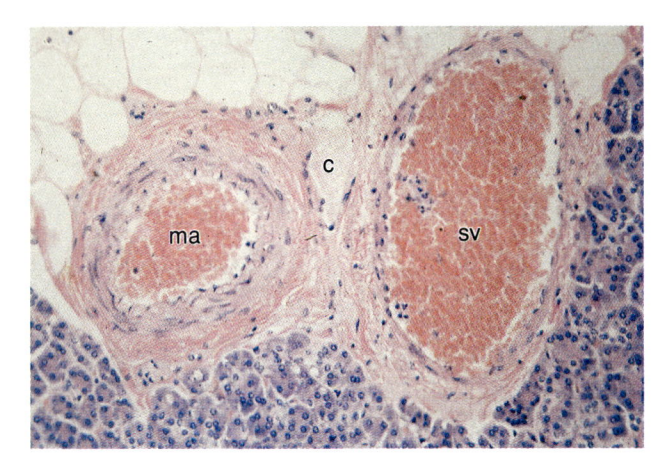

Fig. 10-29. LM illustrating small muscular artery *(ma)*, lymphatic capillary *(c)*, and small vein *(sv)*. Compare to structure of vessel wall shown in Fig. 10-1. (H&E; ×150.)

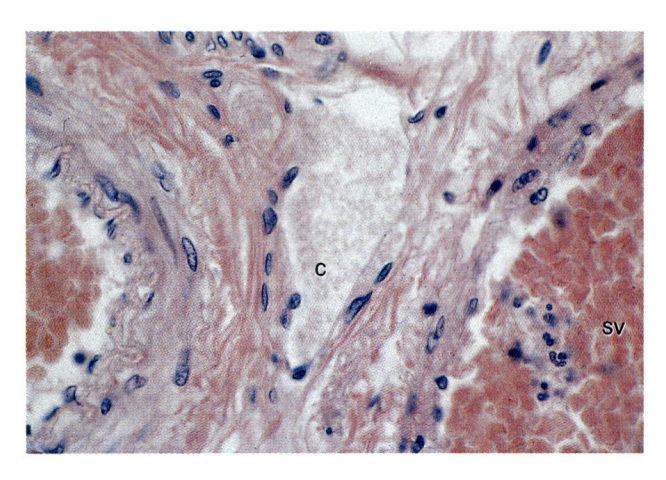

Fig. 10-30. Higher-magnification LM of cluster of vessels seen in Figure 10-29. Compare thickness and composition of walls of artery, lymphatic capillary *(c)*, and small vein *(sv)*. (H&E; ×400.)

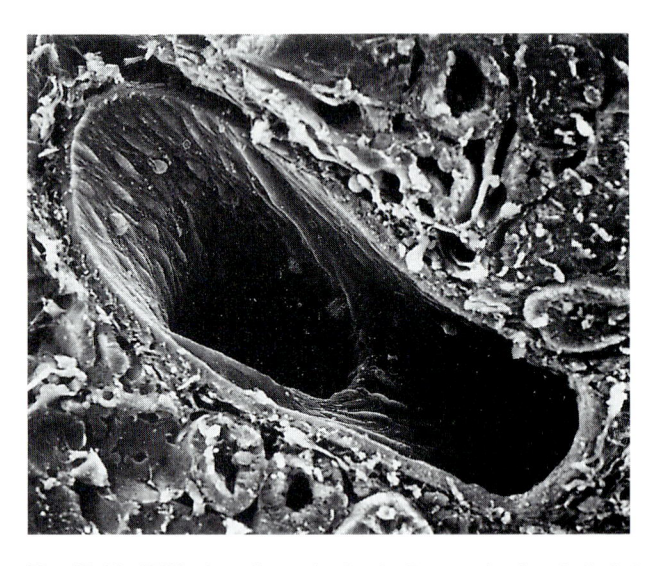

Fig. 10-31. SEM of medium-sized vein. Long axis of endothelial cells parallels flow of blood. Tunica media and tunica adventitia are minimal in thickness. (×350.)

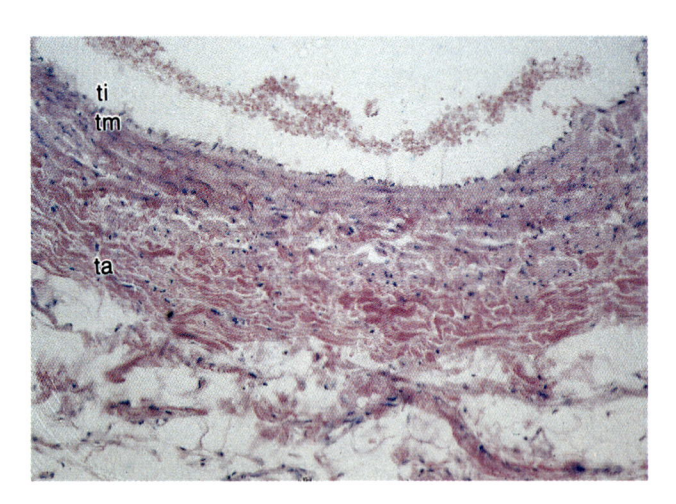

Fig. 10-32. LM of wall of medium-sized vein. Note relative thickness of tunica intima *(ti)*, tunica media *(tm)*, and tunica adventitia *(ta)*. (H&E; ×100.)

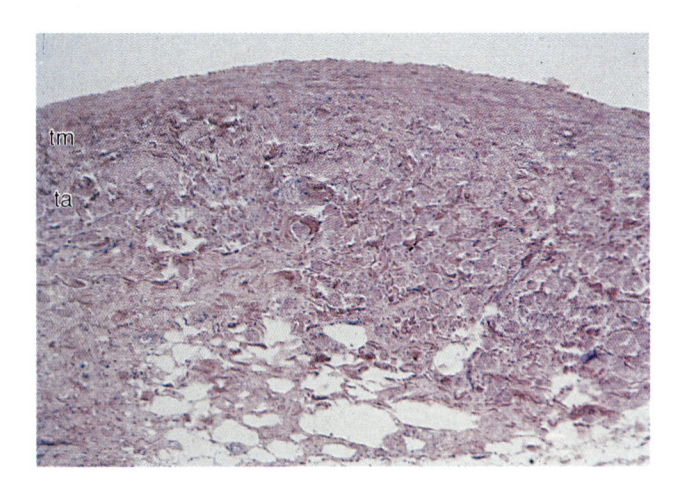

Fig. 10-33. Low-magnification LM of wall of vena cava. There is circularly arranged smooth muscle in tunica media *(tm)* and longitudinally arranged smooth muscle in tunica adventitia *(ta)*. See Fig. 10-1. (H&E; ×70.)

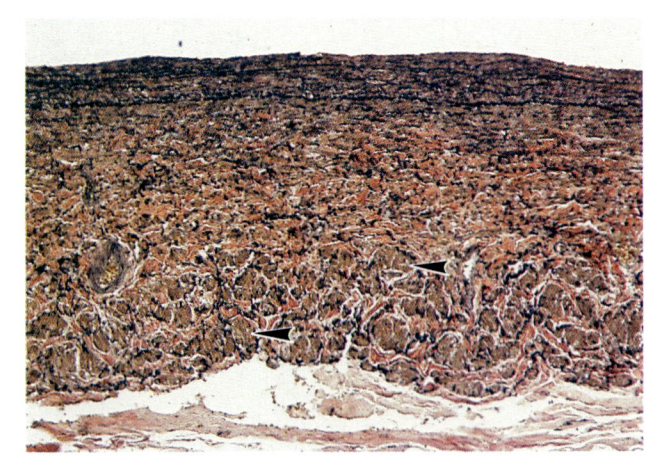

Fig. 10-34. Low-magnification LM of wall of vena cava as seen with Verhoeff stain. Observe distribution of elastin within vessel walls and compare with that seen in walls of aorta in Fig. 10-10 and muscular artery in Fig. 10-13. Longitudinally arranged smooth muscle seen in cross-section *(arrowheads)*, in tunica adventitia is also obvious. (×70.)

CHAPTER 11

LYMPHOID SYSTEM

THE LYMPHOID SYSTEM is involved with immunologic defense mechanisms of the body that defend it against invading organisms (i.e., bacteria, viruses) or foreign (nonself) antigens and is comprised principally of **lymphocytes.** Each lymphocyte is programmed to respond to a single antigen: this is called **specificity.** Other cells (see drawing of immune response) involved with immunologic defense are **macrophages** (MO), **antigen presenting cells** (APC), and **plasma cells.** Lymphocytes circulating in the blood stream may follow chemical attractants (chemotaxis) into connective tissues to form diffuse cellular infiltrations indicative of an inflammatory process. Different types of lymphocytes exist, although it is impossible to distinguish among them by light microscopy unless special immunologic methods are used.

B-lymphocytes differentiate within the bone marrow from lymphoid stem cells. Leaving the bone marrow they recirculate in the blood through lymphoid organs and tissues. Upon contact with antigen (Agn), B-lymphocytes proliferate, may form lymphoid nodules, and further differentiate into plasma cells that produce antibodies that interact with antigen. Because antibodies enter the blood and circulate, B-cells are responsible for what is called **"humoral immunity."**

In contrast, activated T-lymphocytes provide **"cell-mediated immunity,"** killing target cells by direct contact or through the secretion of products called lymphokines, which may also modulate immune reactions or macrophage function (i.e., macrophage inhibitory [MIF] or activating [MAF] factors). Several subtypes of T-lymphocytes are found. Natural killers (NK) cells, which require no assistance from other immune system cells or factors, and T-cytotoxic (Tc) lymphocytes both kill target cells by direct contact. Other activated T-lymphocytes (T-helpers [Th] and T-suppressors [Ts]) secrete products called lymphokines that act on T- or B-lymphocytes and macrophages to modulate the immune response. Both T- and B-lymphocytes, when activated, undergo clonal expansion and produce both **effector** and **memory** cells (primary response). Memory cells recirculate and await the next challenge by the same antigen to which they respond with vigor and speed (secondary response). T-lymphocytes usually have antigen presented to them by macrophages or antigen presenting cells before they can differentiate into lymphocytes (Tc, Th, Ts) that can influence the immune response.

DIFFUSE LYMPHATIC TISSUE

Diffuse infiltration of lymphocytes, common in the connective tissue beneath the mucous membranes of the body, is particularly prominent in the digestive and respiratory systems. In these locations lymphocytes respond to antigen entering the body through the epithelial interface with the outside environment. Plasma cells differentiating in these locations produce secretory immunoglobulins (IgA, IgM) that are transported across the mucosa to interact with antigens in the luminal environment.

LYMPHATIC NODULES

Arrangement of lymphocytes into spherical masses called **lymphatic nodules** indicates an immunologic (B-lymphocyte) response. Nodules are found within tonsils, Peyer's patches and the mucosal linings of tubular organs, and lymphoid organs such as spleen and lymph nodes. Lymphatic nodules are transitory, lasting for only 1 or 2 weeks, which reflects the life span of plasma cells. A pale-staining center (sometimes called a germinal or reaction center) is present during clonal proliferation of B-lymphocytes as the cells enlarge, divide, differentiate into **plasma cells,** and produce additional RER for synthesis of **antibody.**

TONSIL

Groups of lymphatic nodules, in combination with other dense lymphatic tissue, lie beneath the epithelial surfaces of the respiratory and digestive tracts, where they are called **tonsils.** Because they are not completely encapsulated, tonsils are not classified as organs. In the neck several pairs of tonsils (pharyngeal, palatine, tubal, lingual) surround the openings into the respiratory and digestive tracts and are collectively called **Waldeyer's ring.** Clusters of nodules in connective tissues beneath intestinal epithelium are called **Peyer's patches.**

LYMPHATIC VESSELS

Very tiny vessels with incomplete endothelium and basement membrane, called **lymphatic capillaries,** originate in the tissue spaces of the body. They carry excess tissue fluid through a network of lymphatic vessels of increasing size to join the subclavian veins in the neck, where their contents **(lymph)** empties into venous blood. En route lymphatics pass through a series of lymph nodes where filtration occurs. As lymphatic vessels increase in size, they resemble veins and usually possess valves that assist in the movement of lymph against gravity.

LYMPH NODE

Lymph nodes are bean-shaped encapsulated organs with a stroma of reticular fibers produced by reticular cells and a parenchyma composed of lymphocytes. Antigen presenting cells and macrophages are also present. Afferent lymphatic vessels enter a node through the convex surface opposite the hilum, which is an indentation where arteries enter, and where veins and an efferent lymphatic leave the organ. Within the node are a cortex containing lymphatic nodules; a paracortex, or T-dependent zone; and a medulla made up of cords of lymphocytes and plasma cells with intervening sinuses spanned by macrophages. Lymph flows from subcapsular sinuses into radial sinuses that flow through the cortex and into the medullary sinuses; it leaves the node by a single efferent lymphatic vessel. Lymphocytes enter the cortex through postcapillary venules or by way of the afferent lymphatics. In response to antigenic challenge, proliferation of committed cells produces both effector and memory B- and T-lymphocytes.

SPLEEN

The spleen, located in the upper left quadrant of the abdomen, is a large lymphoid organ enclosed in a dense connective tissue **capsule.** It is incompletely divided by partitions, called **trabeculae,** that extend inward from the capsule. Within a reticular fiber stroma, lymphocytes are organized into **white pulp** adjacent to central arteries. **Red pulp** consists of sinusoids and the **cords of Billroth,** the latter composed of hemopoietic and connective tissue cells located between adjacent sinusoids.

The **splenic artery** enters at the hilum of the spleen and divides into **trabecular arteries.** These in turn give off **central arteries of the white pulp,** which are surrounded by **periarteriolar lymphatic sheaths** (PALS) consisting of T-lymphocytes. Central arteries also pass through lymphatic nodules, typically in an eccentric position. Macrophages and lymphocytes are present in both the white and red pulp and in a **marginal zone** between them.

The spleen is a filter for blood. After leaving the white pulp via **penicillar arterioles,** blood may pass into splenic sinusoids by one of two mechanisms. In the **closed circulation** model, blood passes from arterioles into splenic sinusoids where, depending on the intravascular pressure, exchange between cells in the sinusoid and the cords of Billroth (or intrasinusoidal exchange) can take place. In the **open circulation** model, arterioles terminate and release blood into spaces in the red pulp cords. Here it may interact with macrophages as it passes between endothelial cells of splenic sinusoids to reenter the circulation. In both models, sinusoidal blood is drained in succession through **pulp veins, trabecular veins,** and the **splenic vein.** Aged red blood cells whose membranes are too inflexible to allow their movement between the endothelial cells into the sinusoid are trapped and removed by macrophages.

THYMUS

In young people, the thymus lies within the anterior superior mediastinum. With age it involutes, until in the older individual it is little more than fat and connective tissue. In humans, the thymus is seeded with lymphoid stem cells and is responsible for their differentiation into **T-lymphocytes.** The organ has a delicate connective tissue **capsule** and **trabeculae** that subdivide it into incomplete **lobules.** Because the thymus is committed to T-lymphocyte production and development, it has no lymphatic nodules, but the lymphocytes are arranged into a cortex and a medulla. In the cortex, a stroma of **epithelial reticular cells** supports the developing T-lymphocytes and secretes **thymic factors** essential to their differentiation. Epithelial cell processes, along with continuous capillaries, contribute to the **blood-thymus barrier,** which protects the evolving cells in the cortex from premature antigenic challenge. Arteries enter the thymus through the capsule and course through trabeculae to distribute blood to cortex and medulla. Differentiated T-lymphocytes enter the circulation through postcapillary venules at the corticomedullary junction. The thymic medulla is apparently inactive but possesses unique epithelioid structures called **Hassall's corpuscles** whose function is unknown.

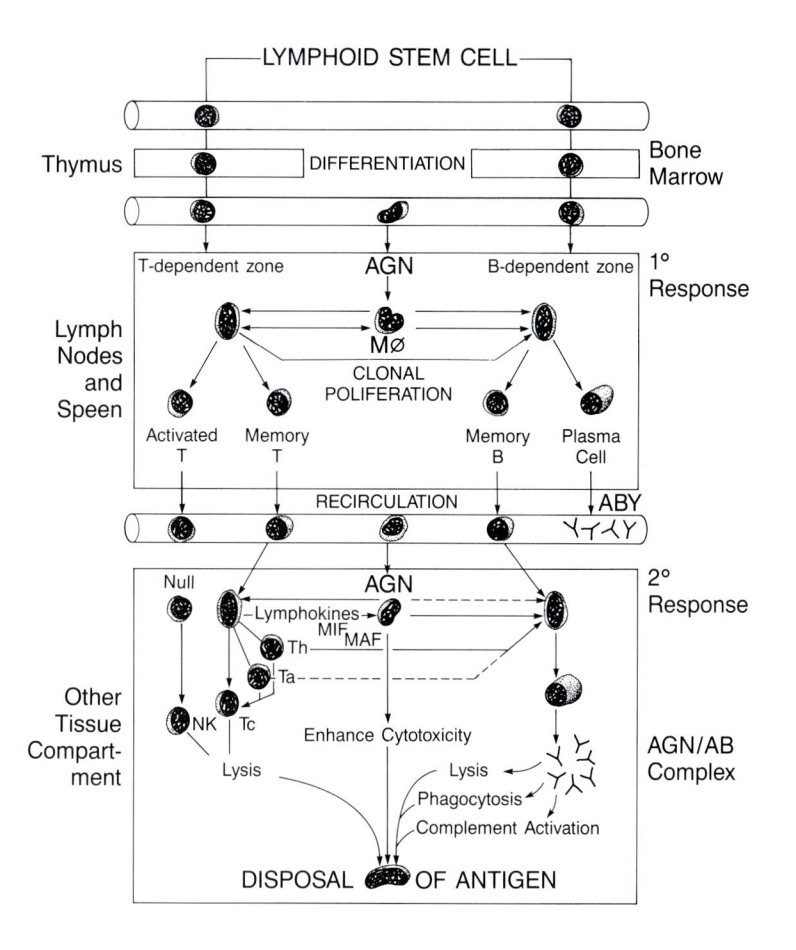

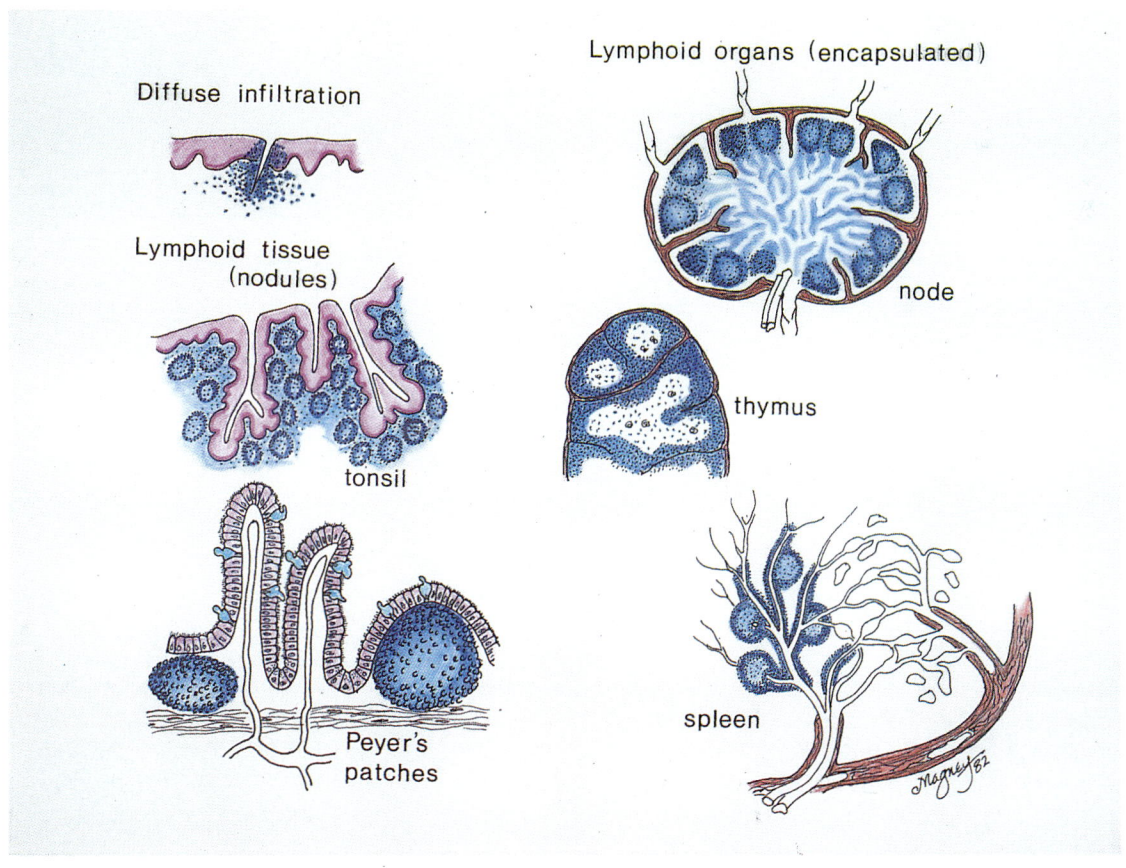

Fig. 11-1. Arrangements of lymphatic tissue and types of lymphatic organs. Foci or accumulations of lymphoid cells in tissue or even clustering of B-lymphocytes into nodules for B-cell proliferation are classified as lymphatic tissue. Lymphoid organs are encapsulated and consist of lymph nodes, spleen, or thymus.

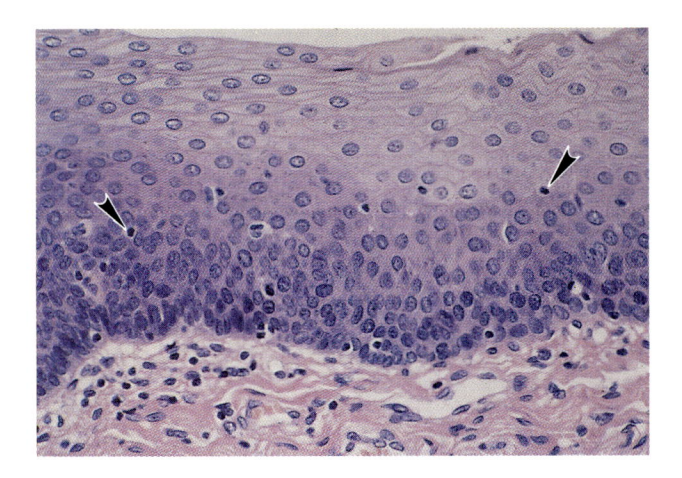

Fig. 11-2. LM of statified squamous nonkeratinized epithelium in vagina. Diffuse infiltration of lymphocytes (arrowheads) is seen in epithelium. (H&E; ×350.)

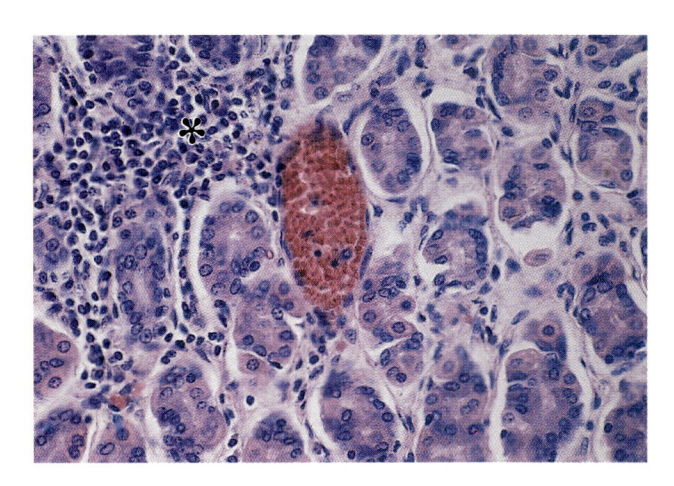

Fig. 11-3. LM of intestinal crypts in small intestine showing dense infiltration of lymphocytes (asterisk) within focal region of connective tissue. (H&E; ×350.)

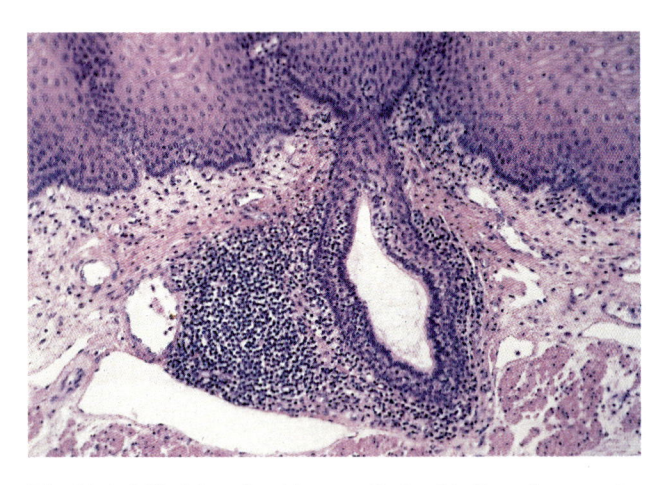

Fig. 11-4. LM of duct lined by stratified epithelium that empties onto esophageal epithelium. Small lymphatic nodule lies adjacent to duct and is classified as dense lymphatic tissue. (H&E; ×150.)

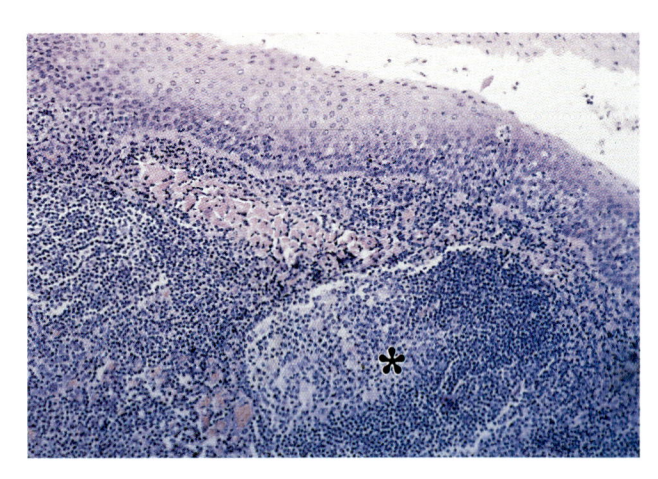

Fig. 11-5. LM of palatine tonsil showing stratified squamous nonkeratinized epithelium, diffuse and dense lymphatic tissue within connective tissue, and presence of secondary lymphatic nodules (*). (H&E; ×150.)

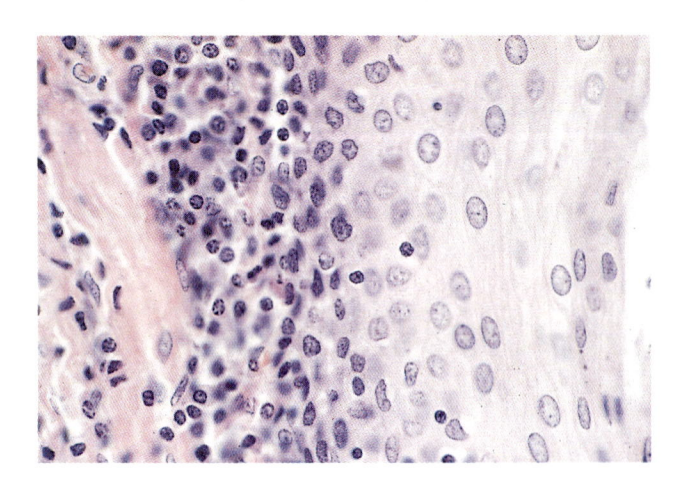

Fig. 11-6. LM of tonsilar epithelium at higher magnification. Diffuse infiltration of lymphocytes into epithelium obscures boundary between epithelium and connective tissue. (H&E; ×500.)

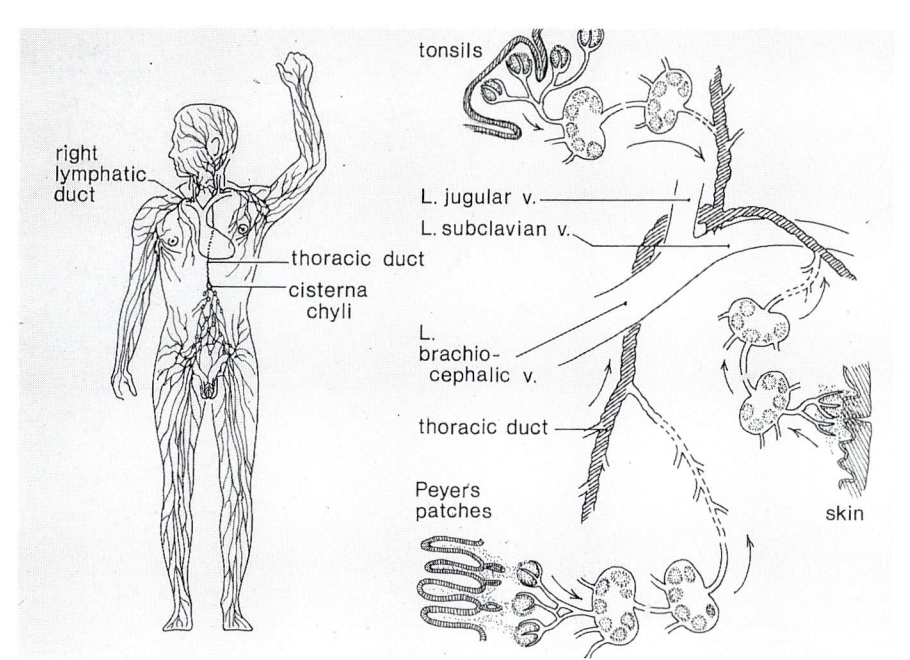

Fig. 11-7 Lymphatic drainage within body. By way of thoracic duct, three quarters of lymphatic drainage is emptied into left subclavian vein, while lymphatic drainage of right upper quarter of body drains into right subclavian vein. In expanded view at right, note that lymph passes through one or more lymph nodes in series, as it is collected from either visceral organs, tonsils, or skin en route to vascular system.

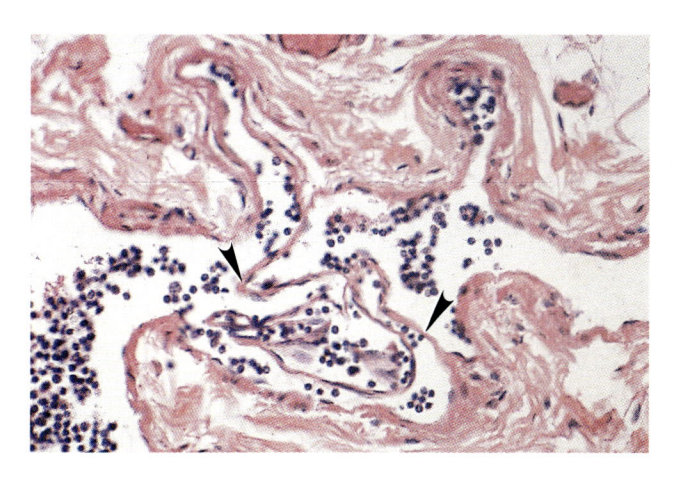

Fig. 11-8. LM of lymphatic capillary in longitudinal section demonstrating a valve *(arrowheads)* within vessel. (H&E; ×300.)

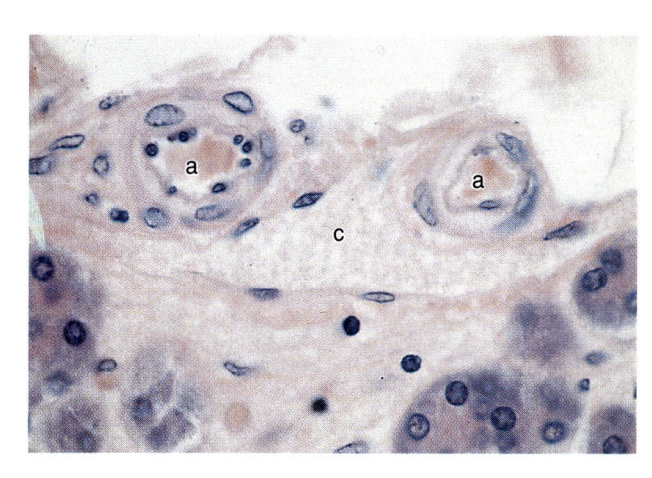

Fig. 11-9. LM of lymphatic capillary *(c)* and adjacent arterioles *(a)*. Compare relative thickness of walls of these vessels. (H&E; ×900.)

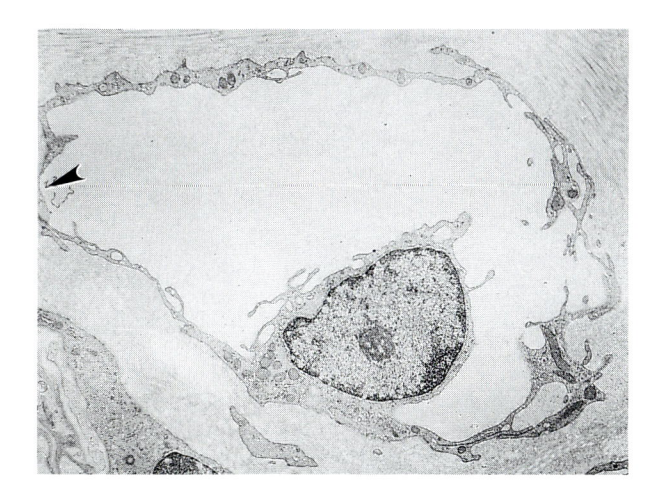

Fig. 11-10. TEM of lymphatic capillary. Basement membrane is discontinuous and endothelial cell lining is incomplete *(arrowhead)*. (×3,000.)

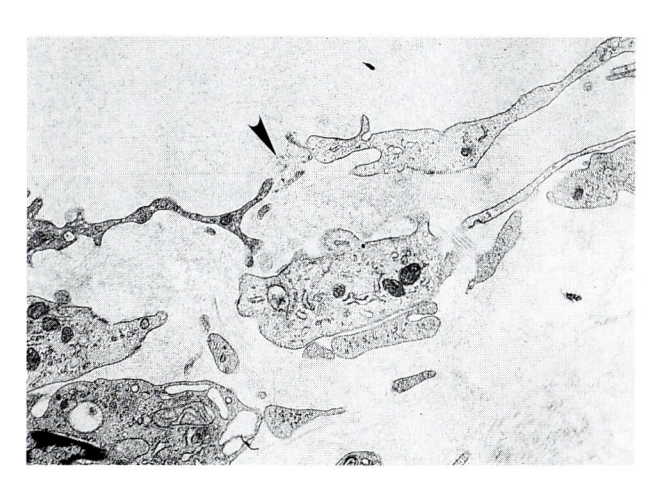

Fig. 11-11. High-magnification TEM of lymphatic capillary demonstrating gap *(arrowhead)* between adjacent endothelial cells. Lumen is at top of image. (×7,500.)

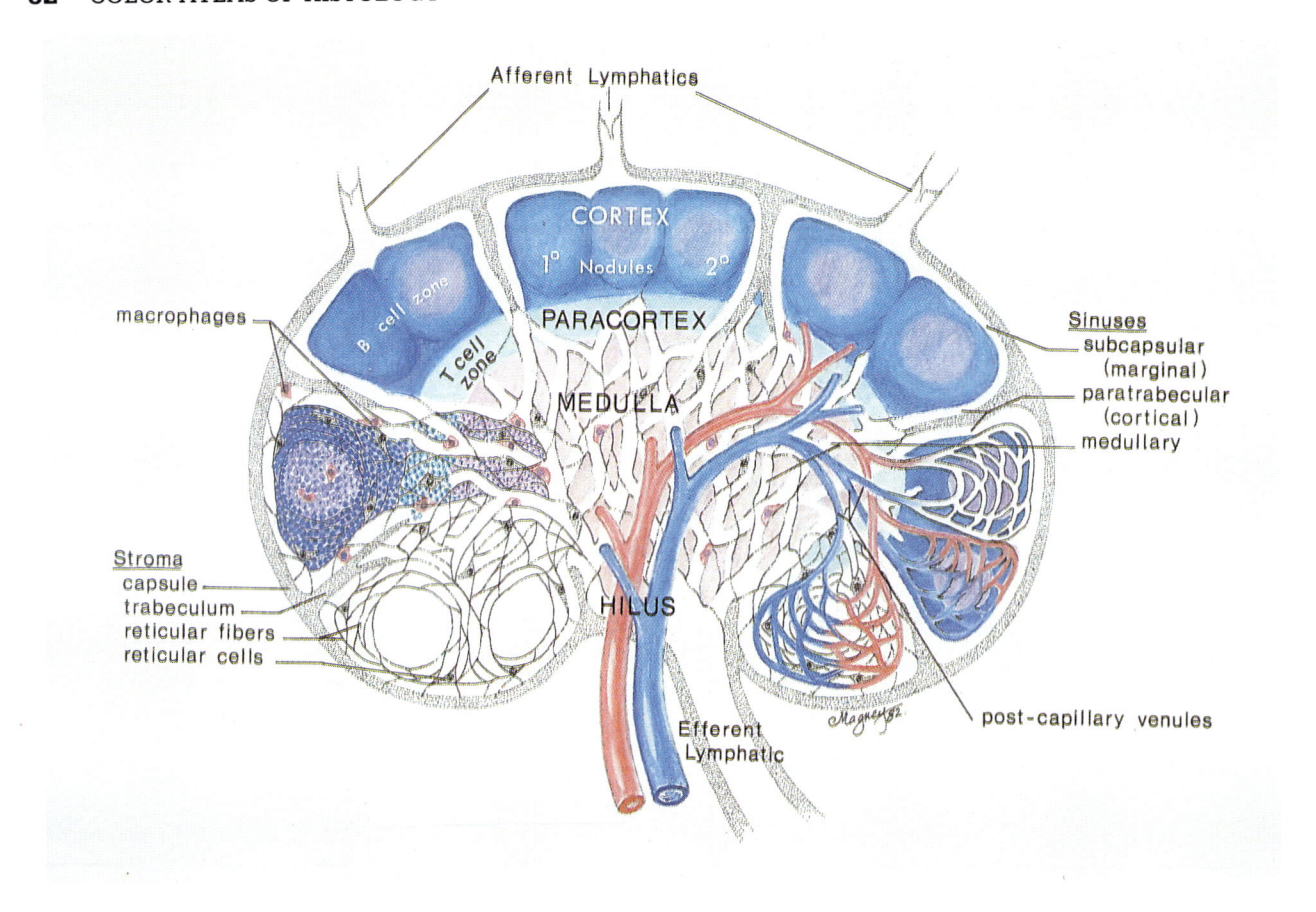

Fig. 11-12. Lymph node showing capsule, stroma, and parenchyma. Lymph enters organ through afferent lymphatic vessels and percolates through sinuses (spaces without endothelial lining) of cortex and into medulla. Lymph leaves organ through efferent lymphatics. Lymph nodes filter lymph, provide for interaction of macrophages and T- and B-lymphocytes, and serve as site for formation of plasma cells.

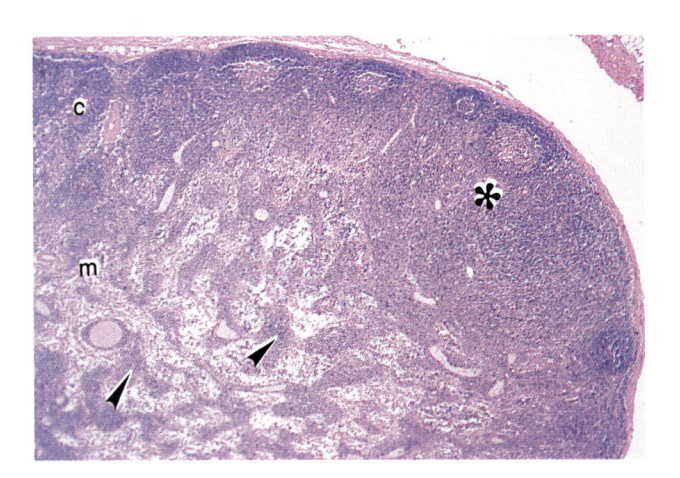

Fig. 11-13. Low-magnification LM of lymph node showing cortex (c), medulla (m), and medullary cords (arrowheads). Secondary lymphatic nodules can be seen in cortex just beneath capsule and are separated from medulla by paracortex (also called tertiary or deep cortex [*]). (H&E; ×40.)

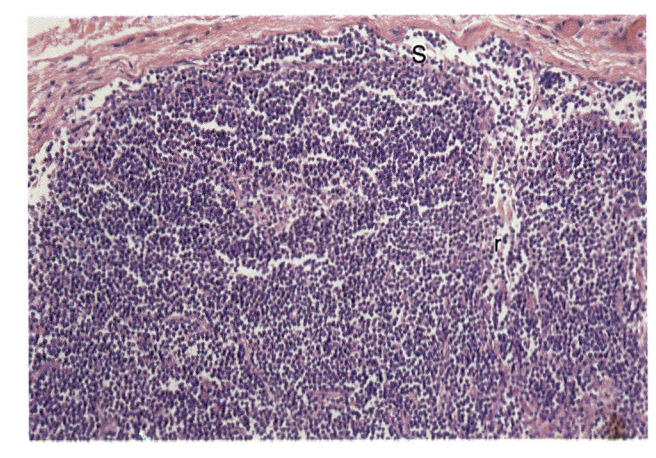

Fig. 11-14. High-magnification LM of secondary nodule lying immediately beneath capsule of lymph node. Note orientation of subcapsular (s) and radial (r) sinuses. (H&E; ×100.)

LYMPHOID SYSTEM   83

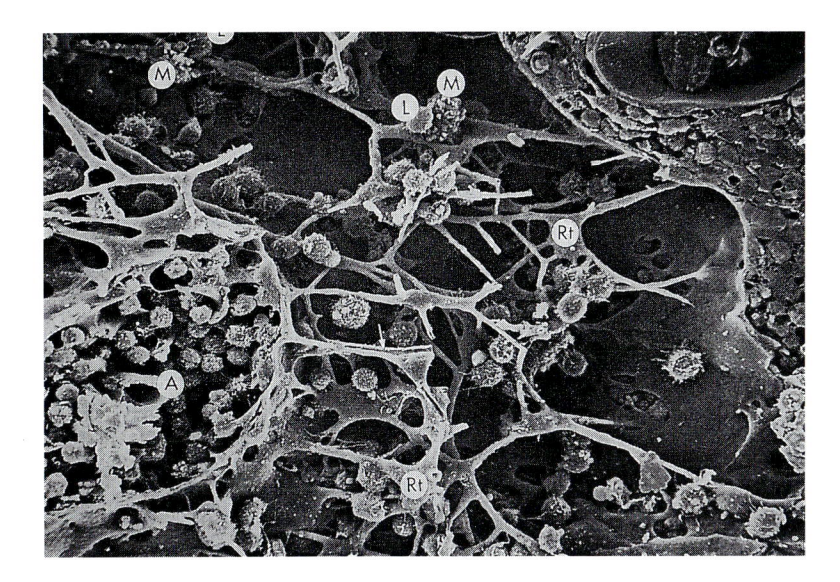

Fig. 11-15. SEM of a lymphatic nodule *(left)* and adjacent radial sinus. Lumen of sinus is spanned by reticular cells, and macrophages can be seen adhering to their surface. *A,* arteriole; *Rt,* reticular cells; *M,* macrophages; *L,* lymphocytes. Arrow indicates long processes of reticular cells. (×500.)

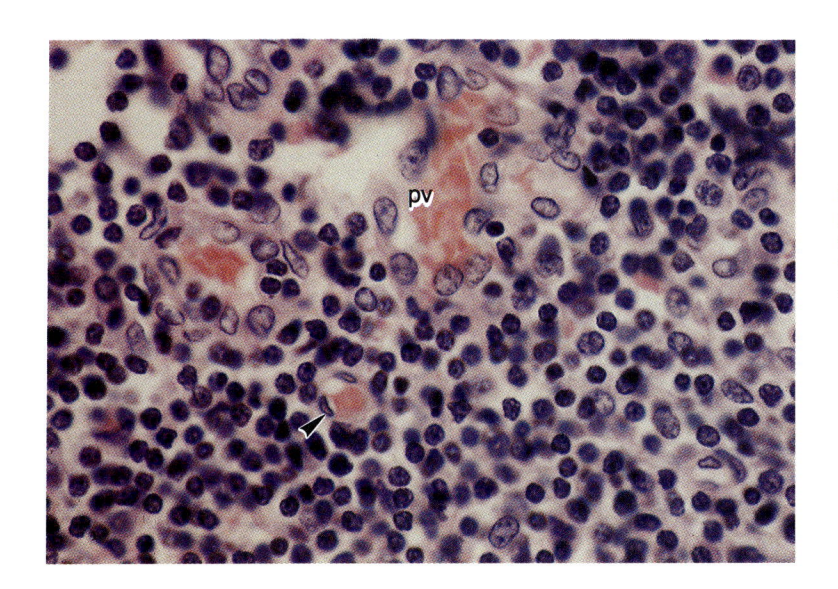

Fig. 11-16. Postcapillary venule *(pv).* Observe lymphocytes within cuboidal endothelial wall of venule. Compare cuboidal endothelium of postcapillary venule to squamous endothelium of capillary *(arrowhead).* (H&E; ×600.)

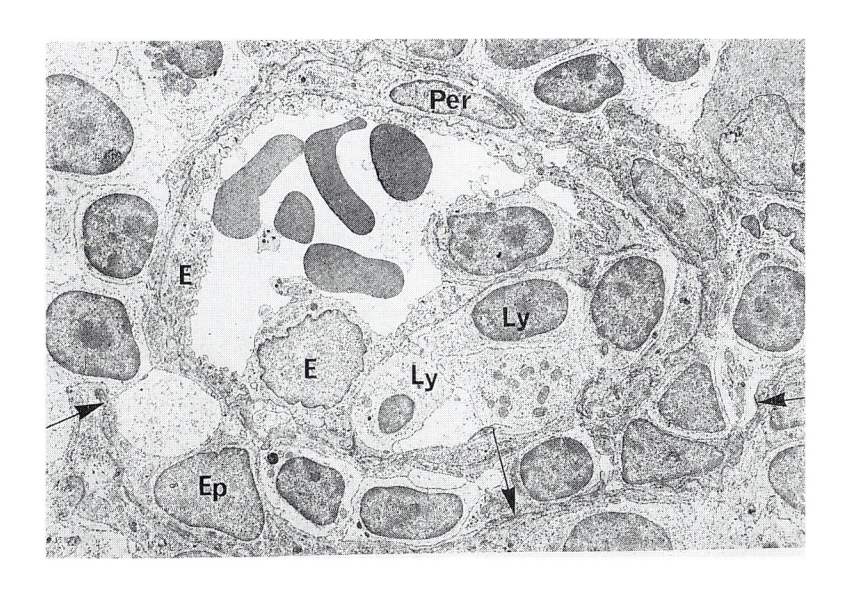

Fig. 11-17. TEM of postcapillary venule in thymus. Notice endothelial cell wall and lymphocytes in transit through the endothelium. *E,* endothelial cell; *Ly,* lymphocytes; *Per,* pericytes; *Ep,* epithelial cell. Arrows indicate periphery of postcapillary venule. (×2,000.)

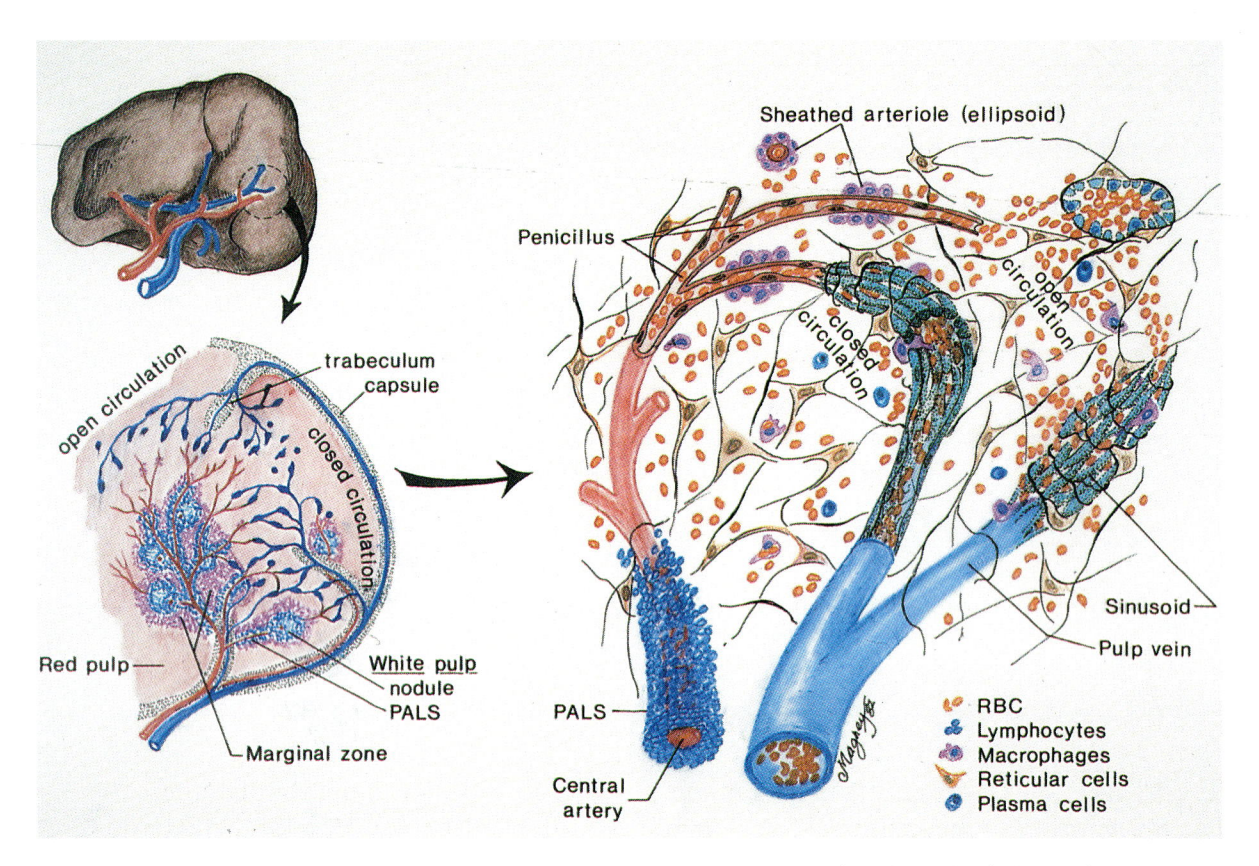

Fig. 11-18. Spleen, showing gross structure, open and closed models for splenic circulation, and microscopic structure.

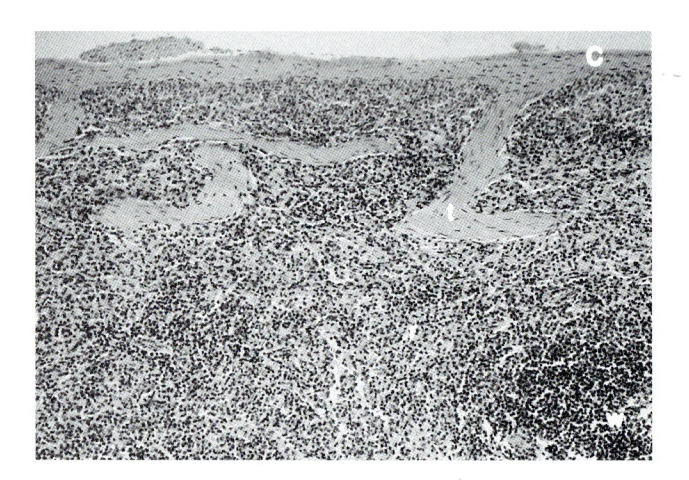

Fig. 11-19. LM of surface of spleen illustrating capsule (c) and trabeculae (t). Examples of red (r) and white (w) pulp are also visible. (H&E; ×100.)

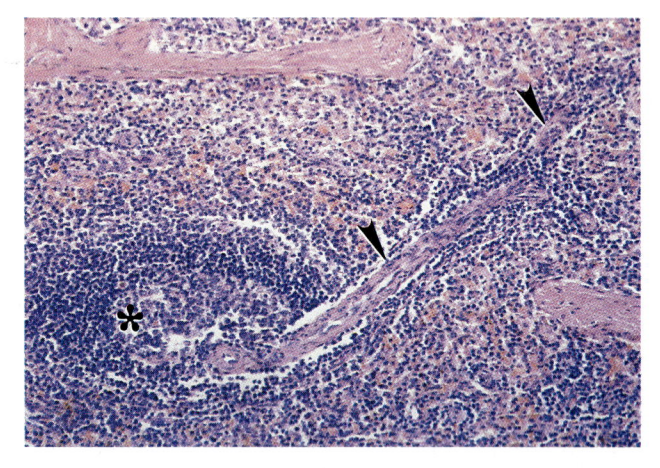

Fig. 11-20. High-magnification LM of splenic parenchyma showing course of central artery of white pulp (arrowheads). Periarteriolar lymphatic sheath (T-lymphocytes) is visible along this vessel. Secondary nodule (*). (H&E; ×150.)

LYMPHOID SYSTEM 85

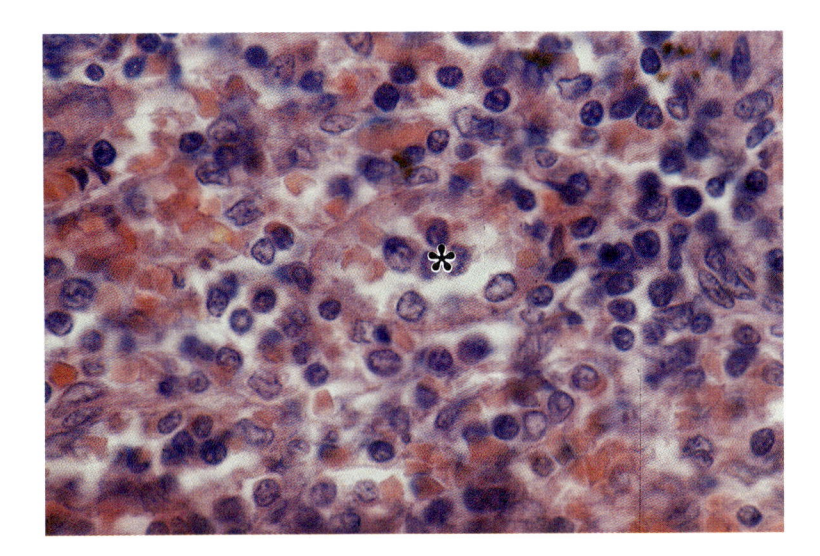

Fig. 11-21. High-magnification LM of red pulp within spleen. Splenic sinusoid (*) is in center of field. (H&E; ×1,000.)

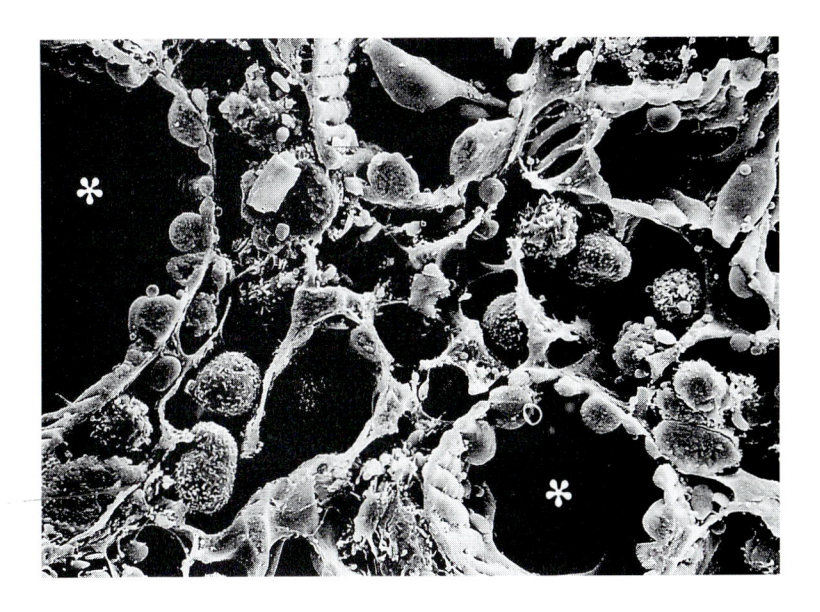

Fig. 11-22. SEM of splenic red pulp including three sinusoids (*). Red pulp between sinusoids constitutes cords of Billroth. Red pulp is supported by reticular cells with extensive processes; lying within their network are macrophages and leukocytes. (×1,100.)

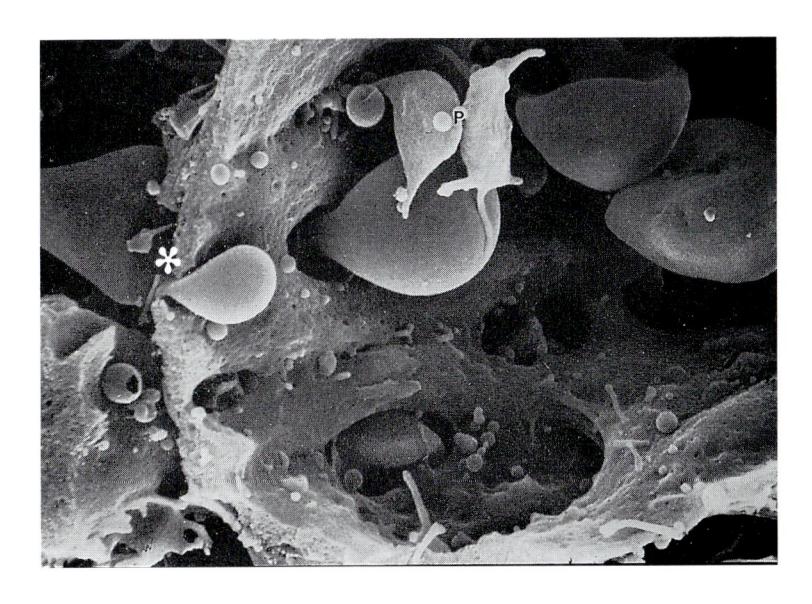

Fig. 11-23. SEM of internal surface of splenic sinusoid illustrating passage of erythrocytes through large gaps in sinusoid wall (*). Increased rigidity of red blood cells with age inhibits their passage, and cells thus arrested may presumably be detected by macrophages and thereby removed from circulation. (×3,000.)

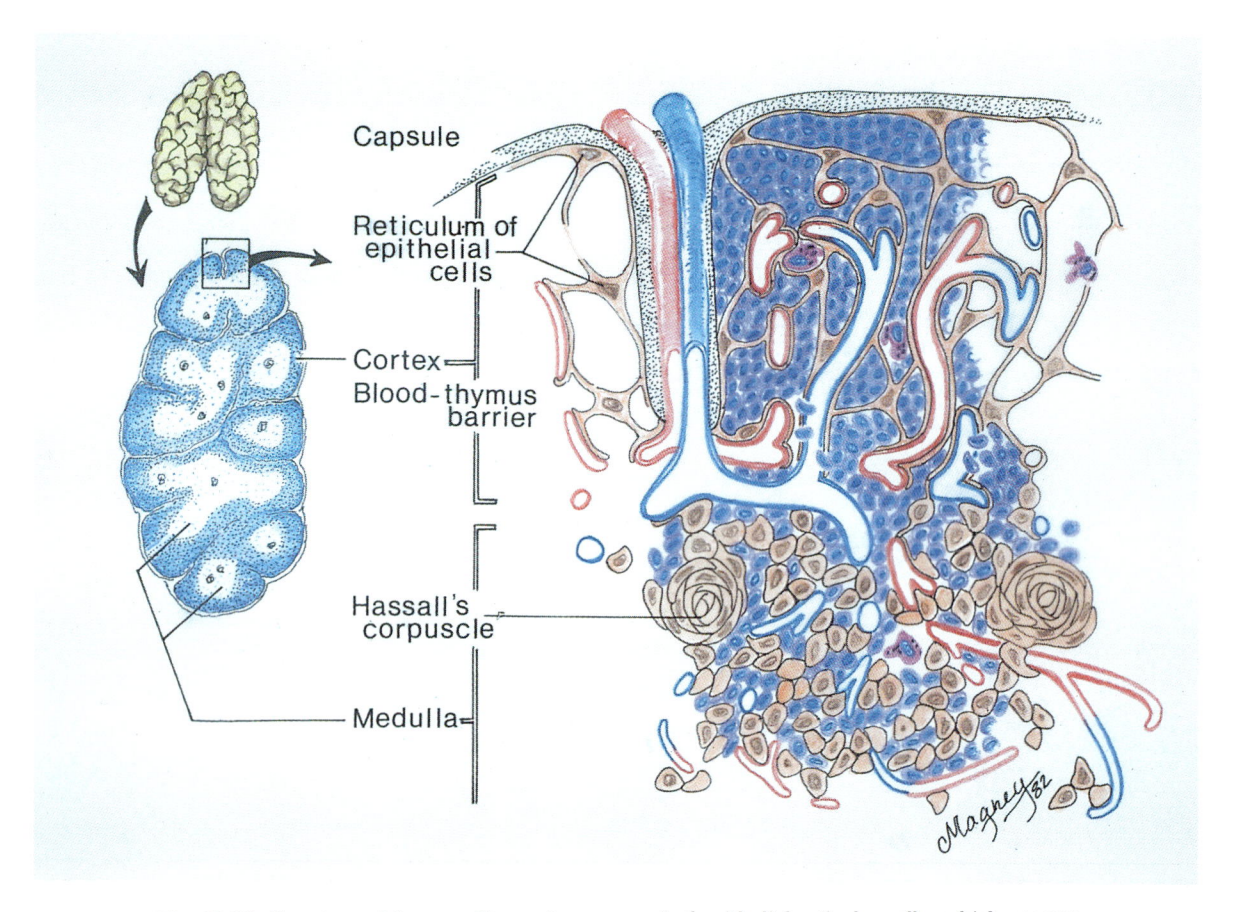

Fig. 11-24. Structure of thymus. Stroma is composed of epithelial reticular cells, which secrete thymic factors. T-lymphoctyes constitute parenchyma of organ and are supported by meshwork of stromal cells. Observe vascular supply and components of blood-thymus barrier.

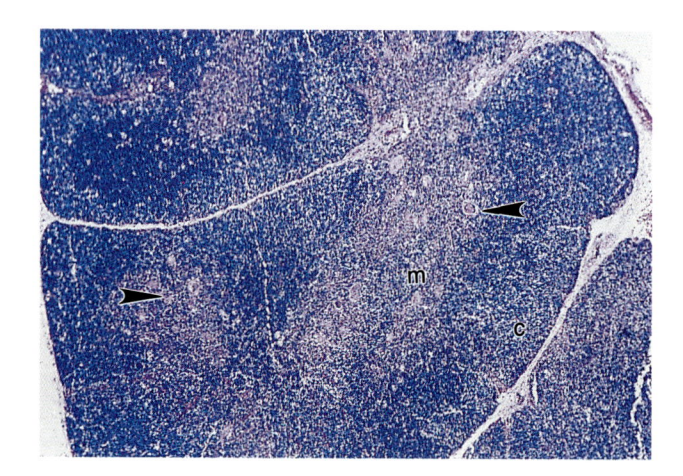

Fig. 11-25. Low-magnification LM of thymus showing lobular nature of gland, presence of continuous medulla (m), and incomplete cortex (c). No lymphatic nodules are found within thymus. Even at this magnification, Hassall's corpuscles (arrowheads) can be seen within medulla. (H&E; ×40.)

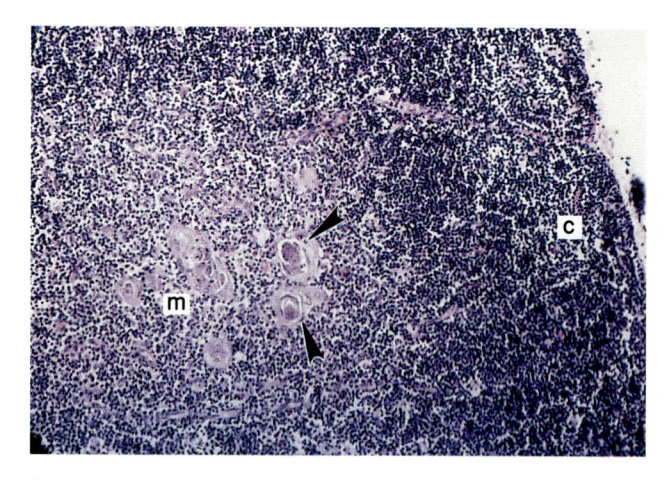

Fig. 11-26. Higher-magnification LM of cortex and medulla in thymus. Thin capsule can be seen on surface. Cortex (c) consists of dense masses of lymphocytes, whereas Hassall's corpuscles (arrowheads) can be seen within medulla (m). (H&E; ×150.)

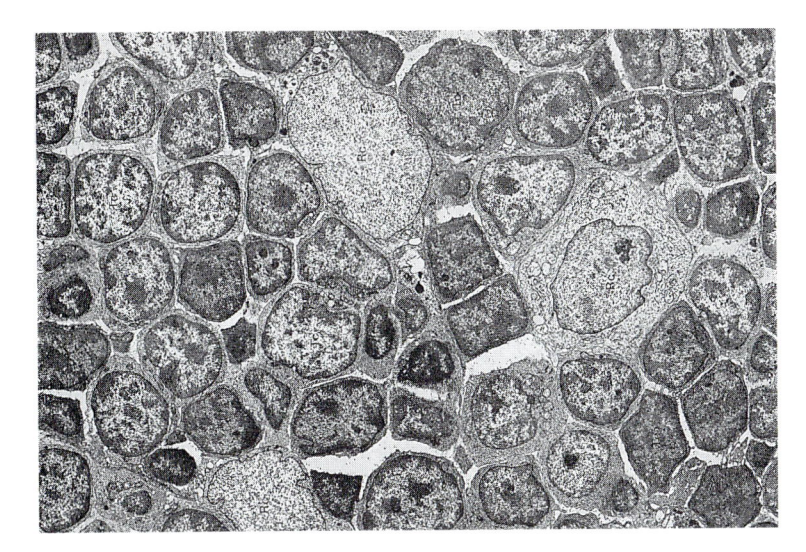

Fig. 11-27. TEM of thymic cortex revealing large numbers of lymphocytes and presence of thymic epithelial cells with large vesicular nuclei. (×1,500.)

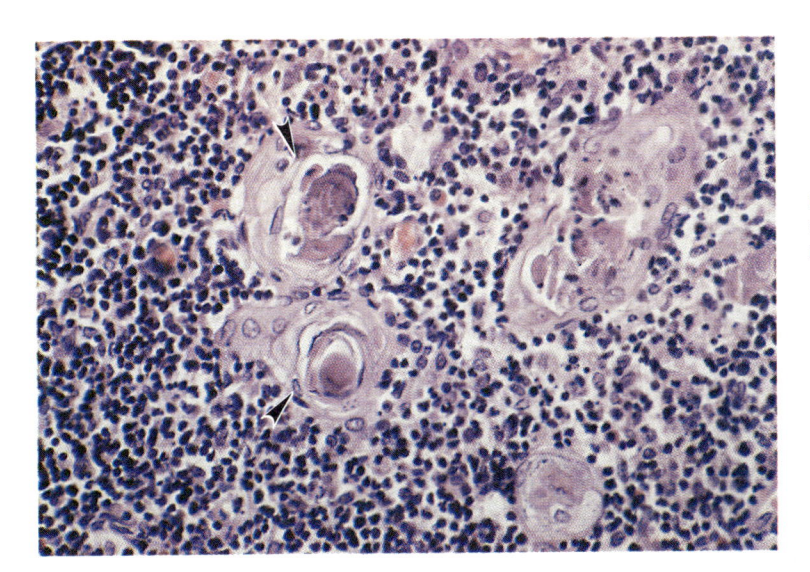

Fig. 11-28. High-magnification LM of thymic medulla illustrating epithelial nature of Hassall's corpuscles *(arrowheads)*. (×350.)

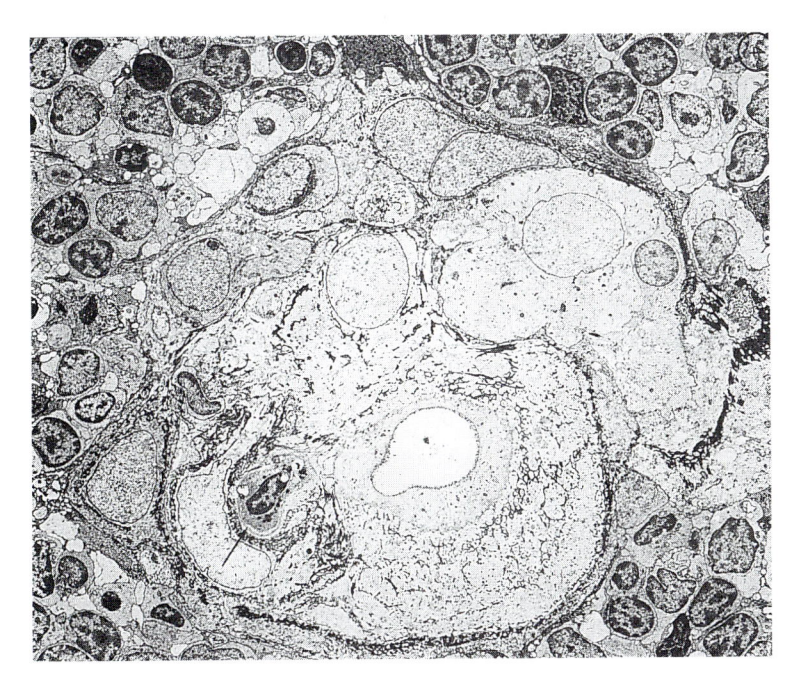

Fig. 11-29. TEM of Hassall's corpuscle in thymus. Prominent tonofilaments are easily seen within corpuscle. Arrow points to degenerating lymphocyte. Center of corpuscle is cystic, and lining epithelial cells have microvilli. However, none of the epithelial cells within corpuscle displays any detectable secretory apparatus. (×1,000.)

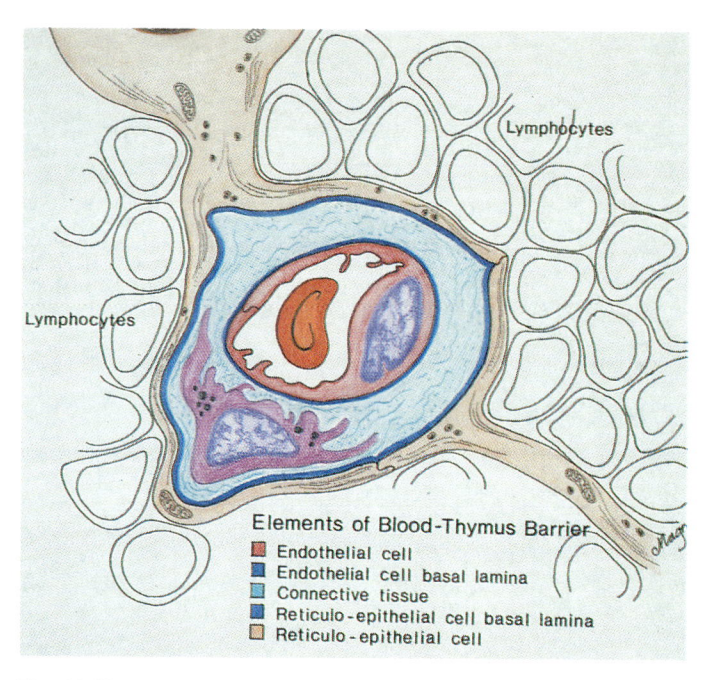

Fig. 11-30. Components of blood-thymus barrier. Cellular components include endothelial and stromal epithelial reticular cells as well as basal laminas of each cell type.

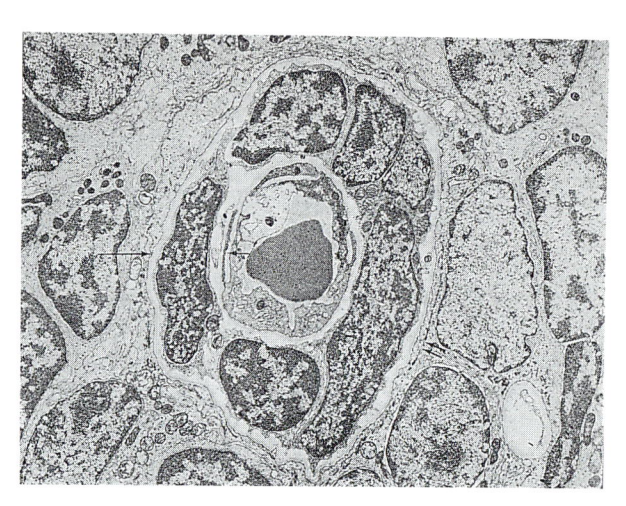

Fig. 11-31. TEM of capillary in thymic medulla surrounded by lymphocytes. Basal lamina of endothelial cell is designated by short arrows; epithelial cell basal lamina, by long arrows. No endothelial fenestrations are present. ($\times 1,900$.)

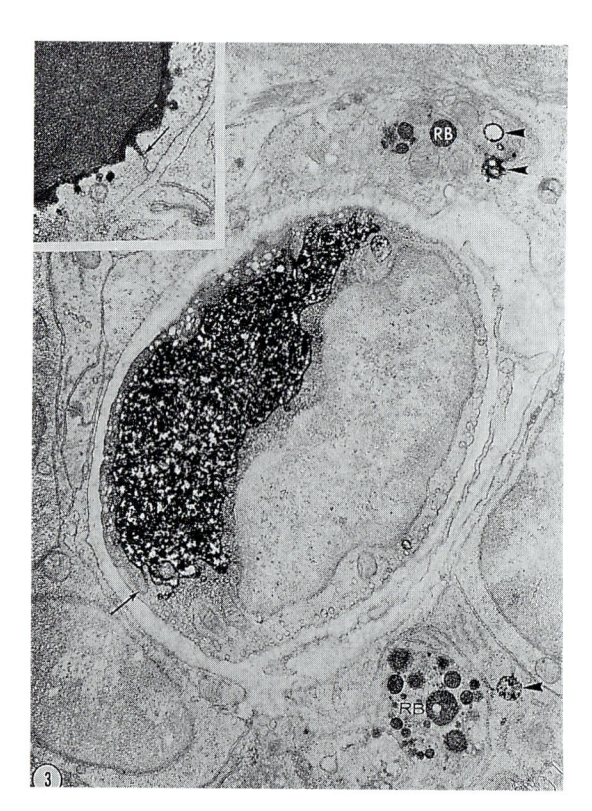

Fig. 11-32. TEM of capillary within thymic cortex 5 minutes after intravenous injection of horseradish peroxidase demonstrating integrity of blood-thymus barrier. Intense staining for peroxidase is seen within lumen of capillary. Endothelial basal lamina, adventitia, and intercellular spaces of surrounding cortical parenchyma are free of peroxidase staining. Nonspecific staining of phagocytic vacuoles within macrophages in adventitia and within residual bodies is also visible. Inset *upper left)* shows part of capillary within thymic cortex 1 minute after intravenous injection of cytochrome C as intravascular tracer. Reaction product for cytochrome C is seemingly arrested at junctional complex between two endothelial cells. Staining of red blood cell in lumen is due to pseudoperoxidase activity of hemoglobin. *RB,* Residual body. Arrowheads indicate phagocytic vacuoles; single arrow, intercellular junctions between endothelial cells. ($\times 10,500$; inset $\times 15,000$.)

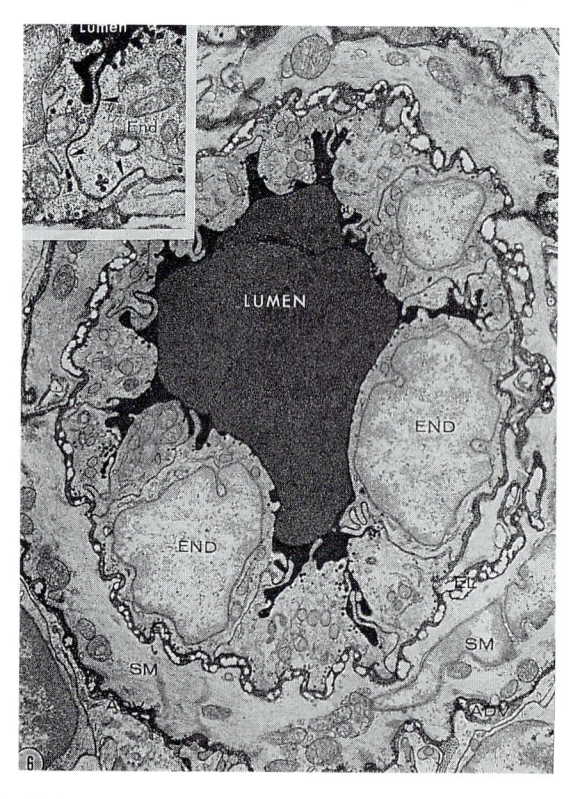

Fig. 11-33. TEM of arteriole wall at corticomedullary boundary in thymus 5 minutes after intravenous injection of horseradish peroxidase illustrating lack of blood-thymus barrier in this zone. Reaction product is seen in clefts of endothelium, within fenestrations of elastic interna, and in adventitia. Inset *(upper left)* illustrates that cleft between adjacent endothelial cells stains throughout its length with same intensity as blood plasma, indicating that this is a route for diffusion of peroxidase from lumen into surrounding adventitial space. Similar staining is also observed within postcapillary venules of medulla. ($\times 6,200$; inset $\times 10,600$.)

CHAPTER 12

EXOCRINE GLANDS

EXOCRINE GLANDS ARE invaginations of epithelial tissue into the underlying connective tissue. These glands produce secretory products that are discharged and transported through a duct system to the epithelial surface, where they are discharged onto the epithelium from which the gland was derived. Exocrine glands can be classified as follows.

A. Cell number
1. **Unicellular.** The simplest exocrine glands are composed of individual glandular cells scattered within an epithelium. These are typified by goblet cells within the gastrointestinal and respiratory tracts.
2. **Multicellular.** Most exocrine glands are multicellular, and the secretory cells are often arranged in either tubules or clusters of cells (acini), or a combination of both. Multicellular glands must have **ducts** to transport the secretion from the **secretory unit** to the surface.

B. Nature of secretory product. This classification is based on the relative abundance of carbohydrate and protein in the secretory product.
1. **Serous.** The secretory products are primarily proteinaceous and the secretion is watery or of low viscosity.
2. **Mucous.** The secretory product contains an abundance of carbohydrate in the form of sialomucins or sulfomucins. Upon exocytosis these secretions become hydrated and are viscous. The secretory portions of mucous glands may be surrounded by **myoepithelial** cells whose contractile activity is thought to help move the viscous secretory product into and along the duct system.
3. **Seromucous (mixed).** The secretory product contains variable amounts of serous and mucous secretory products.

C. Mode of secretion
1. **Merocrine secretion.** This is the usual mode of exocrine secretion for most glands. The fusion of secretion granules with the cell membrane results in release of the product into the extracellular space, a process known as exocytosis.
2. **Holocrine secretion.** The entire cell is released or discharged in the secretion. An example of holocrine secretion is found in the sebaceous gland of the skin.
3. **Apocrine secretion.** The secretory product is discharged by pinching off blebs of cytoplasm that include the secretory product. This unique form of secretion takes place in the mammary gland and specialized sweat glands.

D. Arrangement of the duct and secretory units
1. **Duct system.** Ducts, as shown in Fig. 12-1, are responsible for transporting the secretory product to the epithelial surface. However, in doing so they may alter the product through additional secretory activity of the duct cells (i.e., granulated duct cells in salivary glands containing kallikreins or lysozyme) or by altering the water and electrolyte content of the secretion (i.e., striated ducts of the salivary glands).
   a. **Simple.** The gland contains only one unbranched duct, which may be either straight or coiled.
   b. **Compound** or **branched.** The ducts of these glands show repeated branching.
2. **Secretory units**
   a. **Tubular.** The gland cells are arranged in tubes that may be straight, coiled, or branched.
   b. **Acinar** (alveolar). The cells are arranged in grapelike clusters that open into a common secretory channel that is continuous with the duct system.

Important exocrine glands in the body include the major **salivary glands (parotid, submandibular, sublingual)** and the **pancreas.** Each of these glands possesses a delicate collagenous capsule and a well-defined duct system that discharges its secretory product into the gastrointestinal tract, and each is innervated by the autonomic nervous system. The histologic characteristics of these glands are as follows.

PAROTID GLAND

This branched compound acinar gland produces a serous secretion that accounts for approximately 25% of the salivary flow. Prominent histologic characteristics of the gland include serous acinar cells, numerous profiles of striated ducts, and fatty infiltration.

SUBMANDIBULAR GLAND

This branched tubuloacinar gland produces about 70% of the salivary flow. Approximately 80% of the gland is composed of serous cells; 5% of the gland consists of mucous tubules capped by clusters of serous cells known as serous demilunes. Because of the large serous secretion of this gland, striated ducts are well developed and numerous within every lobule.

SUBLINGUAL GLAND

The sublingual gland is a branched tubular gland that contributes a mucous secretion comprising about 5% of the salivary flow. The secretory units are composed chiefly of mucous cells arranged in tubules that may possess serous demilunes. Because of the increased viscosity of the secretion (less free water), striated ducts involved in ion transport are greatly diminished within the sublingual gland and are infrequently seen in lobules.

PANCREAS

The pancreas has both exocrine and endocrine function. The exocrine pancreas is a compound acinar gland that produces a variety of digestive enzymes. Histologically, it is similar to the parotid gland in structure. However, intralobular ducts are difficult to detect within pancreatic lobules. Intercalated ducts extend into individual acini, where duct cells are referred to as centroacinar cells. The pancreas does not contain striated ducts, although the ductular system does secrete substantial amounts of bicarbonate.

Exocrine glands associated with major organs systems such as skin and the reproductive system are discussed in later chapters.

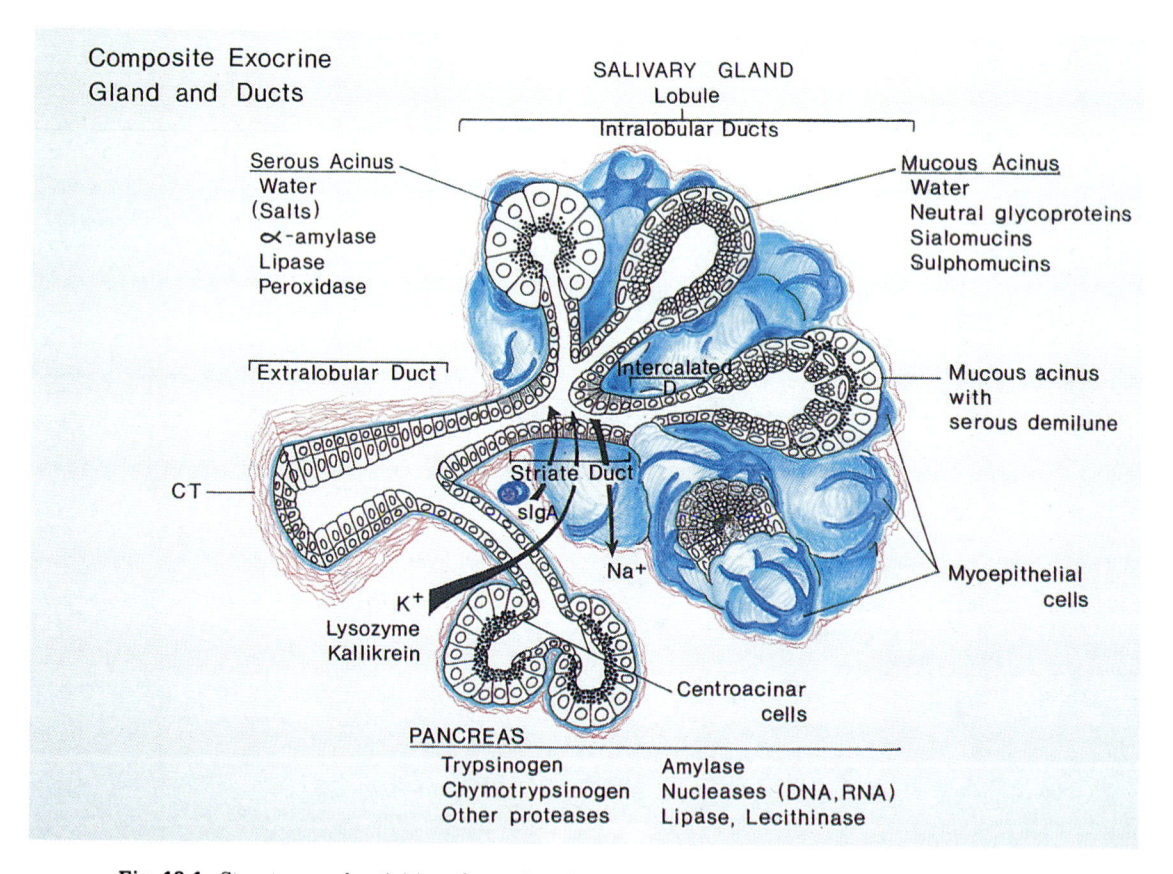

Fig. 12-1. Structure and activities of exocrine glands and duct systems which drain them. Ducts are described as intralobular when they lie within lobule (subdivisions are intercalated and striated ducts), whereas interlobular ducts are located in connective tissue between lobules and drain secretions from several adjacent lobules. Salivary glands may have serous secretions (parotid gland) or mixed seromucous secretions (submandibular and sublingual glands). The serous product of acini may be modified by ion exchange (striate duct), secretory activity of granulated intralobular duct cells, and transport of secretory IgA into lumen through its binding to receptors on acinar and/or duct cells.

EXOCRINE GLANDS 91

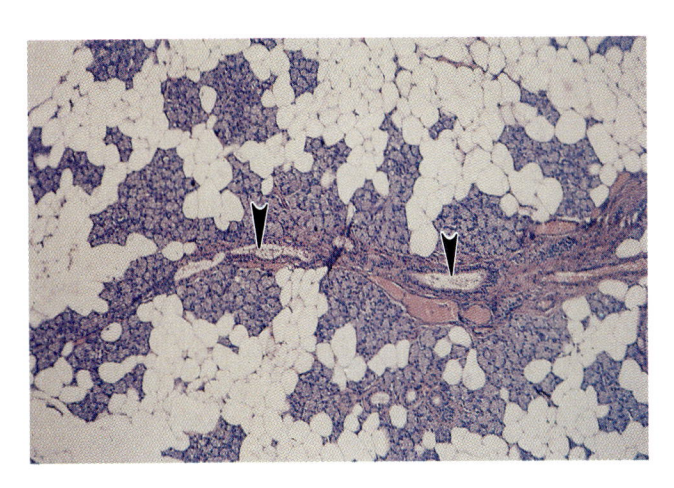

Fig. 12-2. Low-magnification LM of parotid gland showing serous acini and their ducts surrounded by large numbers of adipocytes. Intralobular ducts *(arrowheads)* are seen in center of lobule. (H&E; ×100.)

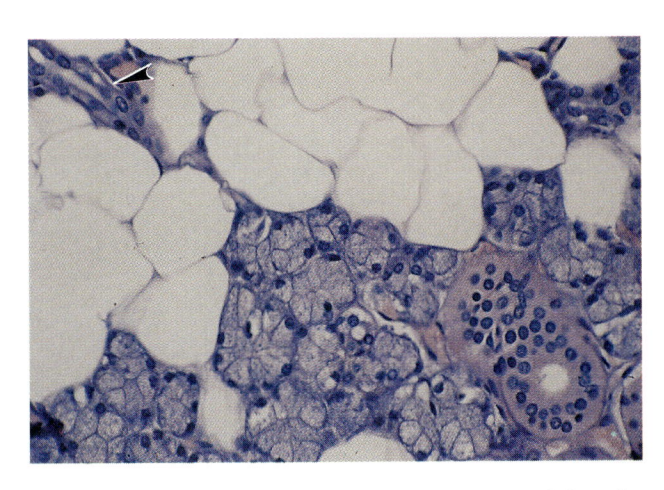

Fig. 12-3. LM of parotid lobule showing intercalated duct *(arrowhead)* and striated duct *(lower right)*. Nuclei of basophilic serous cells can be seen at periphery of acini. Numerous adipocytes are present. (H&E; ×400.)

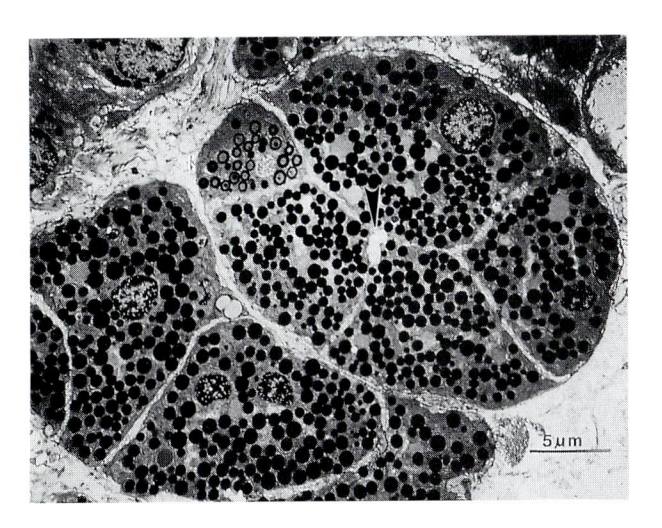

Fig. 12-4. TEM of parotid acini from unstimulated gland, showing serous cells with numerous secretory granules in apical cytoplasm adjacent to central lumen of excretory channel *(arrowhead)*. (×2,200.)

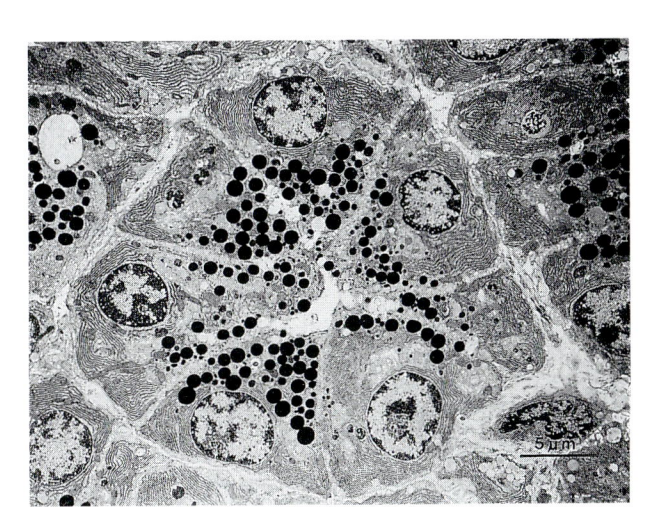

Fig. 12-5. TEM of parotid acini from gland stimulated to secrete. By comparison to unstimulated acini shown in Fig. 12-4, stimulated acinar cells contain fewer secretion granules as a result of their earlier discharge into duct system. (×2,200.)

92 COLOR ATLAS OF HISTOLOGY

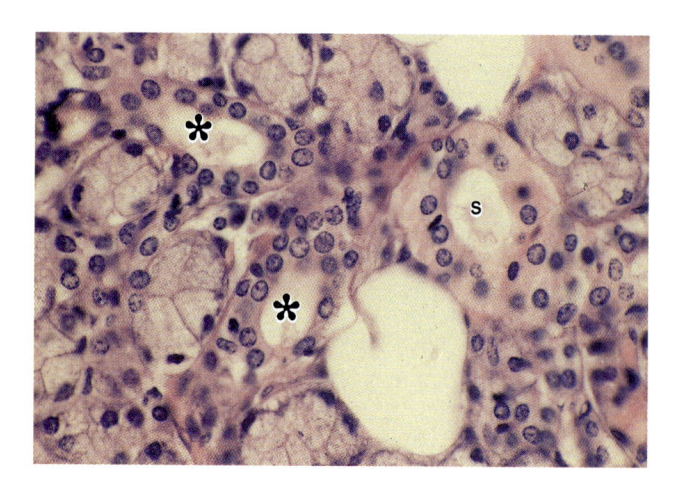

Fig. 12-6. LM of parotid lobule showing intercalated (*) and striated (s) ducts intermixed between serous acini. Several adipocytes are also present. (H&E; ×500.)

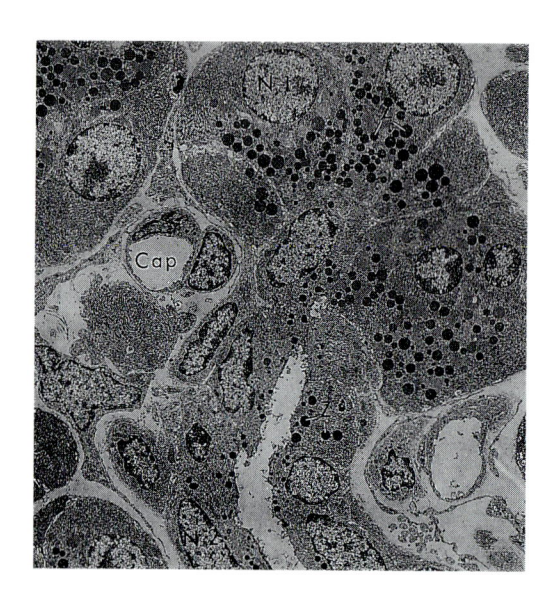

Fig. 12-7. TEM of exocrine acinus–intercalated duct junction. Observe connection of intercalated duct cells to acinus. Compare this with LM of intercalated ducts in Fig. 12-6. Cap, capillary; N, nucleus. (×1,500.)

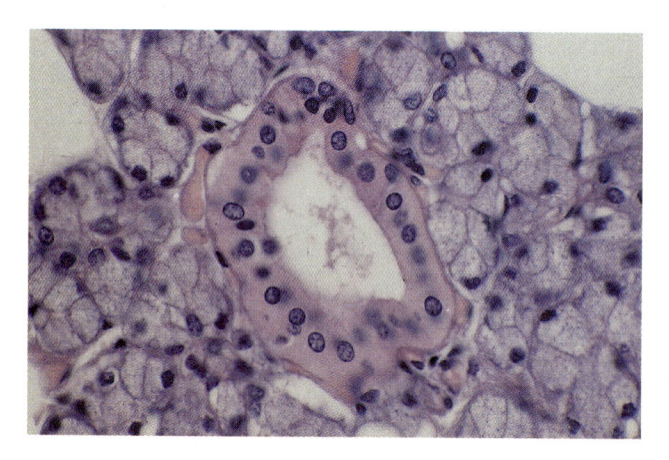

Fig. 12-8. LM of striated duct. Cells forming duct are columnar and contain centrally located nucleus because of basal infoldings associated with ion transport. Acidophilia of duct cells is due to large numbers of mitochondria (see Fig. 12-9). (H&E; ×500.)

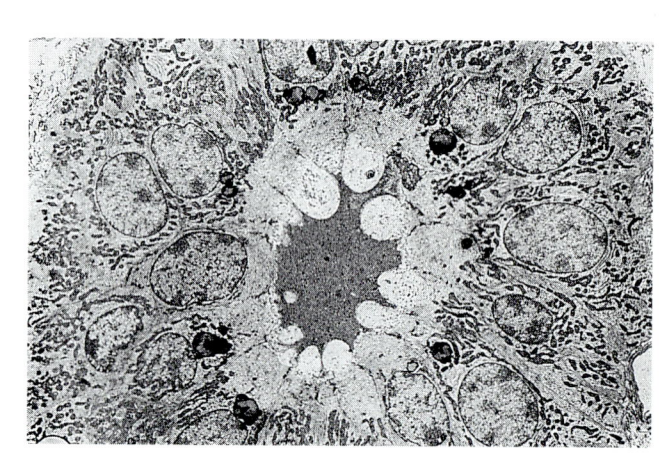

Fig. 12-9. TEM of striated duct in parotid gland. Tall columnar duct cells possess numerous mitochondria within infoldings of basal plasmalemma. (×2,500.)

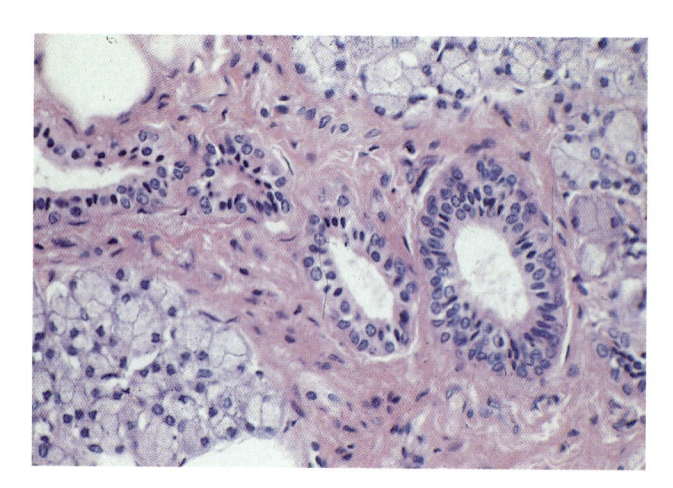

Fig. 12-10. LM of interlobular ducts. Large amounts of collagen invest interlobular ducts as they course between adjacent lobules of glandular tissue. Epithelium of these ducts is usually stratified cuboidal or columnar. (H&E; ×300.)

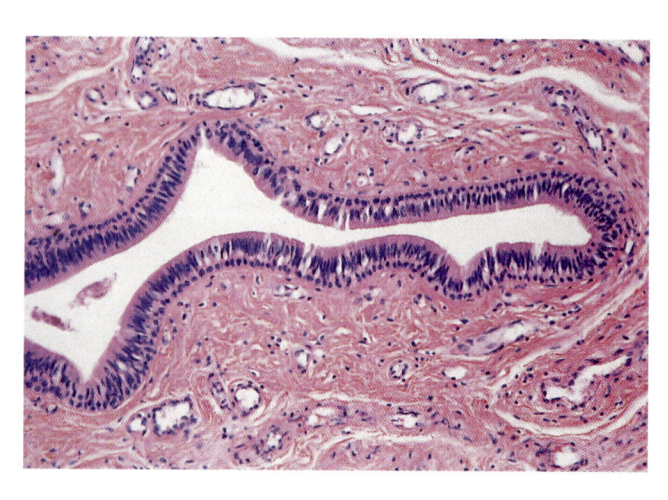

Fig. 12-11. LM of main excretory duct with stratified columnar epithelium surrounded by increased amounts of collagenous connective tissue. (H&E; ×150.)

EXOCRINE GLANDS 93

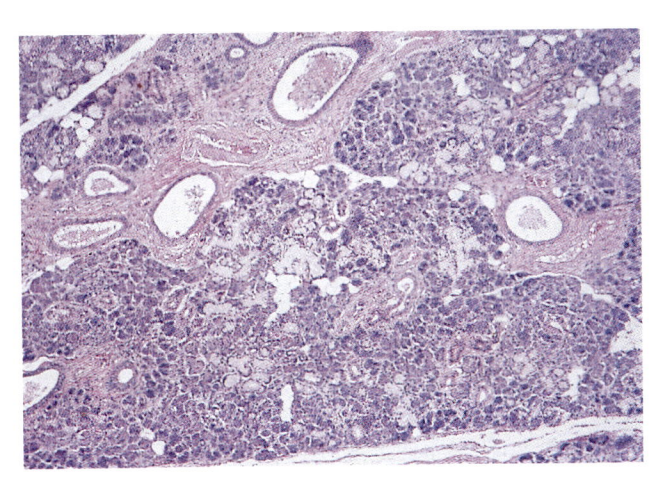

Fig. 12-12. Low-magnification LM of submandibular gland showing interlobular ducts and secretory lobules. (H&E; ×75.)

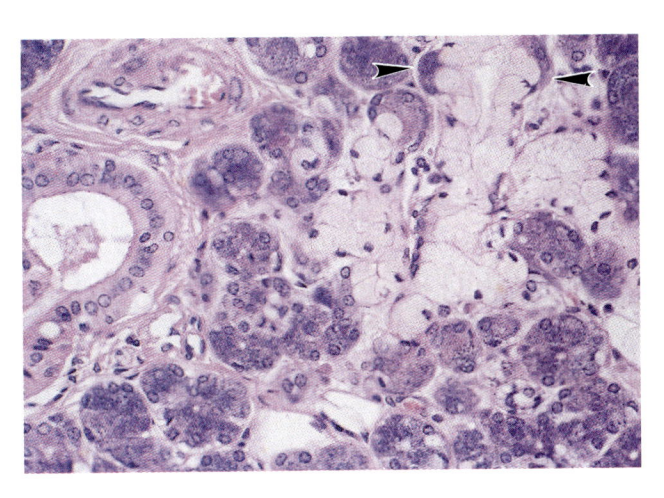

Fig. 12-13. Higher-magnification LM illustrating serous and mucous secretory units within lobule of submandibular gland. Portion of striated duct can be seen at left. Note presence of serous demilunes *(arrowheads)*. (H&E; ×300.)

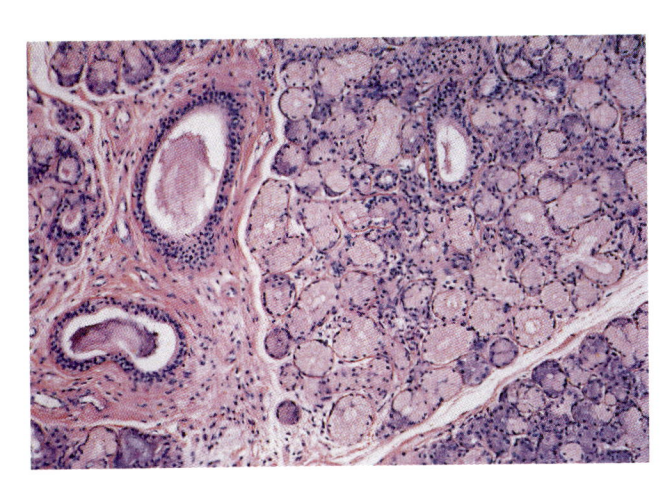

Fig. 12-14. Low-magnification LM of sublingual gland illustrating interlobular ducts and presence of intralobular ducts within the glandular lobule. (H&E; ×300.)

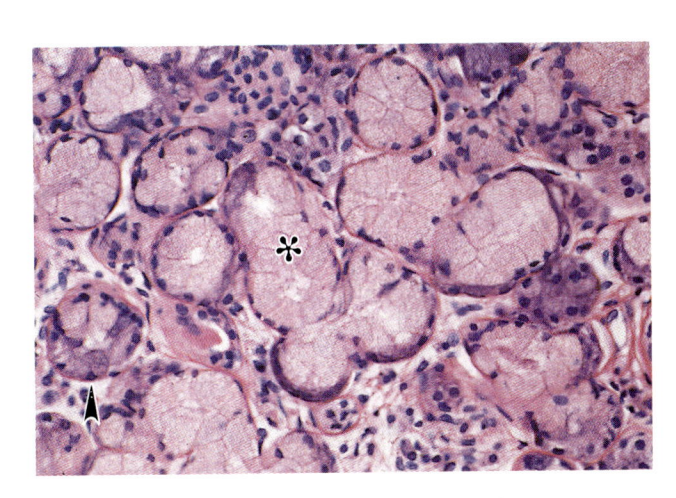

Fig. 12-15. LM of sublingual gland at higher magnification showing mucous acini (*) surrounded by myoepithelial cells. A few serous cells *(arrowhead)* are present in some acini. (H&E; ×100.)

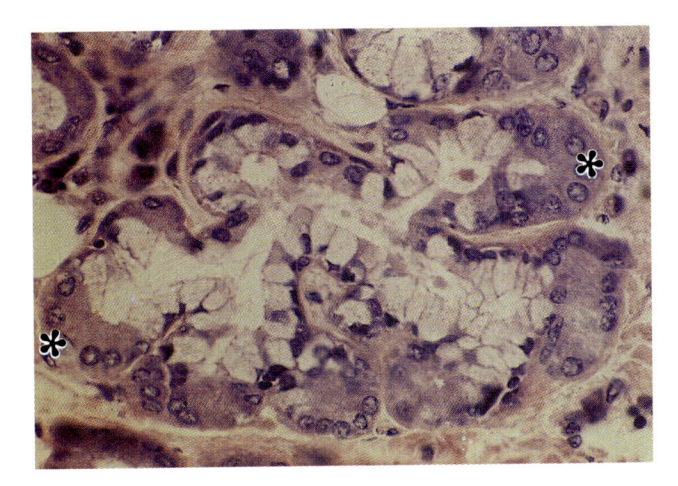

Fig. 12-16. LM of mixed seromucous gland. Serous demilunes are basophilic clusters of cells (*) arranged in crescent at ends of mucous tubules. (H&E; ×500.)

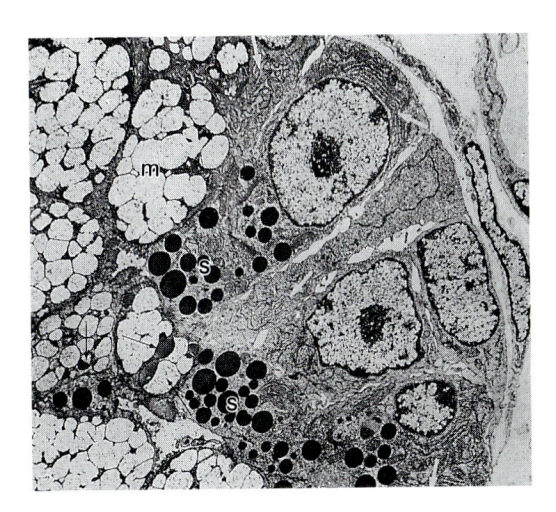

Fig. 12-17. TEM of sublingual gland acini showing both mucous-secreting cells *(m)* and serous-secreting cells *(s)*. Mucous granules have high carbohydrate content and are electron-lucent, whereas serous secretion granules have higher protein content, making them more electron-dense. Myoepithelial cell (*) is visible at periphery of acinus. (×3,500.)

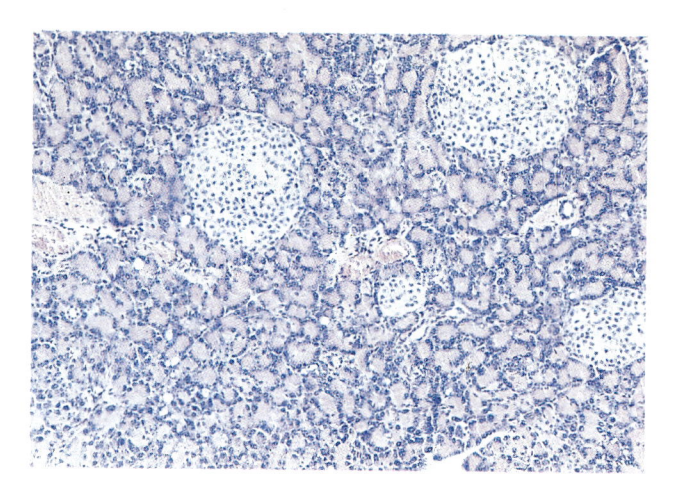

Fig. 12-18. Low-magnification LM of pancreas. Pale clusters of endocrine cells comprising islets of Langerhans can be seen interspersed among serous acini. (H&E; ×100.)

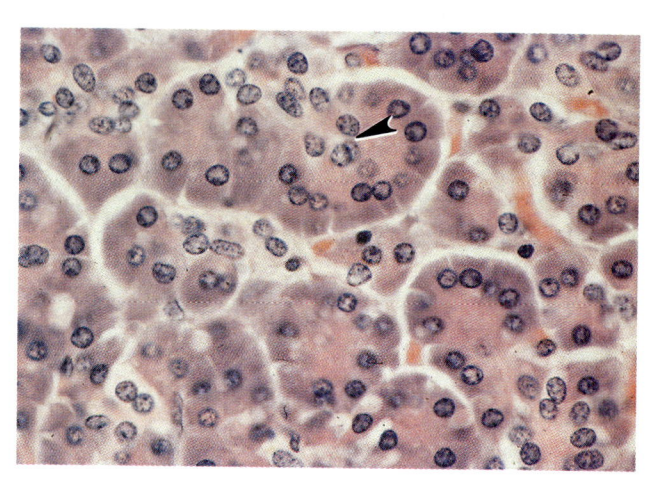

Fig. 12-19. High-magnification LM illustrating structure of pancreatic acinus. Acinus at top contains centrally located nuclei *(arrowhead)* of cells that are beginnings of intercalated duct. These cells are referred to as centroacinar cells. (H&E; ×500.)

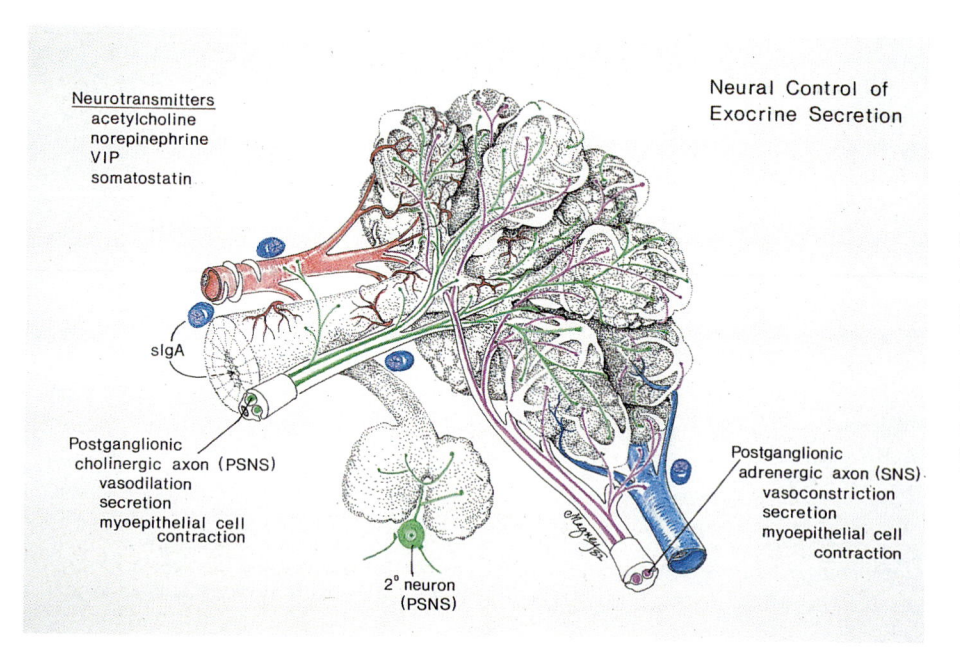

Fig. 12-20. Neural regulation of exocrine secretion. Autonomic nervous system innervates exocrine glands through its sympathetic and parasympathetic divisions. Sympathetic blood vessels, whereas those of parasympathetic division follow ducts. Nerve fibers terminate as small dilated endings that are intimately associated with depressions in basal surface of acinar cell (see Fig. 12-21).

Fig. 12-21. TEMs showing innervation of parotid acinar cell by autonomic nervous system. **A** shows an unmyelinated nerve terminal beneath basal lamina. In **B** unmyelinated nerve terminal has also penetrated basal lamina and lies within indentation of acinar cell. Arrows indicate subsurface cisternae. *LV*, Large vesicle. (A, ×19,500; B, ×25,600.)

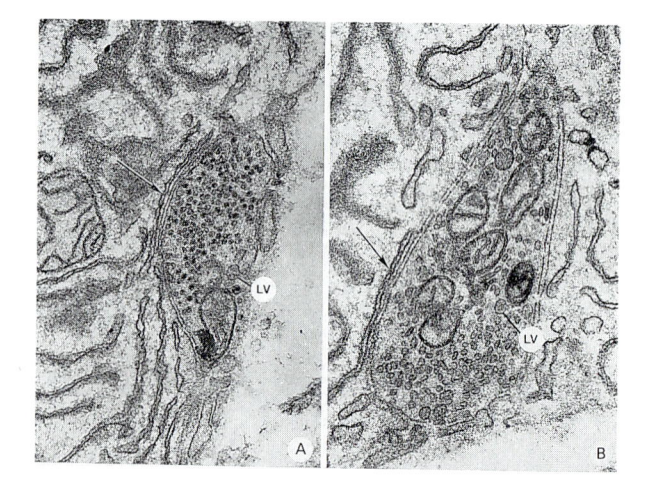

CHAPTER 13

ENDOCRINE GLANDS

ENDOCRINE GLANDS ARE usually comprised of epithelial cells that have grown into connective tissues and then lost their continuity (via ducts) with the surface epithelium from which they were derived. Their secretions, called **hormones,** are released into the bloodstream for distribution to distant **target organs.** As a consequence, endocrine glands are profusely supplied with fenestrated capillaries, which facilitate the diffusion of hormones into the blood in response to chemical or nervous stimuli.

Hormones are chemical substances that have well-defined effects on various parts of the body; in general, they **integrate, correlate,** and **control** body processes by chemical means. Hormones may consist of modified **amino acids, peptides, proteins,** or **steroid** molecules. Endocrine glands have a connective tissue capsule and a reticular fiber stroma within which the parenchymal cells are situated. These glands, which are widely distributed throughout the body, are described in this chapter. Other endocrine tissue found in a variety of organs such as kidney, testis, ovary, and the gastrointestinal epithelium are discussed in later chapters.

PITUITARY GLAND

The pituitary gland **(hypophysis)** has a dual derivation. The anterior pituitary **(adenohypophysis** or **pars distalis)** arises from pharyngeal epithelium (ectoderm) while the posterior pituitary **(neurohypophysis** or **pars nervosa)** is derived from neuroectoderm of the forming hypothalamus. Neurosecretions of neurons in the **paraventricular** and **supraoptic nuclei** of the hypothalamus are transported down their axons, which pass through the infundibulum (via **hypothalamohypophyseal tract**) to the pars nervosa, where they are stored until released in axonal dilatations called **Herring bodies.** A **hypophyseal portal system** of venules carries releasing or inhibitory hormones, produced by other hypothalamic neurons, to cells of the pars distalis, where they regulate the production and secretion of hormones that have trophic effects on other endocrine glands or tissues of the body. **Pars intermedia,** between pars distalis and pars nervosa, and **pars tuberalis,** which forms a sleeve around the infundibular stalk and through which the hypophyseal portal system passes, are thought to be (functional) parts of the pars distalis.

The pituitary gland lies within the sella turcica of the sphenoid bone and is surrounded by a capsule that blends with the dura mater. A reticular fiber stroma supports the parenchymal cells of the gland and the surrounding sinusoids. The gland receives its blood supply from hypophyseal branches of the internal carotid artery.

THYROID GLAND

The thyroid gland has two lobes joined by an isthmus and is covered by a double-layered connective tissue capsule. The thyroid lies adjacent to the lower larynx and upper trachea and is richly supplied with blood by thyroidal arteries from the thyrocervical trunk and external carotid artery. Parenchymal cells of the thyroid gland are derived embryonically from pharyngeal epithelium and are arranged into hollow cellular clusters called **follicles.** The wall is composed of follicular cells that vary from low cuboidal to columnar, depending on their functional state. The follicular lumen is filled with a gelatinous **"colloid,"** the stored form of the gland's product, a glycoprotein called **thyroglobulin** containing the iodinated amino acid tyrosine. Under the influence of **thyroid stimulating hormone (TSH)** from the anterior pituitary gland, follicular cells produce and store thyroglobulin as colloid. Simultaneously, lamellipodia on the apical membranes of the follicle cells surround colloid and internalize it by endocytosis.

Within the follicle cell, thyroglobulin is degraded by the lysosomal apparatus into forms of iodinated tyrosines, which are released through the basal membrane as **thyroid hormone (thyroxine [tetraiodothyronine] and triiodothyronine).** Thyroid hormone regulates the metabolic rate, stimulates cell metabolism, and, in conjunction with growth hormone, ensures proper brain cell formation and myelination of axons. Associated with the basal part of the follicular epithelium are **parafollicular** or **C cells,** which are the source of **thyrocalcitonin,** a hormone that lowers blood calcium (an action opposite to that of parathyroid hormone) and increases osteogenesis.

PARATHYROID GLAND

Four small parathyroid glands lie on the posterior aspect of the thyroid gland within the thyroid capsule and are richly supplied with blood by vessels coursing through the thyroid. The parathyroid gland secretes **parathyroid hormone (PTH),** which regulates calcium absorption/reabsorption and, through production of an **osteoclast stimulating factor,** raises blood calcium levels by osteolysis. **Principal** or **chief cells,** arranged in compact masses or anastomosing cords, are the source of parathyroid hormone, a polypeptide synthesized and released immediately in response to low blood calcium levels. Also present are **oxyphil cells,** which are larger than chief cells and appear singly or in small acidophilic clusters, and **Wasserhelle** or **clear cells,** which contain large amounts of glycogen. The preparation of tissue for light microscopy extracts glycogen and makes the cytoplasm of the Wasserhelle cell appear clear. The functional roles of oxyphil and Wasserhelle cells have not been determined.

SUPRARENAL GLAND

A thick connective tissue capsule attaches a suprarenal gland to the superior pole of each kidney. The gland itself is divided into an outer, solid **cortex,** derived from **embryonic mesoderm,** and a **medulla,** with origin from the **neural crest.** Branches of the suprarenal, inferior phrenic, and renal arteries penetrate the capsule and form capillary plexuses. Sinusoidal capillaries carry blood that percolates between cord of cortical parenchymal cells into the medulla, while other (arteriolar) vessels pass directly into the medulla. From the medulla, blood is drained by suprarenal veins.

Cortical tissue is subdivided into zones with names that describe the arrangement of parenchymal cells. The **zona glomerulosa,** immediately beneath the capsule, produces the **mineralocorticoid aldosterone,** which acts on the kidney to regulate sodium and potassium in the body. Aldosterone secretion is regulated by the kidney via the **renin-angiotensin system.** The **zona fasciculata** synthesizes **glucocorticoids** (i.e., **cortisol, corticosterone**), which is important in controlling the inflammatory response. Located adjacent to medullary tissue, the **zona reticularis** also produces glucocorticoids and small amounts of **androgens.** Secretion of glucocorticoids and androgens is regulated by **adrenocorticotropic hormone (ACTH).** The medulla, which comprises about 10% of the suprarenal gland, consists largely of **chromaffin cells,** so named for their reaction with potassium dichromate. Chromaffin cells are regulated by the sympathetic division of the autonomic nervous system and produce **norepinephrine, epinephrine,** and **enkephalins.**

ISLETS OF LANGERHANS

Clusters of endocrine cells, the **islets of Langerhans,** are dispersed throughout the parenchyma of the pancreas. The islets of Langerhans comprise about 1%

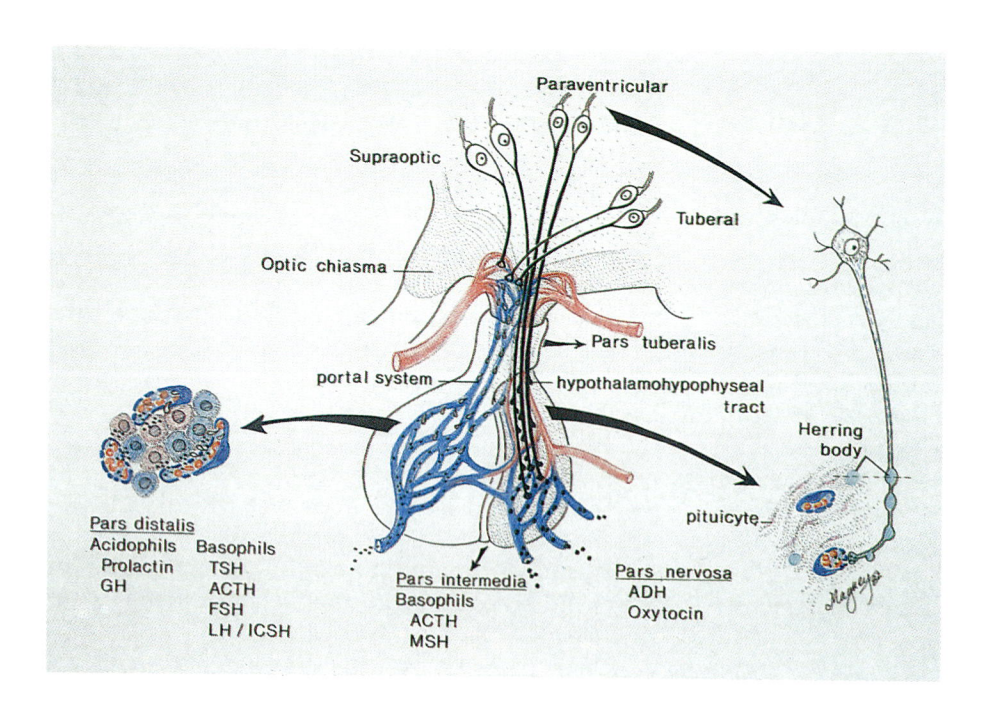

Fig. 13-1. Relationships between hypothalamus and anterior and posterior lobes of pituitary gland. Note hypothalamic-hypophyseal portal system, which transports releasing hormones from median eminence to anterior lobe, where they stimulate acidophils or basophils. Note also pathway for neuronal fibers from hypothalamic nuclei to posterior lobe, (hypothalamohypophyseal tract) for release of hypothalamic hormones in a site where blood-brain barrier does not exist.

ENDOCRINE GLANDS 97

to 2% of the pancreatic volume and are approximately 100 to 200 μm in diameter. Different populations of islet cells are involved in the production of **insulin (beta cell—B), glucagon (alpha cell—A), somatostatin (delta cell—D),** and **pancreatic polypeptide (PP cell).** Beta cells account for 60% to 70% of islet volume and are arranged in cord-like clusters. Alpha cells account for 15% of the islet volume and, together with D and PP cells (less than 5% of islet volume), are located on the periphery of beta cell clusters. Elevated levels of blood glucose cause **insulin secretion** and storage of glucose as glycogen following a meal; low levels of blood glucose cause **glucagon secretion,** which stimulates the breakdown of stored glycogen in the liver into glucose for energy utilization between meals. Somatostatin inhibits insulin secretion, but the role of pancreatic polypeptide is not well defined.

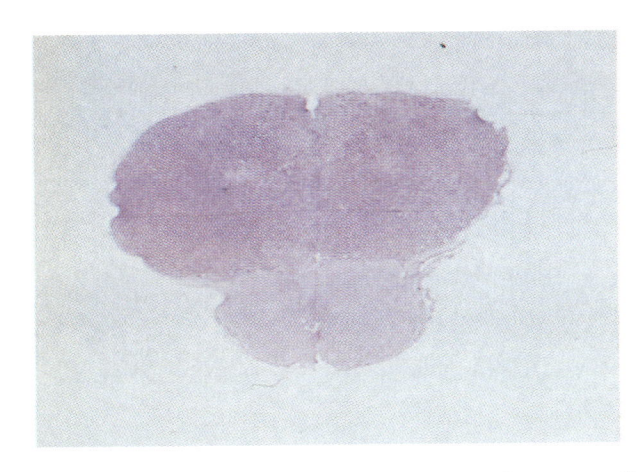

Fig. 13-2. Macrophotograph of pituitary gland. Large pars distalis portion of pituitary gland consists of acidophilic and basophilic cells and is easily distinguished from pale-staining pars nervosa. (H&E; ×5.)

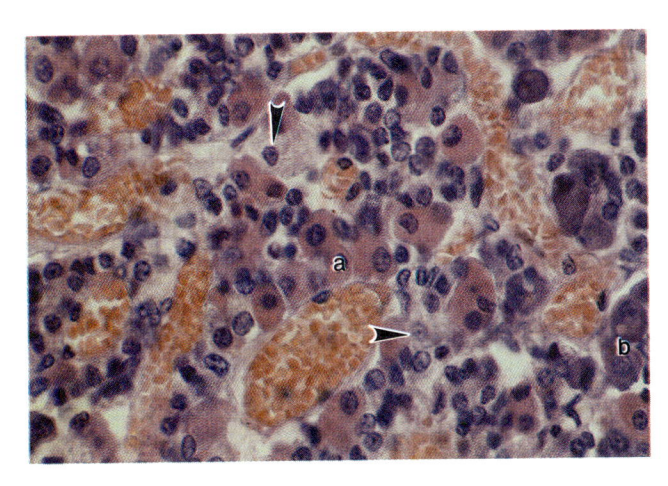

Fig. 13-3. LM of pars distalis illustrating cordlike arrangement of cells and sinusoidal vessels. Three cell types can be recognized: acidophils (a), basophils (b), and chromophobes (arrowheads). First two cell types are recognized by tinctorial staining properties of their secretion granules and produce six different hormones. Chromophobes, characterized by lack of staining, are now known to represent degranulated acidophils/basophils. (H&E; ×400.)

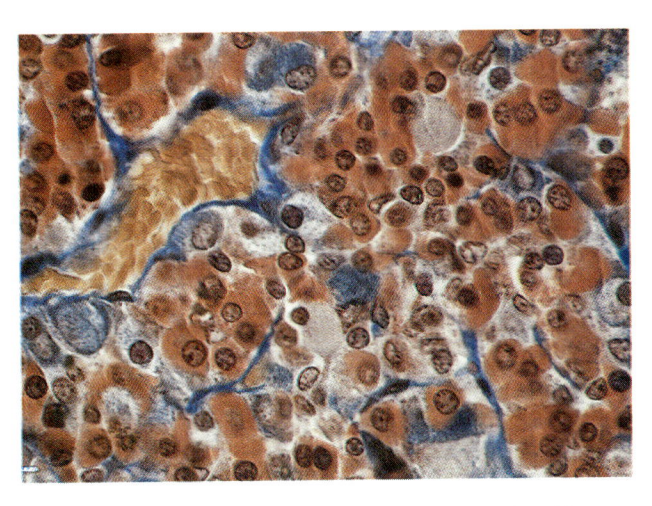

Fig. 13-4. LM of pars distalis stained with Masson's trichrome. Distinction between acidophils and basophils is easily made. Nonstaining chromophobes are also seen. (×400.)

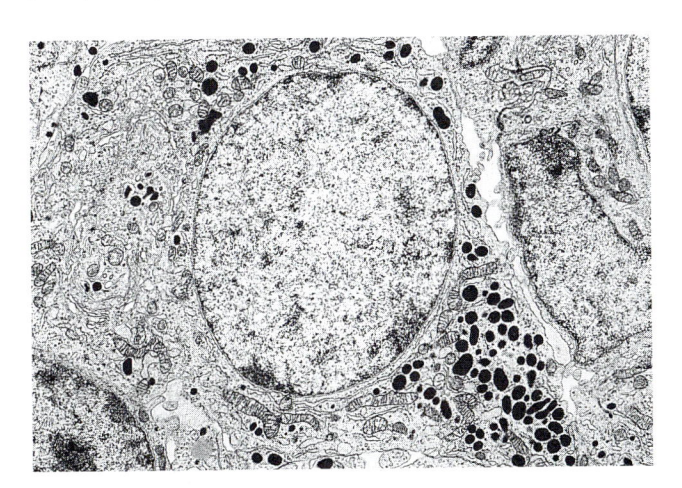

Fig. 13-5. TEM of pars distalis showing somatotropes. These cells are characterized by large round secretory granules that contain growth hormone. (×5,100.)

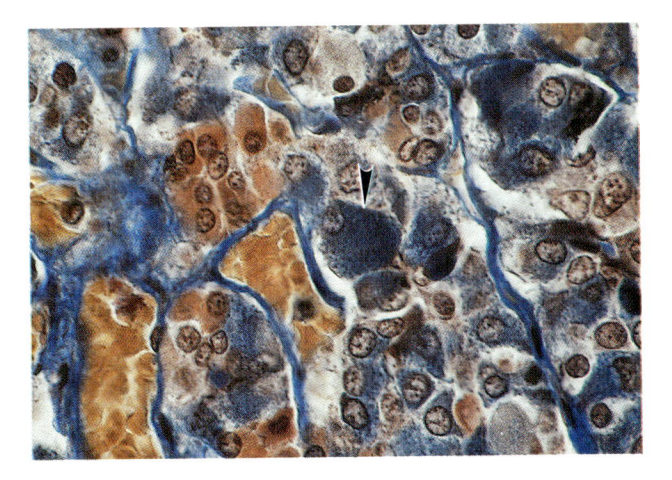

Fig. 13-6. LM of pars distalis. This pituitary gland was obtained from woman who had been both ovariectomized and adrenalectomized. Since target organs for both ACTH and gonadotrophic hormones were removed, basophilic gonadotropes and ACTH cells underwent hypertrophy in attempt to stimulate missing glands. These enlarged cells form what are called, respectively, adrenalectomy or castration cells (arrowhead). (Masson's trichrome; ×500.)

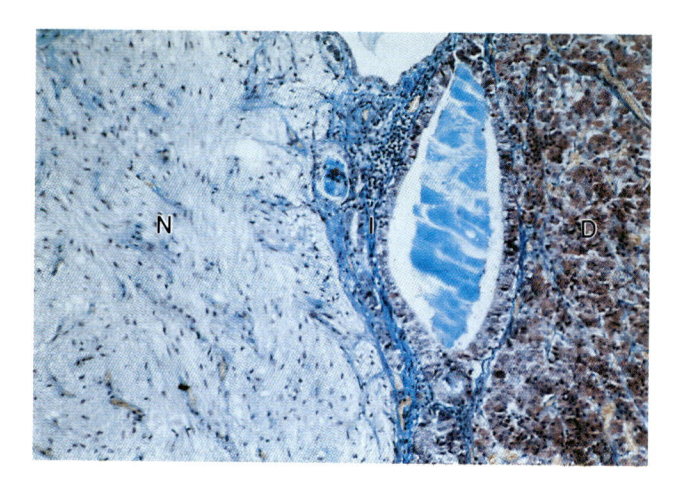

Fig. 13-7. LM showing pars distalis (d), Rathke's cyst, intermediate lobe (i), and pars nervosa (n). That portion of pars distalis posterior to lumen of Rathke's cyst constitutes intermediate lobe. (Masson's trichrome; ×100.)

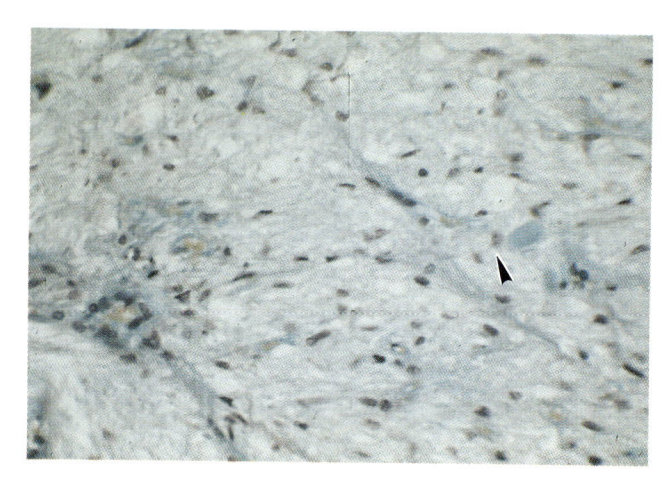

Fig. 13-8. Higher-magnification LM of pars nervosa demonstrating pituicytes (glial cells), endothelial cells, and Herring bodies (arrowhead). With Masson's trichrome stain, Herring bodies can be recognized by their smooth, homogeneous blue-staining appearance. (×400.)

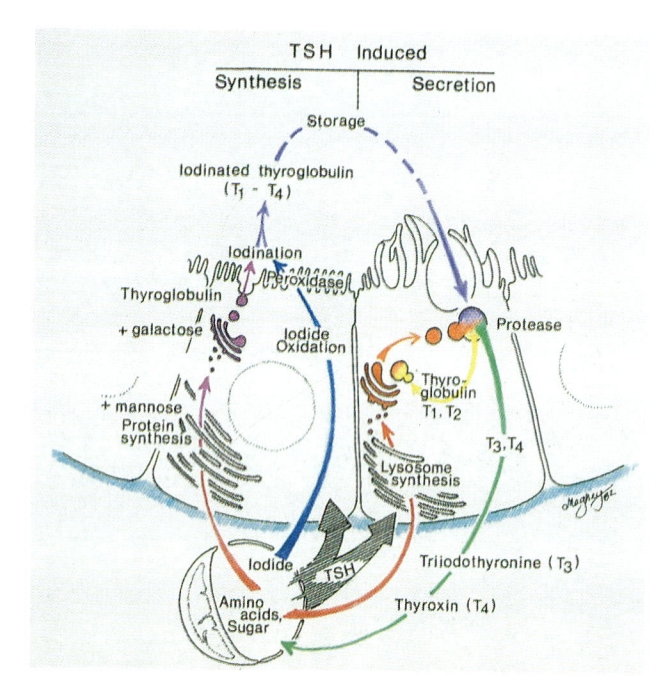

Fig. 13-9. Using precursor molecules taken up from bloodstream, thyroid gland synthesizes thyroglobulin and stores it in common colloidal pool within a lumen formed by sphere-shaped clusters of follicular cells. Secretion of hormone involves TSH stimulation of cellular uptake of stored colloid by endocytosis, its breakdown within cell's lysosomal system, and subsequent release of thyroxine into bloodstream.

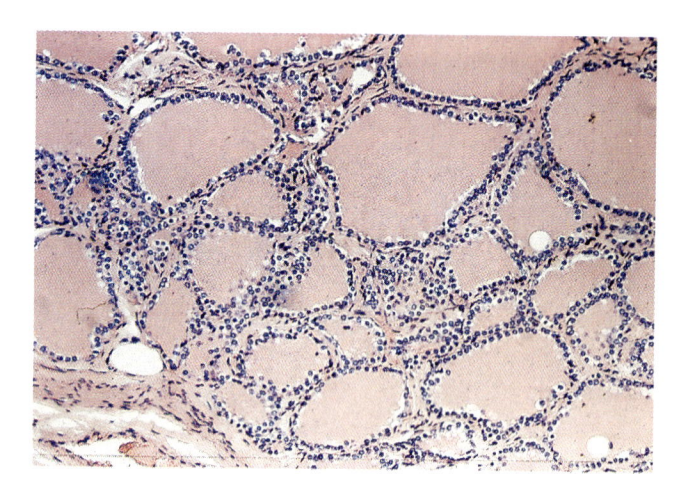

Fig. 13-10. LM of thyroid gland showing ball-like arrangement of follicular cells and colloid within central lumen. (H&E; ×200.)

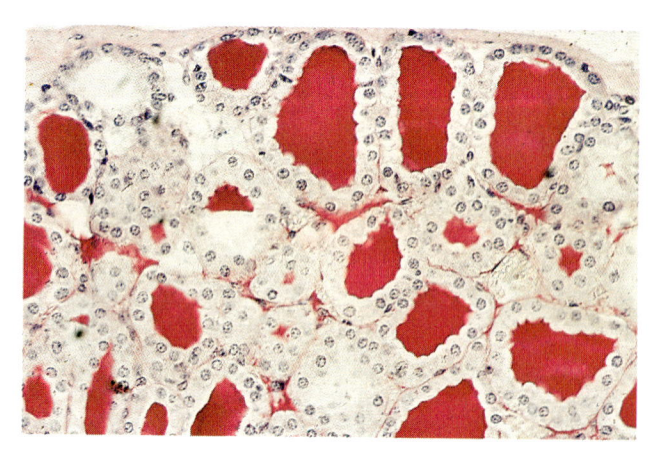

Fig. 13-11. LM of thyroid gland stained with PAS technique. Thyroglobulin is glycoprotein stored in follicular lumen; it therefore appears intensely red with this staining method. (×300.)

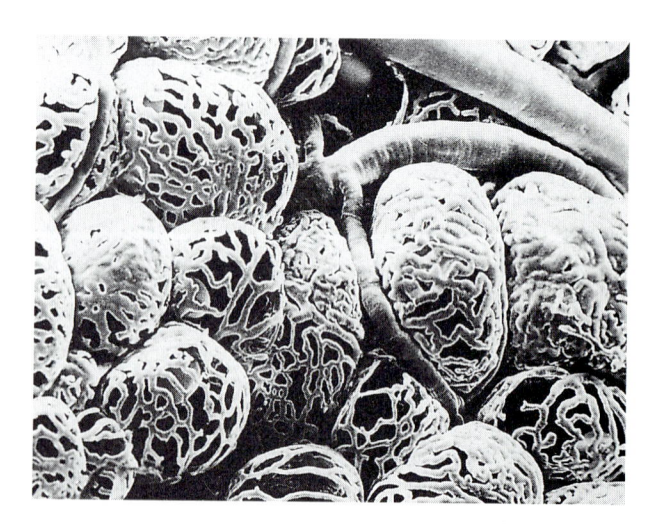

Fig. 13-12. SEM of vascular cast of thyroid gland. Note tortuous arrangement of capillaries around follicle, indicative of high vascularity of thyroid gland. (×400.)

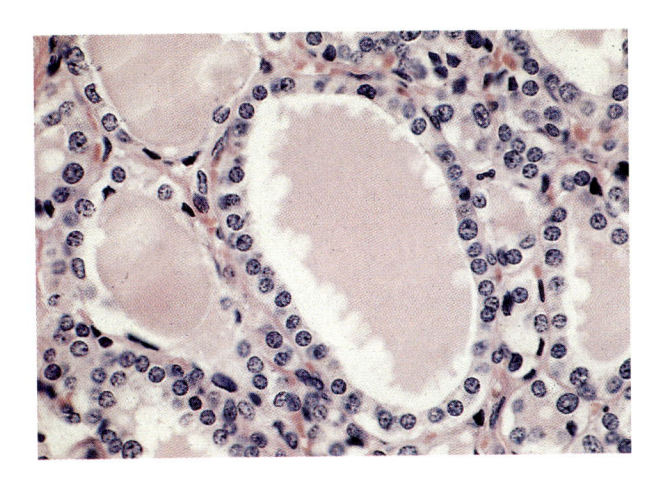

Fig. 13-13. LM of thyroid gland. Observe that within large central follicle, edge of colloid appears scalloped. This appearance indicates increased endocytic activity of columnar follicular cells, which ultimately results in release of thyroxine after colloid is degraded in lysosomal apparatus. In contrast, cells of inactive follicle immediately to left are low cuboidal to squamous, and periphery of colloid appears smooth. (H&E; ×500.)

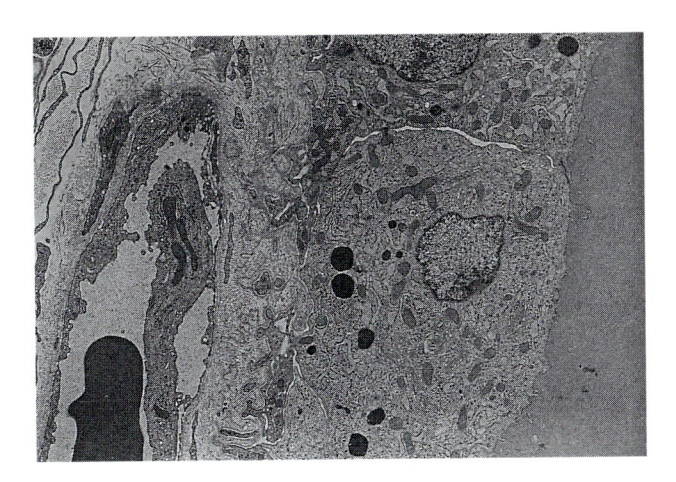

Fig. 13-14. TEM of thyroid follicle. Colloid can be seen *(left)* within luminal pool. Follicular cells forming wall are cuboidal and relatively inactive. Several dense bodies are visible in basal regions of follicular cells. Fenestrated capillary lies in surrounding connective tissue. (×3,500.)

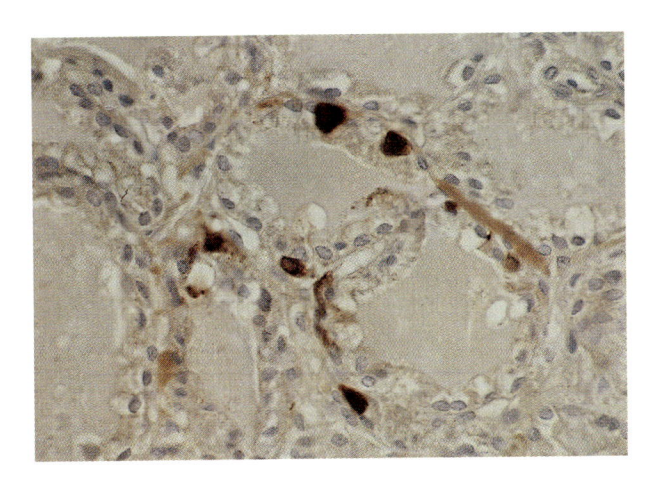

Fig. 13-15. LM of thyroid gland stained immunocytochemically for hormone thyrocalcitonin. Cells stained dark brown contain thyrocalcitonin and are located in wall of thyroid follicle, but do not abut the lumen of the follicle. (×500.)

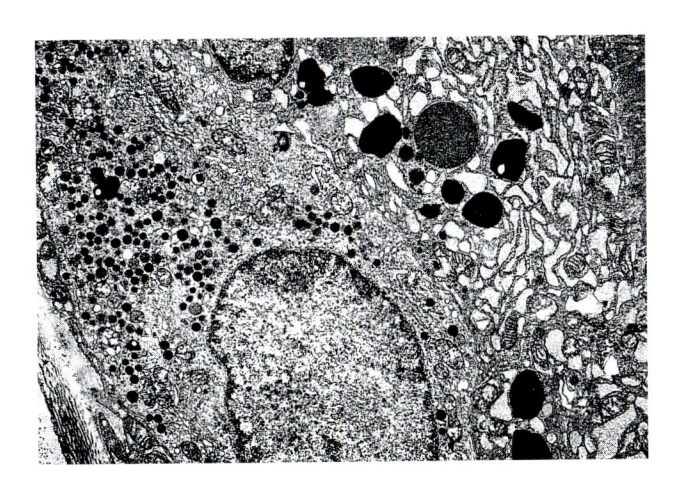

Fig. 13-16. TEM of thyrocalcitonin (parafollicular) cell. Observe small dark secretory granules that are polarized toward connective tissue face of follicle. (×5,500.)

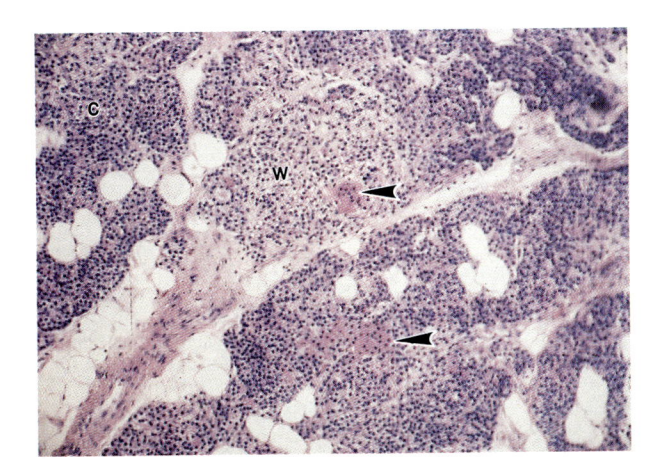

Fig. 13-17. LM of parathyroid gland. Parenchyma consists of three cell types: small, dark-staining chief cells *(c)*; larger, pink-staining oxyphil cells *(arrowheads)*; and Wasserhelle *(w)* or clear cells. This gland often shows fatty infiltration. (H&E; ×100.)

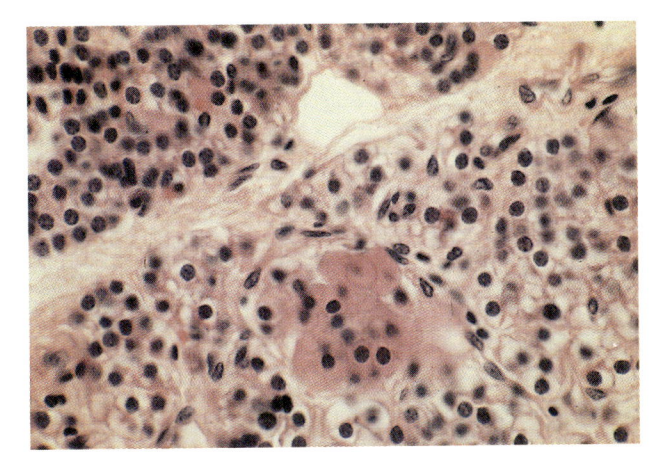

Fig. 13-18. Higher-magnification LM of parathyroid gland showing chief cells, oxyphil cells, and Wasserhelle (or clear) cells. (H&E; ×500.)

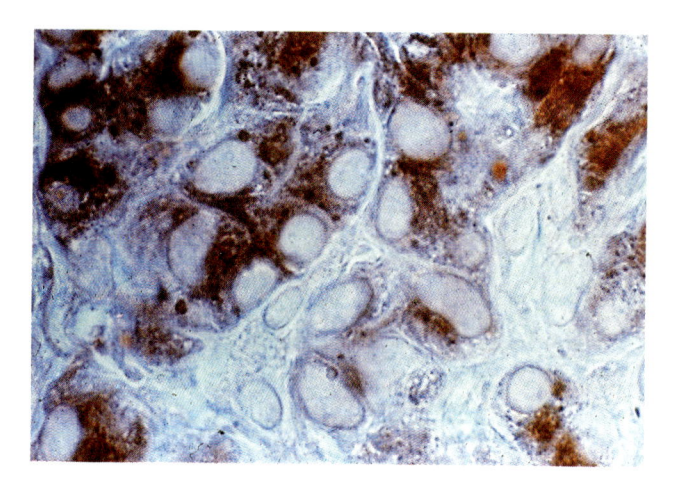

Fig. 13-19. LM illustrating immunocytochemical localization of parathormone in chief cells of parathyroid gland. (×1,200.)

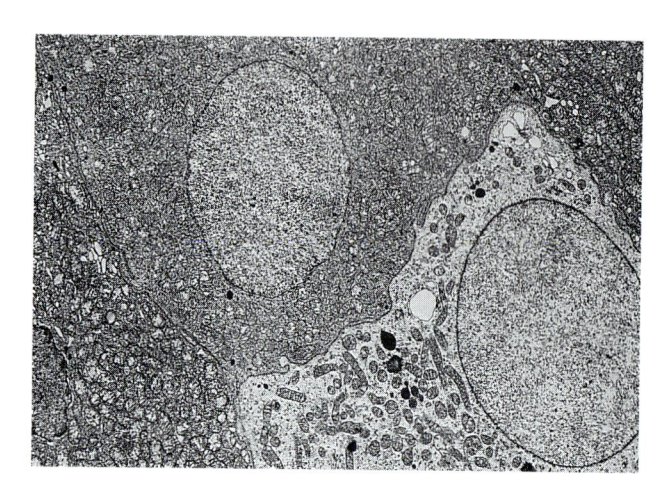

Fig. 13-20. TEM of oxyphil cells in parathyroid gland. Note abundant mitochondria, which almost completely fill cytoplasm of this cell type and account for the acidophilia seen by LM. (×4,800.)

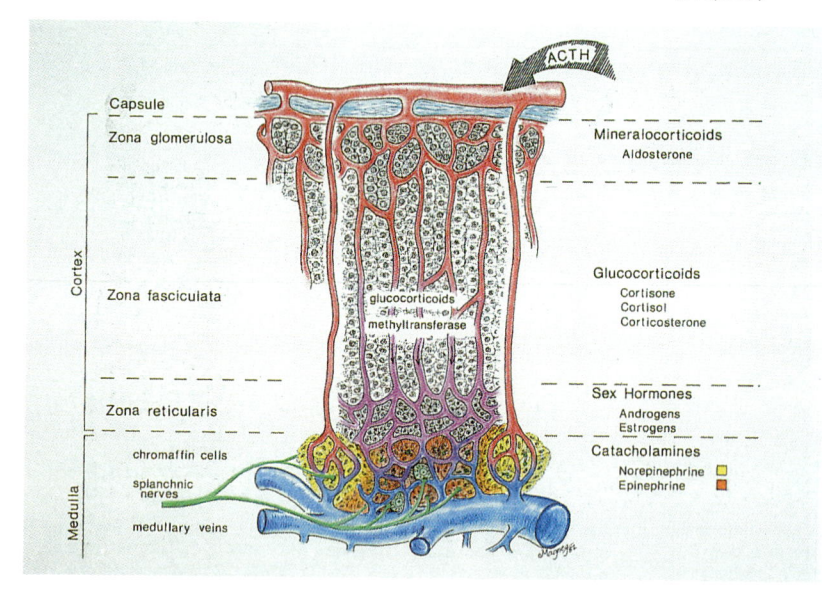

Fig. 13-21. Cellular zonation of adrenal cortex and blood flow through cortex to collecting veins in medulla. Steroid hormones produced by adrenal cortex include mineralocorticoids (aldosterone), glucocorticoids (cortisol, corticosterone), and androgens. Stimulation of glucocorticoid secretion by ACTH and its release into sinusoids supplying adrenal medulla result in induction of methyltransferase enzyme in chromaffin cells that leads to production of epinephrine. Chromaffin cells supplied by direct flow of blood from adrenal capsule (lacking glucocorticoids) do not produce methyltransferase enzyme and therefore secrete norepinephrine. Chromaffin cells also synthesize and secrete enkephalins. Hormonal secretion in adrenal gland is regulated by ACTH from anterior pituitary gland (zona fasciculata and zona reticularis), by renin from kidney (zona glomerulosa), and by preganglionic sympathetic neurons (medullallary chromaffin cells). Occasional postganglionic neuron may be found in adrenal medulla, while chromaffin cells of medulla are modified postganglionic sympathetic neurons of neural crest derivation.

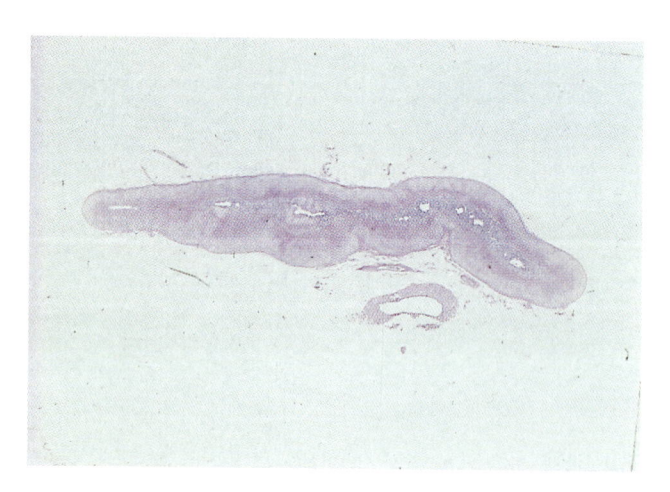

Fig. 13-22. Macrophotograph of adrenal gland. Zonation of cortex and presence of medulla can be easily distinguished. Large collecting veins are also recognizable within medulla. (H&E; ×5.)

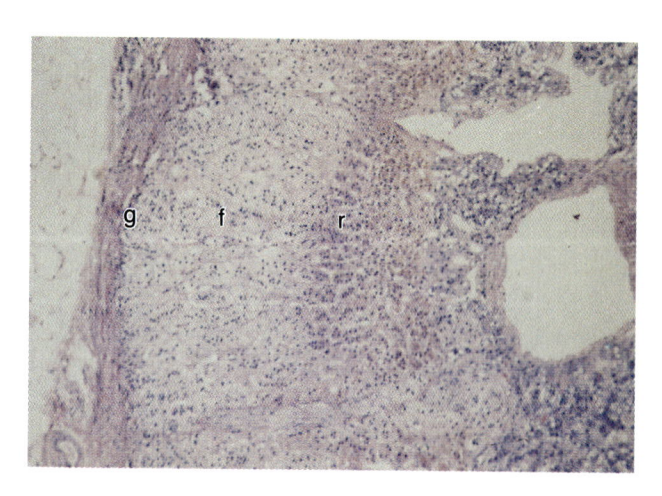

Fig. 13-23. Low-magnification LM of adrenal gland. At left is capsule containing small amount of pericapsular fat. Immediately beneath capsule is zona glomerulosa (g), then zona fasciculata (f) and acidophilic zona reticularis (r). At right is basophilic medulla in which several large collecting veins are present. (H&E; ×75.)

ENDOCRINE GLANDS 101

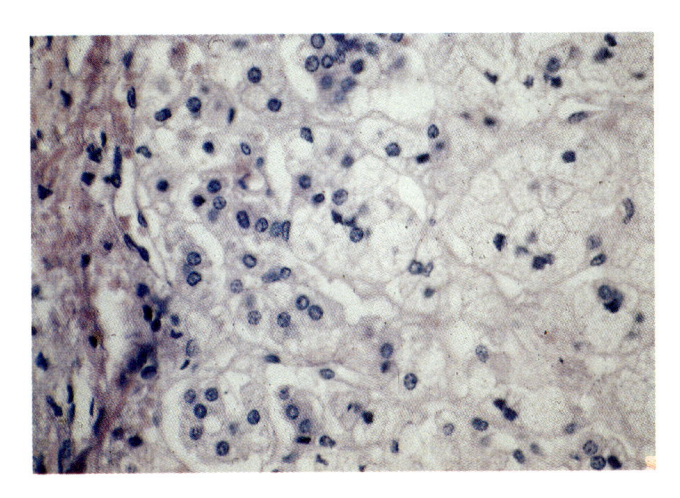

Fig. 13-24. Higher magnification of zona glomerulosa of adrenal gland. Capsule of gland is seen at left. Parenchymal cells arranged in round clusters constitute zona glomerulosa in center of field, while on right, parallel plates of cells form zona fasciculata. (H&E; ×400.)

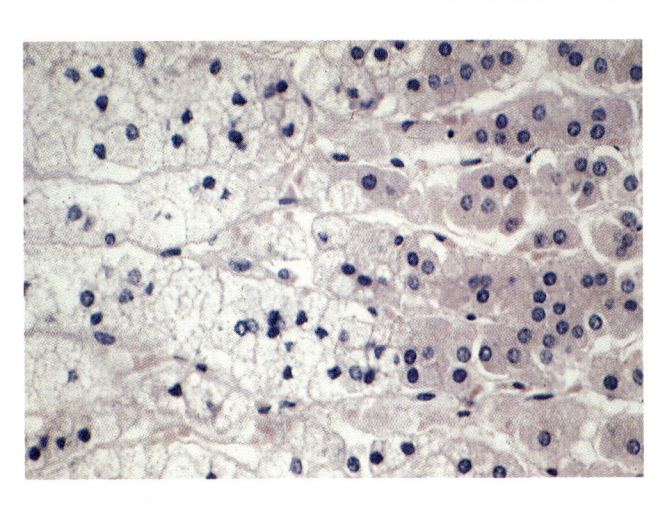

Fig. 13-25. LM of adrenal cortex illustrating junction between zona fasciculata *(left)* and zona reticularis *(right)*. Note vacuolated cytoplasm in zona fasciculata, indicating presence of large amounts of lipid. (H&E; ×400.)

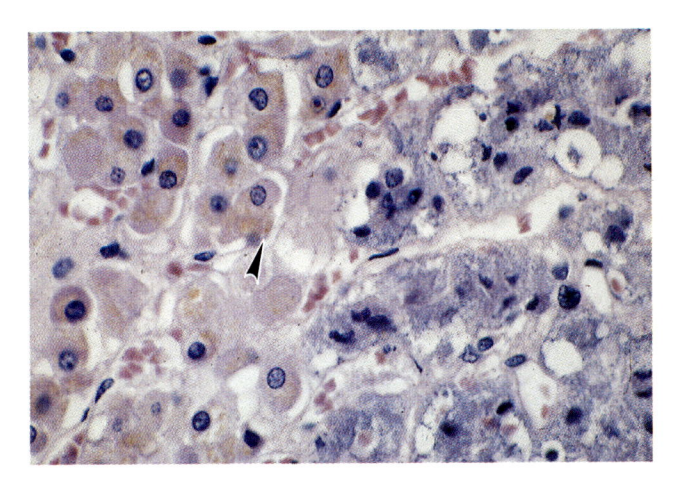

Fig. 13-26. LM illustrating junction between zona reticularis and adrenal medulla. Cells in zona reticularis are compact and more intensely stained than those in zona fasciculata. These cells also contain lipofuscin pigment, which is visible as gold-brown granules *(arrowhead)* near nuclei. (H&E; ×500.)

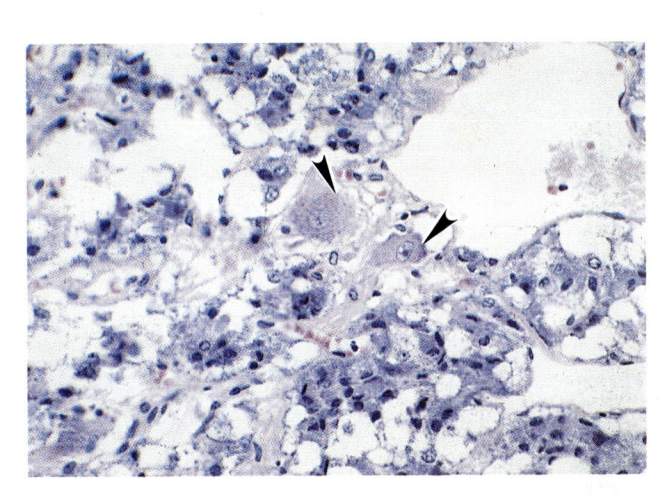

Fig. 13-27. LM of adrenal medulla showing chromaffin cells and two sympathetic postganglionic neurons *(arrowheads)* in center of figure. (H&E; ×400.)

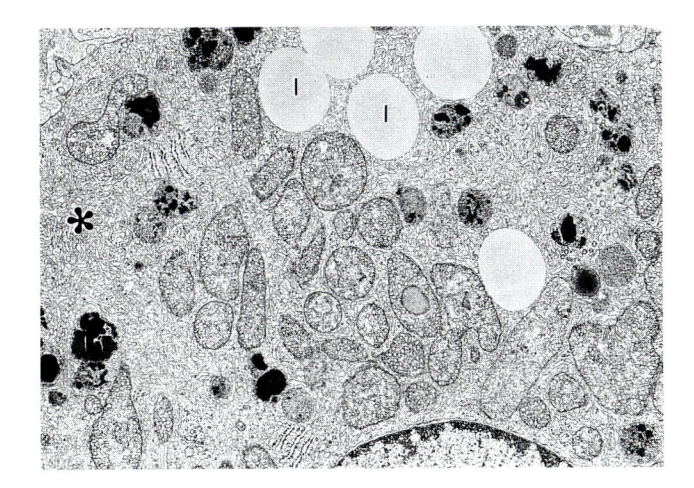

Fig. 13-28. TEM of cells of zona fasciculata at high magnification. These cells are characterized by large numbers of lipid droplets *(l)* and distinctive mitochondria containing short tubular cristae. Their cytoplasm also contains well-developed smooth endoplasmic reticulum (*), electron-dense lysosomes, and occasional patches of rough endoplasmic reticulum. (×12,000.)

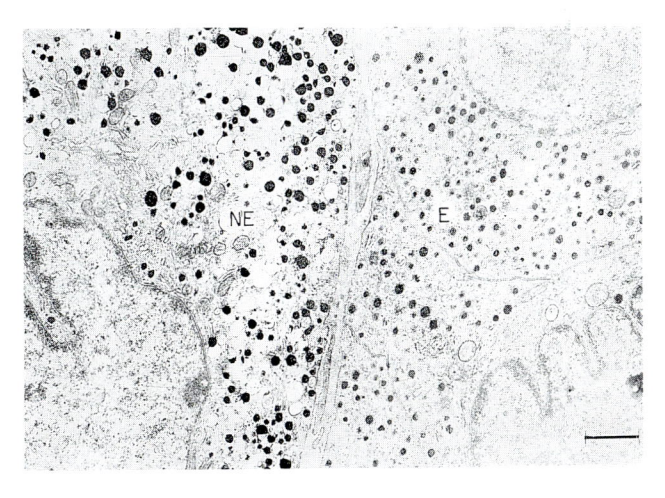

Fig. 13-29. TEM of adrenal medulla showing different granule types within adjacent cells. Because of effects of fixation on adrenal medulla, epinephrine-secreting cells contain granules that exhibit only slight to moderate electron density, while norepinephrine cells possess electron-dense secretion granules. *NE*, Norepinephrine; *E*, epinephrine. (×5,300.)

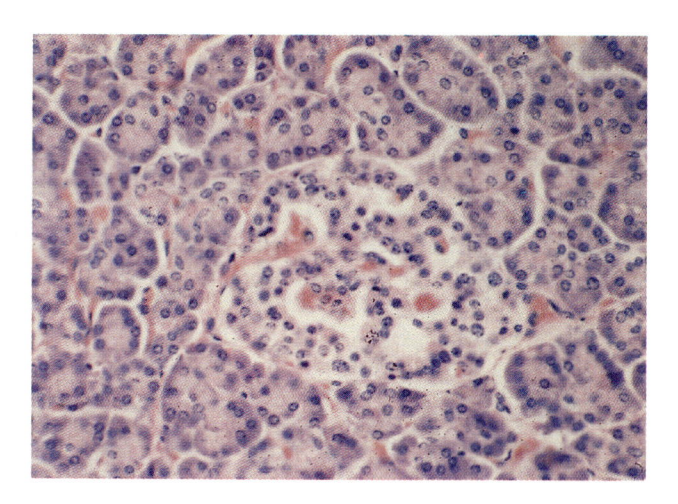

Fig. 13-30. High-magnification LM of pancreas showing well-vascularized islet of Langerhans *(center)* surrounded by serous acini. (H&E; ×250.)

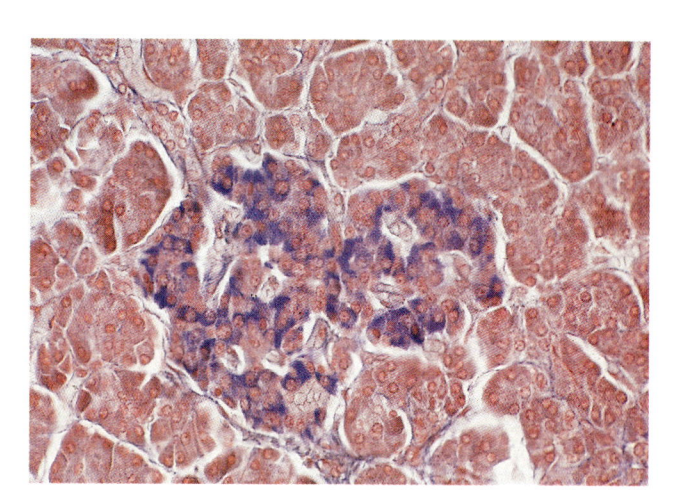

Fig. 13-31. LM of aldehyde fuchsin–stained pancreas demonstrating selective staining for insulin within beta cells of islets of Langerhans. Cells within islet unstained with this procedure most likely represent either alpha cells (responsible for glucagon secretion) or delta cells (produce somatostatin). (×250.)

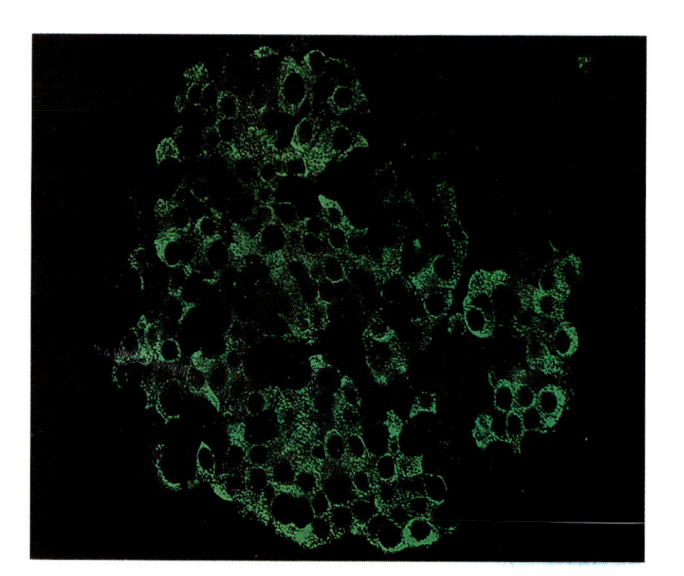

Fig. 13-32. Immunofluorescent localization of insulin in beta cells *(green)* in islet of Langerhans as seen by laser scanning confocal microscopy. Beta cells account for approximately 60% to 70% of islet cells and are coupled by gap junctions. (×400.)

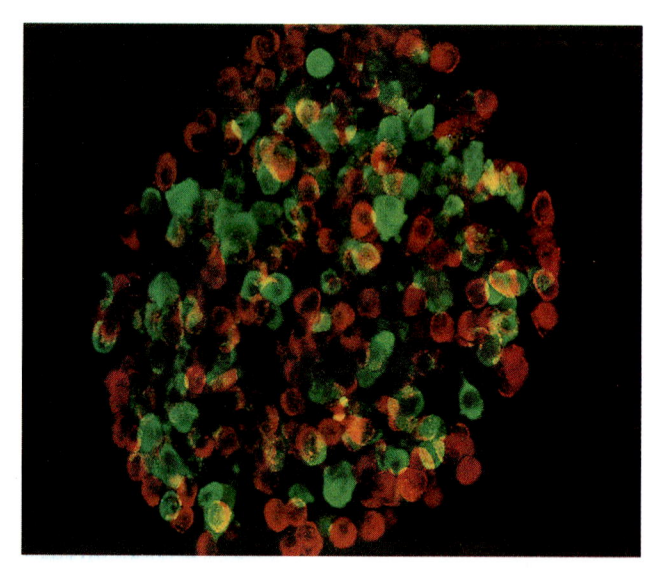

Fig. 13-33. Immunofluorescent localization of alpha (glucagon-producing) cells *(green)* and delta somatostatin-producing cells *(red)* in islet of Langerhans as seen by three-dimensional reconstruction using confocal microscopy. Alpha and delta cells are located at periphery of clusters of beta cells (not shown). (×400.)

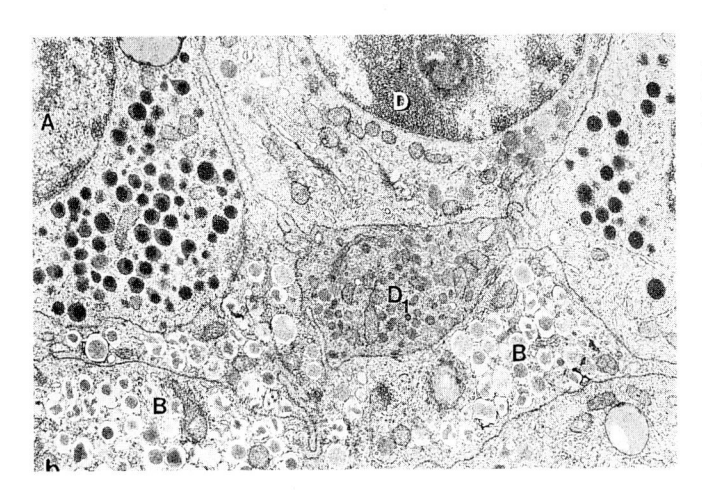

Fig. 13-34. TEM of adjacent cells in islet of Langerhans in pancreas. Each cell type in pancreatic islet has distinct granular morphology. Beta cell *(B)* granules contain a core with moderate electron density and a nonstaining halo. Alpha cell *(A)* granules contain an electron-dense core and an eccentric halo. Somatostatin-producing cell (labeled *D-1*) contains granules with moderate electron density and no halo. Cell labeled D (now called the PP cell) (top) produces pancreatic polypeptide. (×9,000.)

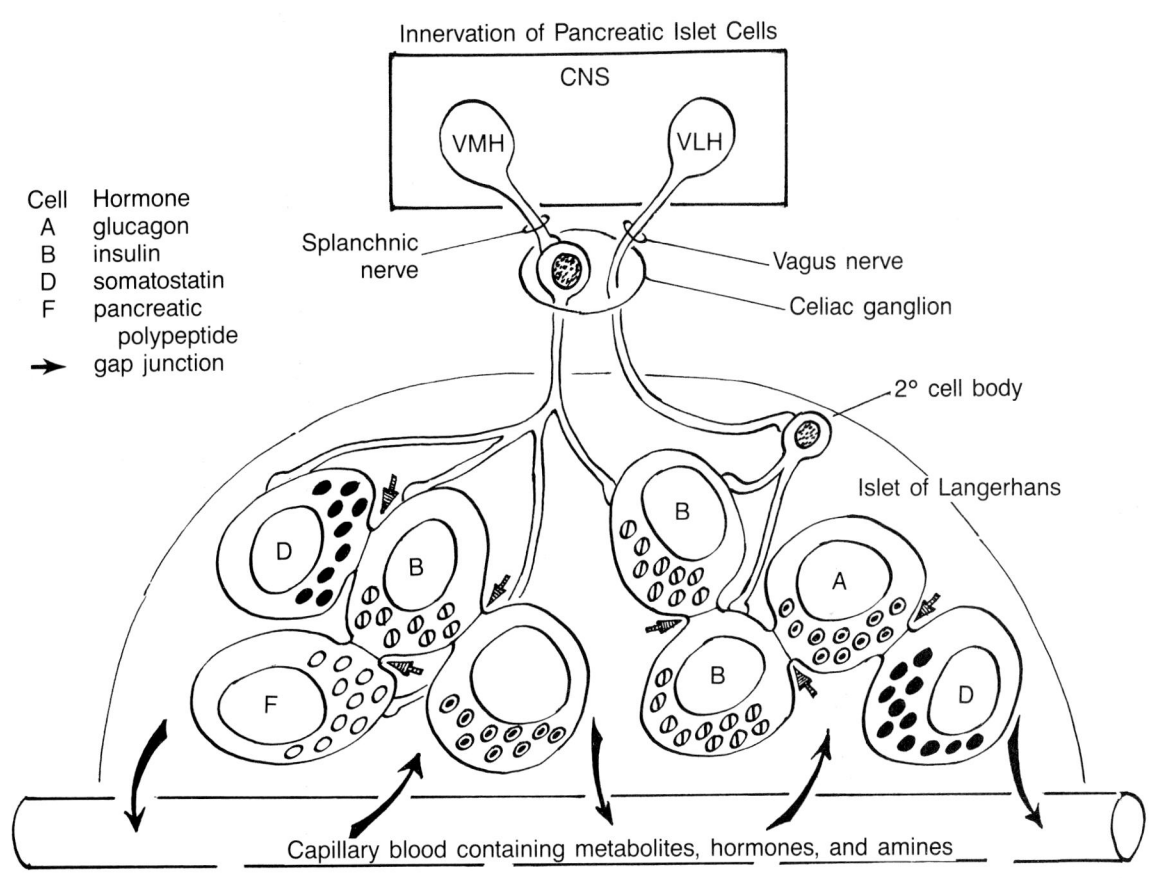

Fig. 13-35. Relationship between gap junctions and innervation of pancreatic islet cells. Adjacent beta cells are coupled by gap junctions and function as multicellular units for release of insulin in response to elevated glucose levels. Decoupling of beta cells leads to abnormally lowered secretion of insulin.

CHAPTER 14

SKIN

SKIN, THE LARGEST organ in the body, has many functions:
1. Regulates body temperature through heat exchange and fluid loss
2. Prevents dehydration
3. Prevents invasion by chemicals or microorganisms
4. Protects the body from ultraviolet light
5. Produces vitamin D
6. Participates in the immune response
7. Assists in blood pressure regulation
8. Provides sensory contact with the environment

Skin is divided into **epidermis,** a stratified squamous, keratinized epithelium, and **dermis,** an underlying connective tissue that contains specialized structures such as **glands** and **hair follicles** derived from epithelium and **sensory receptors** of the nervous system. Skin is attached to deep fascia by a loose areolar layer called the **hypodermis** (also called subcutaneous connective tissue), which stores fat, gives the body its contour, provides insulation, and permits the skin to move easily over underlying structures. Hypodermis is not a subdivision of skin.

Thin skin covers most of the body except for the palmar and plantar surfaces of the hands and feet, which, because of frequent abrasive contact with the environment, are covered with **thick skin.** The epidermis of thin skin is 70 to 150 μm thick and is thinly keratinized, while the epidermis of thick skin is 400 to 600 μm thick and is thickly keratinized.

Epidermis consists of several strata that differ in structure and function. The principal cells of the epithelium, **keratinocytes,** divide in the basal layer of the epithelium **(stratum basalis** or **stratum germinativum),** lose contact with the basement membrane, and migrate toward the surface. En route, the cells increase the number of desmosomal contacts **(stratum spinosum)** and their cytoplasm accumulates the protein keratin. Secretion of lipid-containing granules **(stratum granulosum)** forms a waterproof barrier and prevents fluid loss from the body. Eventually, the keratinized remnants of keratinocytes form a tough protective outer layer **(stratum corneum)** from which surface cells are continuously sloughed as the epithelium is renewed from below. Specialized cells within the epithelium **(melanocyte, Langerhans cell, Merkle cell)** are involved with pigmentation, immune function, and sensation.

The underlying dermis is divided into a **papillary layer** of loose connective tissue that interdigitates with epidermal invaginations to provide an expanded area for attachment. Capillary beds in the papillary layer provide nutrients to the avascular epidermis and allow for heat conservation or loss by regulating blood flow to the skin. Touch receptors are also present. The papillary layer merges with an underlying **reticular layer,** which consists of dense irregular connective tissue with elastic fibers. **Sweat glands** participate in thermal regulation by secreting a watery fluid onto the skin, where it evaporates. **Sebaceous** and **apocrine glands** are also found in skin, but their function is not well understood. **Hair follicles,** formed by the invagination of epidermis into the dermis, are found in thin skin. A variety of sensory receptors (pressure, temperature, vibration) are located in the dermis; naked pain endings are found in the epidermis.

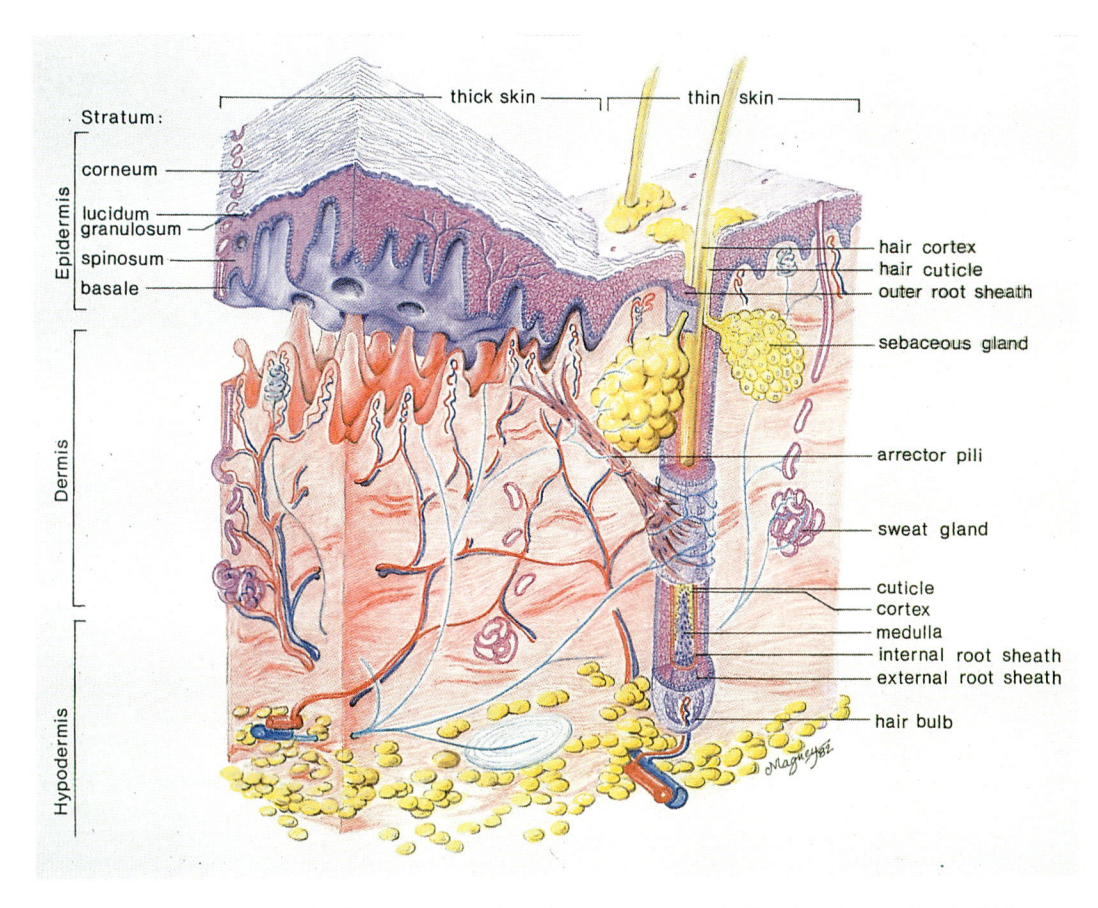

Fig. 14-1. Thick skin *(left)* and thin skin *(right).* Skin is composed of epidermis and dermis. Hair follicles are only associated with thin skin, but sweat glands exist in both types. Skin is avascular, so nutrients cross into epidermis by diffusion. Sensory receptors are present only in dermis or hypodermis, except for naked nerve endings, which penetrate epidermis.

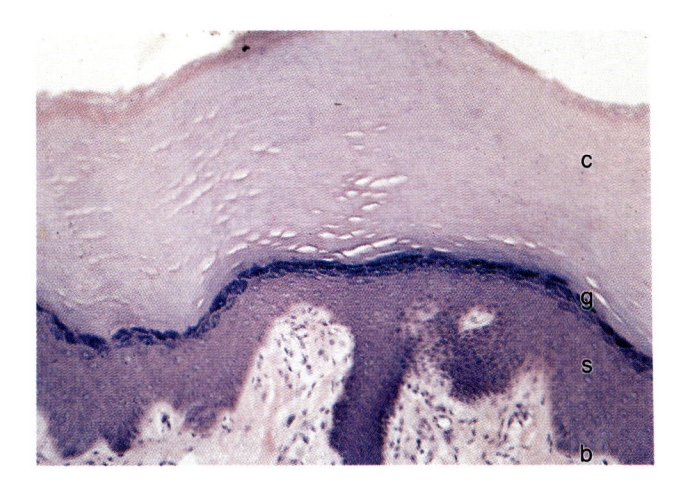

Fig. 14-2. Low-magnification LM of thick skin. Observe thickness of each layer: strata basalis *(b)*, spinosum *(s)*, granulosum *(g)*, and corneum *(c)*. (H&E; ×100.)

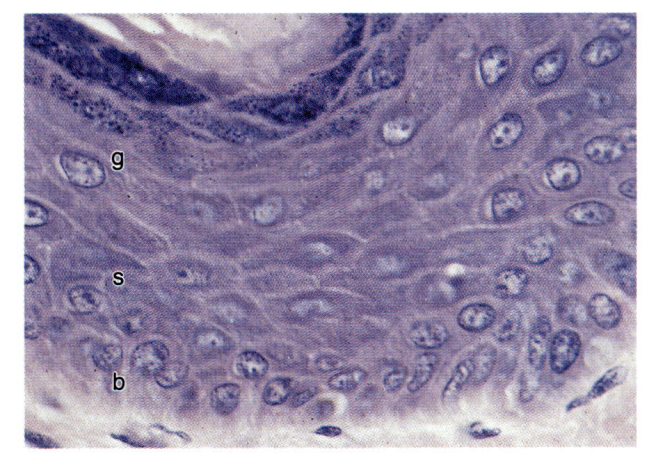

Fig. 14-3. High-magnification LM of thick skin showing stratum basalis *(b)*, stratum spinosum *(s)*, and stratum granulosum *(g)*. (H&E; ×800.)

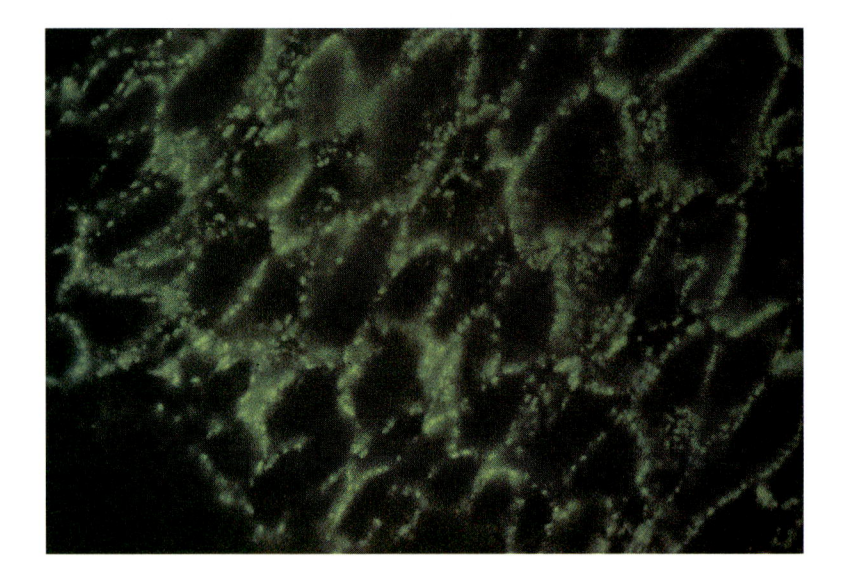

Fig. 14-4. Indirect immunofluorescent staining of frozen sections of stratified squamous epithelium with mouse antiserum prepared against bovine desmosomal glycoproteins. Observe that epithelial cell borders are stained in highly punctate pattern characteristic of distribution of desmosomes (see Fig. 14-8). (×1,200.)

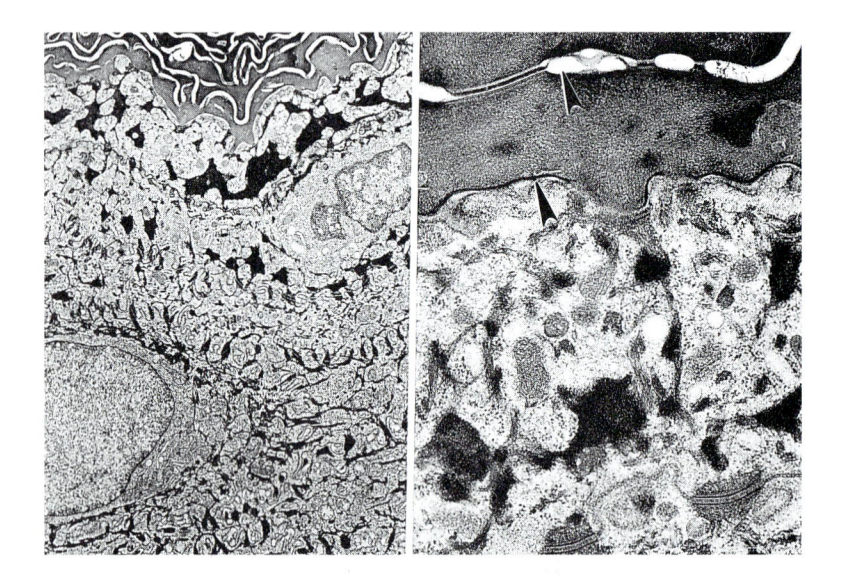

Fig. 14-5. Low-magnification TEM showing cells in strata spinosum, granulosum, and corneum *(left)*. Electron-dense keratohyalin material is deposited between keratin filaments. High-magnification TEM of portions of granular and cornified cells *(right)* shows cornified cell membrane *(arrowheads)*. Lamellar granules present in granulosum cells discharge into extracellular space by exocytosis *(left margin)*. (Left, ×4,800; right, ×11,000.)

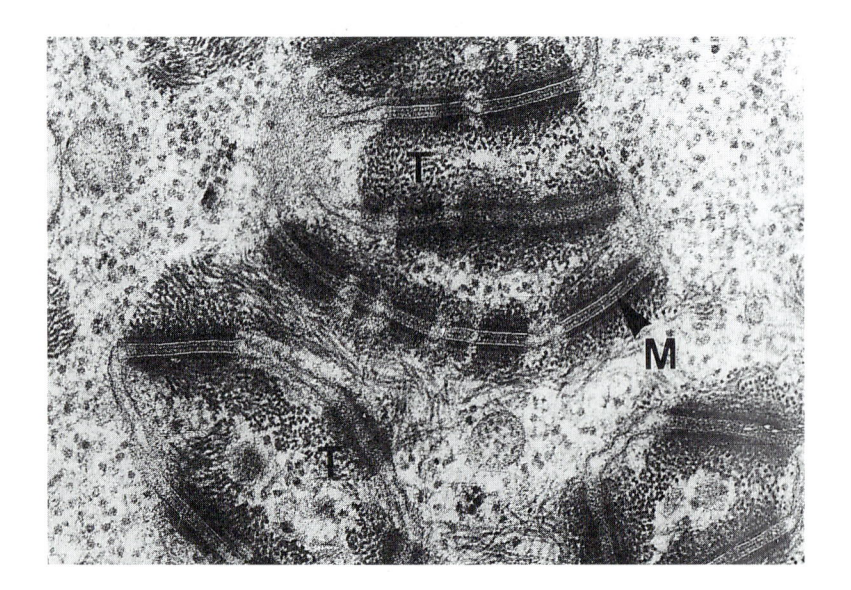

Fig. 14-6. High-magnification TEM of desmosomal complexes in spinous layer of epidermis. Tonofilaments seen in transverse section course toward dense desmosomal plaques. *M*, Midline; *T*, tonofilaments. (×80,000.)

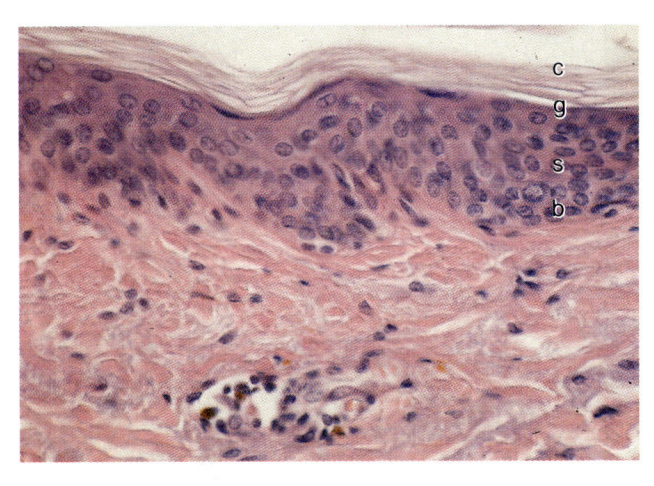

Fig. 14-7. LM of thin skin. Compare thickness of strata basalis *(b)*, spinosum *(s)*, granulosum *(g)*, and corneum *(c)* to that seen in thick skin (Fig. 14-2). (H&E; ×350.)

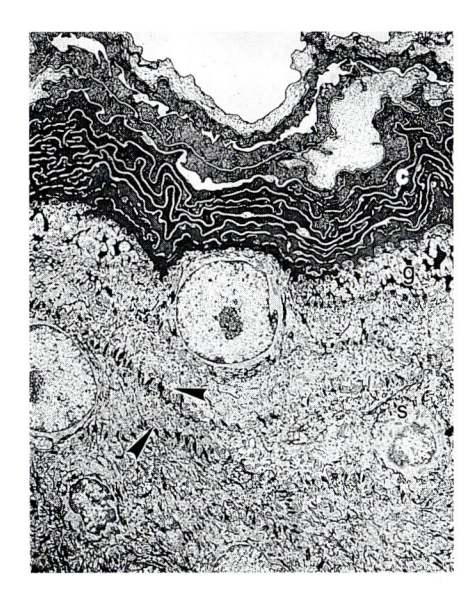

Fig. 14-8. TEM of strata spinosum *(s)*, granulosum *(g)*, and corneum *(c)*. Numerous desmosomes join cells in stratum spinosum. Electron-dense deposits that represent keratohyalin granules are seen in stratum granulosum and stratum corneum. Degradation of cellular organelles occurs in stratum corneum. Desmosomes in cornified layer *(arrowheads)* are modified and fewer in number as compared to those of stratum spinosum. (×3,000.)

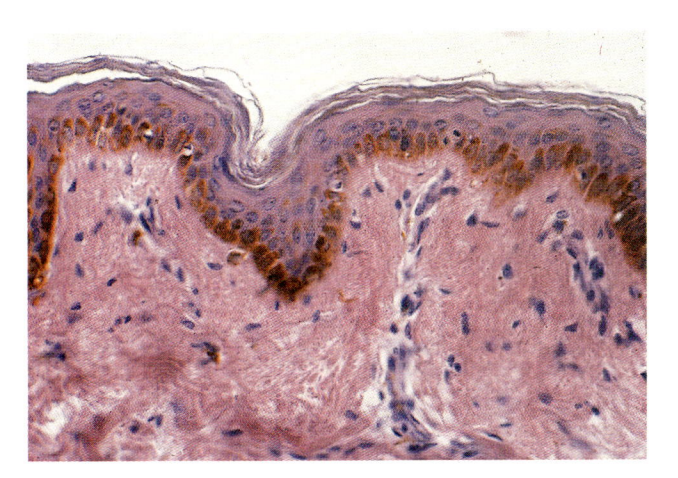

Fig. 14-9. LM of thin skin from black individual. Melanin is evident in keratinocytes of stratum germinativum. (H&E; ×350.)

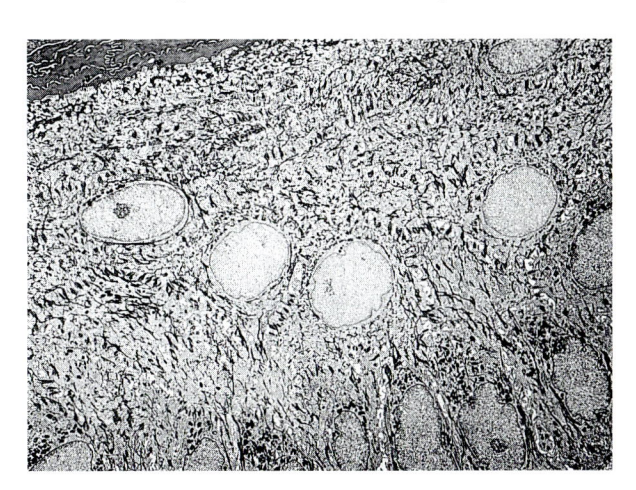

Fig. 14-10. TEM of full-thickness epidermis from black individual. Observe amount of pigmentation in basal keratinocytes and smaller amount of melanin in suprabasal cells. Degradation of pigment occurs in melanosome complexes as differentiation progresses, although some pigment is always retained. (×2,200.)

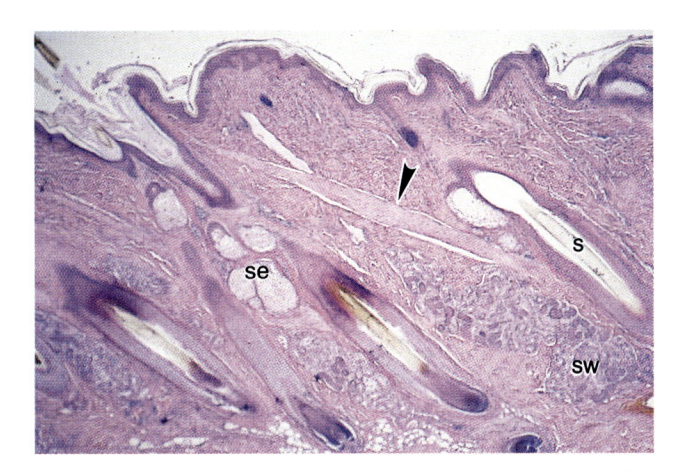

Fig. 14-11. Low-magnification LM of hairy skin showing examples of sebaceous glands *(se)*, sweat glands *(sw)*, and arrector pili muscle *(arrowhead)* as well as shafts of hair *(s)*. (H&E; ×50.)

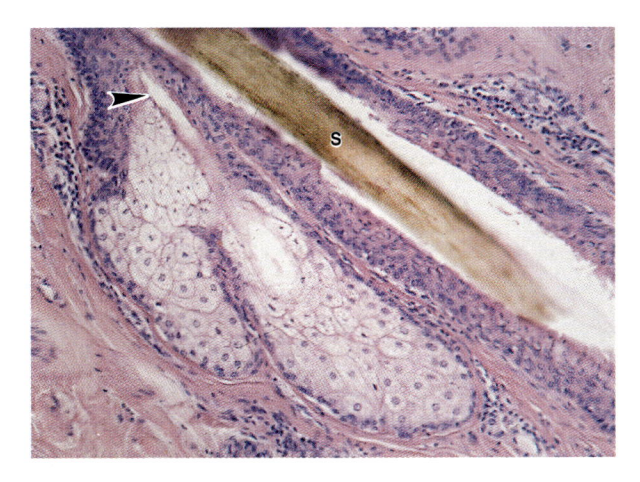

Fig. 14-12. LM showing longitudinal section of hair shaft and opening *(arrowhead)* of sebaceous gland into hair shaft *(s)*. (H&E; ×200.)

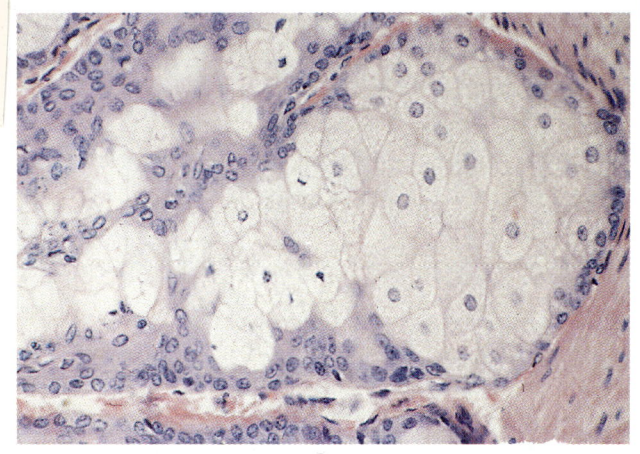

Fig. 14-13. High-magnification LM of sebaceous gland. Outermost cells of gland rest on basal lamina comparable to that of epidermis. The basal cells are germinative cells of gland. As cells migrate toward center of gland, they progressively accumulate lipid within their cytoplasm. Cells continue to enlarge, their nuclei become distorted and disintegrate, and eventually cells lyse, thus forming sebum, the lipid product of glands. (H&E; ×300.)

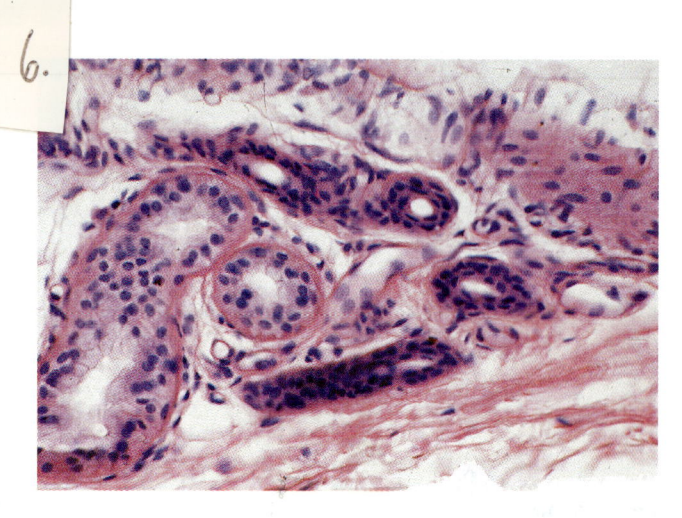

Fig. 14-14. LM of sweat gland showing coiled sweat ducts and secretory portions of gland. Secretory portions have larger diameters than ducts which are smaller and stain more intensely. (H&E; ×300.)

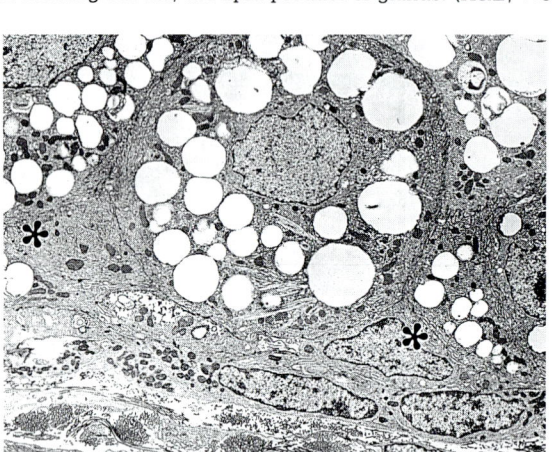

Fig. 14-15. TEM showing periphery of sebaceous gland. Less differentiated germinative cells (*) lie at periphery of gland, while lipogenesis is evident in cells closer to center. (×2,000.)

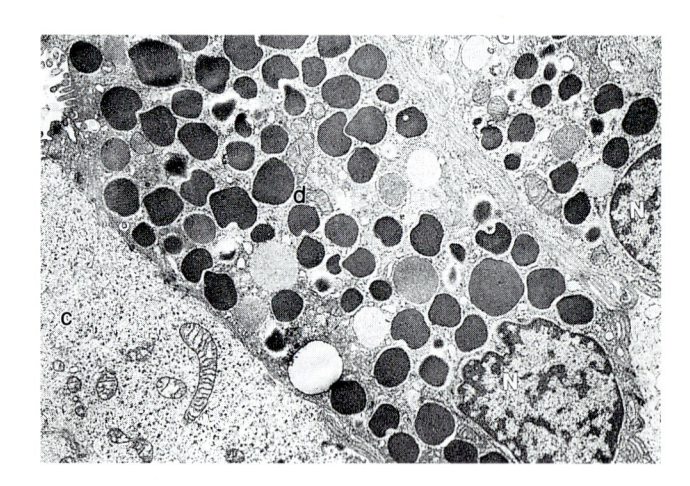

Fig. 14-16. TEM of eccrine sweat gland. Secretory tubule (lumen at upper left) is composed of three distinct cell types: myoepithelial cells (not shown), clear serous cells (c), and dark serous cells (d). Granulated dark cells are believed to secrete mucosubstance. Clear cells contain abundant glycogen particles and are thought to produce most of the watery secretion. (×6,000.)

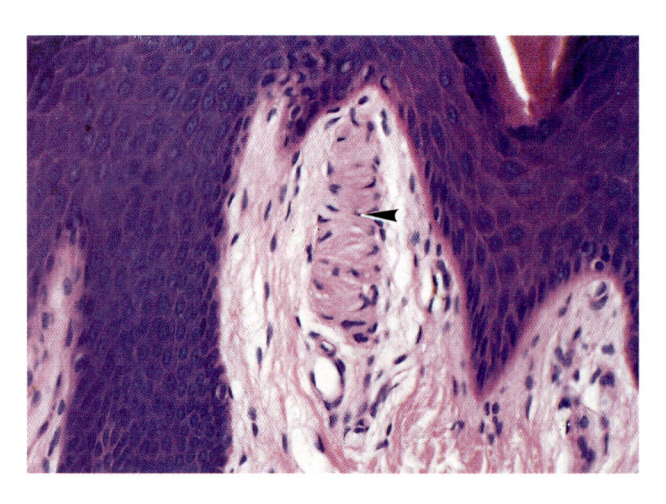

Fig. 14-17. LM of thick skin demonstrating Meissner's corpuscle (arrowhead) in dermal papilla. This corpuscle functions in touch reception. (H&E; ×300.)

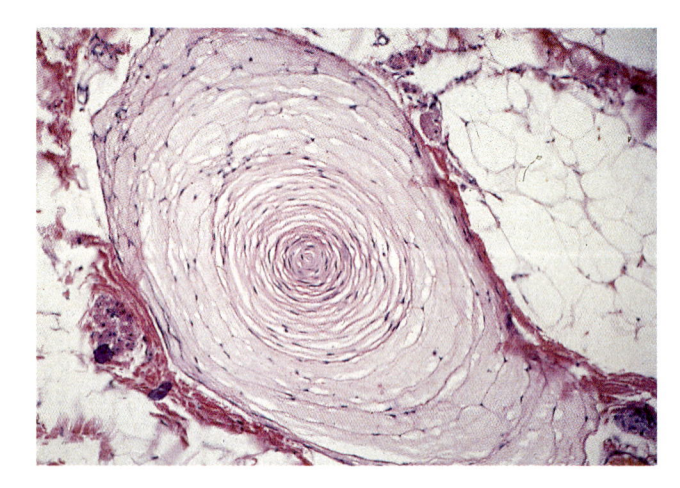

Fig. 14-18. LM of hypodermis containing Pacinian corpuscle, which is a deep pressure receptor. (H&E; ×50.)

CHAPTER 15

DIGESTIVE SYSTEM

THE DIGESTIVE SYSTEM is comprised of a group of organs that ingest food, reduce it to small particles, lubricate it, mix it with digestive juices, absorb usable molecules, and eliminate waste material.

In the oral cavity, teeth and tongue mechanically break down food and shape it into a bolus that can be swallowed. Salivary glands add mucus, which lubricates the bolus, and enzymes, which initiate digestion.

The bolus passes from the oral cavity through the pharynx and into the first part of the alimentary canal, a tubular structure that continues, with functional modifications, to the anus. The walls of the alimentary canal, in spite of regional variation, have a common architecture. Because the canal is continuous with the external environment through both mouth and anus, it is lined throughout by a **mucosa** that has three subdivisions. The **epithelium** lining the lumen of the canal is subtended by a loose areolar connective tissue, the **lamina propria,** which attaches it to smooth muscle of variable thickness called the **muscularis mucosa.** A variety of glands, formed by epithelial invaginations into the lamina propria, discharge mucus, digestive juices, and antibodies into the lumen. Mobility of the mucosa is a function of the muscularis mucosa. The **submucosa** is composed of dense irregular connective tissue, supports the mucosa and provides it with nerves, blood vessels, and lymphatics. Contraction of the **muscularis externa,** two (or more) concentric layers of smooth muscle, mixes luminal contents and propels it along the alimentary canal. This process is called **peristalsis.** A peripheral layer of connective tissue, the **adventitia,** attaches some organs (i.e., esophagus, rectum) to surrounding structures. Alternatively, organs lying within the abdominal cavity are partly or entirely surrounded by **serosa,** a single layer of mesothelial cells (peritoneum) attached to the muscularis externa by delicate connective tissue. The serosa secretes a watery fluid into the peritoneal cavity to lubricate the movement of digestive organs against each other during peristalsis.

ESOPHAGUS

The first segment of the alimentary canal is the **esophagus,** a short, muscular tube that functions principally to convey a bolus of food from the oral cavity and pharynx to the stomach. The mucosa of the oral cavity, pharynx, and esophagus, exposed to material that is only roughly broken down, is lined with **nonkeratinized stratified squamous epithelium** to resist abrasion. Mucus-producing **cardiac** and **submucosal glands** within the wall of the esophagus assist in lubricating the bolus as it is moved toward the stomach by alternating contractions of the thick, inner circular and outer longitudinal layers of the **muscularis externa.** The esophagus is unique in that the upper third of the muscularis externa contains a large proportion of **skeletal muscle** fibers, the middle third is composed of approximately equal amounts of skeletal and smooth muscle, and the lower third is mostly smooth muscle. Although adventitia covers the esophagus in its passage through the thorax, a short (1 inch) distal segment lies within the abdominal cavity and is covered with serosa.

STOMACH

Variations in the design of the stomach reflect its function in producing digestive juices, mixing them with food to break it down into a liquid digesta called **chyme,** and transporting it to the small intestine. Based on the histology of the mucosa, the stomach is subdivided into **cardia** (near the entrance of the esophagus), **body** or **fundus,** and **pylorus,** a distal segment associated with a thick muscular **pyloric sphincter** that controls movement of chyme into the small intestine. The mucosa, thrown into folds called **rugae** that direct food toward the duodenum, is lined with simple columnar **surface mucous cells** whose secretions protect the organ from autodigestion. Epithelial cells invaginate to form **gastric pits,** and from the base of each pit further invaginations form **gastric glands.** Pits and glands lie within the lamina propria, where they are separated by scant amounts of loose connective tissue. A variety of secretory cells within the gastric glands produce **enzymes (chief cell), mucus (mucous neck cell), hydrochloric acid** and **intrinsic factor (parietal cell),** and **hormones (enteroendocrine cell)** essential to the digestive process. The muscularis mucosa exhibits three irregularly arranged layers of smooth muscle instrumental in mixing food with gastric juices. The stomach is covered with serosa.

SMALL INTESTINE

The stomach empties chyme into the first part of the small intestine, the **duodenum,** which is attached to the posterior body wall by adventitia and covered anteriorly with serosa. The duodenum is continuous with the **jejunum** and **ileum,** middle and distal segments of the small intestine that are entirely surrounded by serosa and are supported by a double layer of serosa called the **mesentery.** The duodenum differs from the distal segments in having **submucosal (Brunner's) glands,** which produce an alkaline mucus important in neutralizing the acidic chyme as it enters the small intestine. Also, the bile duct from the liver and the pancreatic duct empty bile and pancreatic juice into the duodenum to assist in digestion and neutralization of acid chyme.

Throughout the small intestine, circular intestinal wall folds **(plicae circulares)** composed of mucosa and submucosal layers increase the surface area of the tube, as do finger-like evaginations (of epithelium and lamina propria) called **villi** and invaginations (of epithelium into lamina propria) called **intestinal glands** or **crypts of Lieberkühn.** The principal epithelial cell of the small intestine, the **absorptive cell,** exhibits numerous apical microvilli **(striate border),** which further increase the area available for absorption. Associated with the microvilli is a **glycocalyx,** which contains enzymes involved in the digestion of disaccharides and small peptides.

In the core of a villus are blood vessels that take up and transport absorbed amino acids and carbohydrates to the liver via the **portal circulation.** Lymphatics (lacteals) transport absorbed lipids via the thoracic duct to the cardiovascular system for distribution. The simple columnar epithelium also includes mucus-producing **goblet cells,** a variety of **enteroendocrine cells** that help to regulate digestion, and, deep in the crypts, **Paneth cells** that produce an antibacterial enzyme, lysozyme. Also within the crypts are stem cells that undergo mitotic renewal to form all of the epithelial cell types, resulting in a resurfacing of the intestine every 2 to 4 days. **Plasma cells,** prominent in the lamina propria between crypts, produce mainly **secretory IgA,** an immunoglobulin that is transported across the mucosa into the lumen by receptors (secretory component) located on the epithelial cells.

Lymphatic nodules become increasingly numerous in the small intestine and form multinodular buldges on the antimesenteric border called **Peyer's patches** that deform the mucosal surface. **M cells** are present in the epithelium overlying Peyer's patches and may function in the transport of certain antigens into the underlying lymphoid tissue. The submucosa and muscularis externa contain intramural nerve plexuses and ganglia (Meissner's and Auerbach's ganglia, respectively) of the parasympathetic division of the autonomic nervous system, which, together with the enteroendocrine system, help to regulate peristalsis, vascular tone, and secretion.

COLON (LARGE INTESTINE)

The ileum terminates by joining the large intestine at the ileocecal valve, a double fold of mucosa and submucosa. The **cecum** is the small initial segment of the colon inferior to the ileocecal valve and gives rise to a slender diverticulum called the **appendix.** The **ascending, transverse, descending,** and **sigmoid** portions complete the colon, and these, along with the cecum, display similar histologic characteristics. Plicae circulares divide the organ into pouchlike **haustra.** The inner layer of muscularis externa is complete, but the outer, longitudinal layer is divided into three equally spaced ribbons called **taenia coli,** which, when they contract, accentuate the segmentation of the colon into haustra.

Internally, the mucosa lacks villi but possesses tightly packed crypts of Lieberkühn. The colonic epithelium absorbs water and thus compacts the waste materials into fecal masses. **Goblet cells** lubricate the feces with their mucous secretions, and lymphatic nodules are abundant in the mucosa. Transverse and sigmoid colons are surrounded by serosa and are suspended by a double layer of serosa called **mesocolon,** similar to the mesentery of the small intestine. Ascending and descending colon are covered anteriorly with serosa but are attached posteriorly to the dorsal body wall by adventitia.

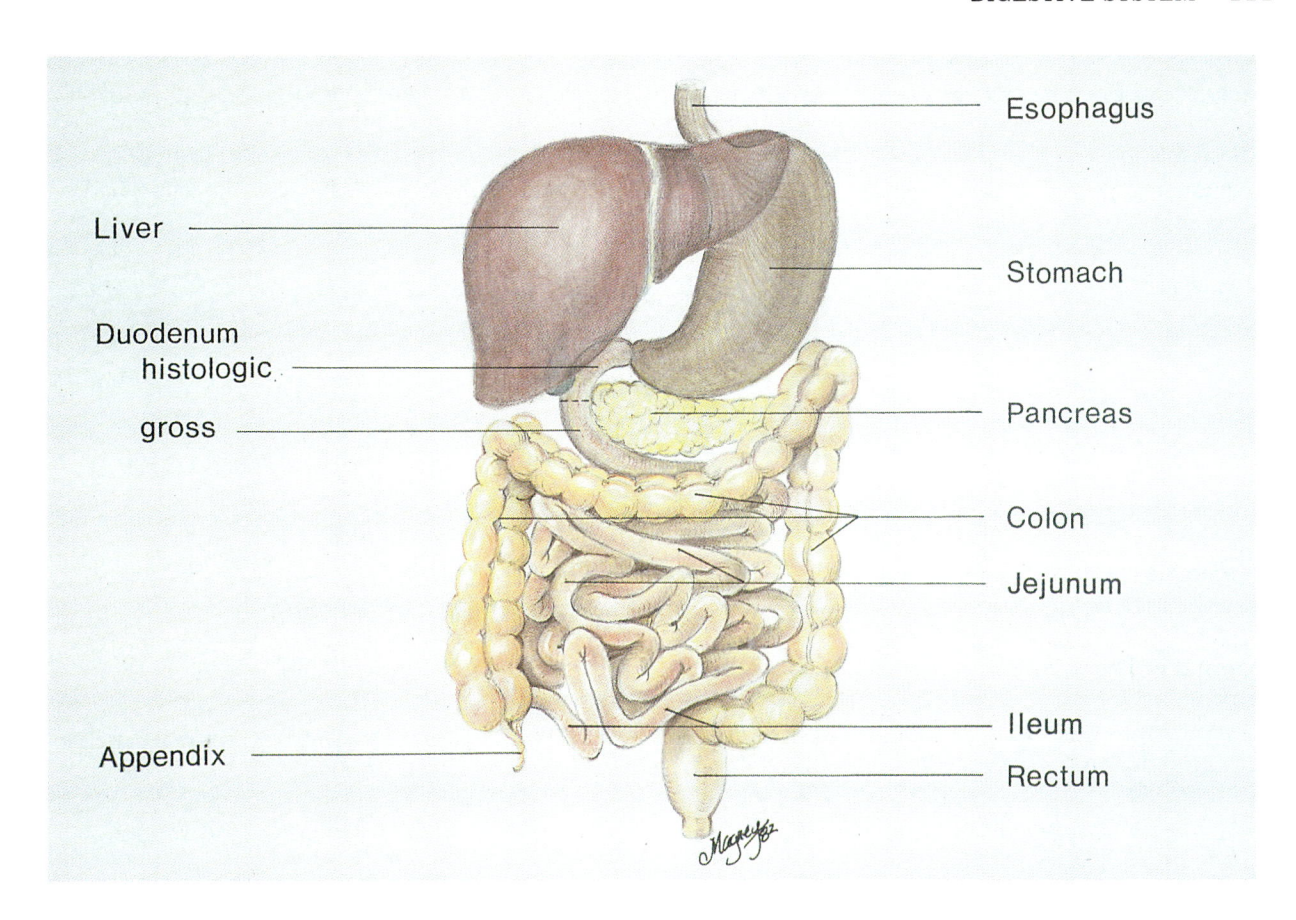

Fig. 15-1. Gastrointestinal tract from esophagus to rectum, and accessory organs of digestion. Duodenum is shorter by histologic examination than by gross anatomic standards, since only the first 3-5 inches of duodenum (up to sphincter of Oddi) contains Brunner's glands in the submucosa.

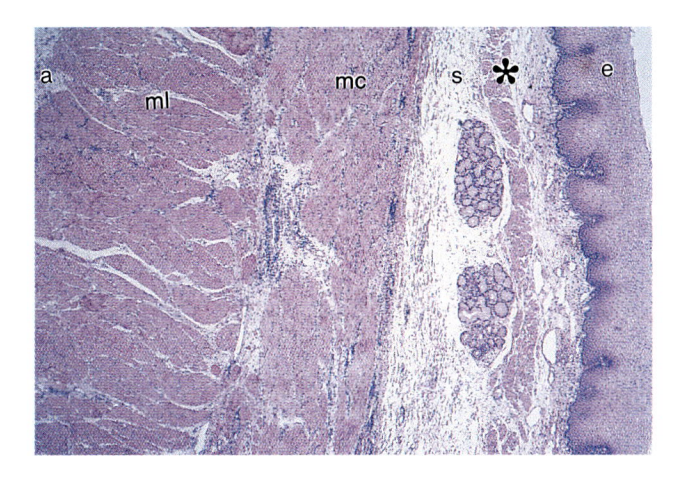

Fig. 15-2. Low-magnification LM illustrating four layers of esophagus. From right to left, these consist of (1) the mucosa, made up of epithelium (e), underlying lamina propria, and muscularis mucosa (*); (2) the submucosa (s), containing two mucous glands; (3) the muscularis, consisting of inner circular (mc) and outer longitudinal (ml) layers of smooth muscle; and (4) a portion of adventitia (a). (H&E; ×50.)

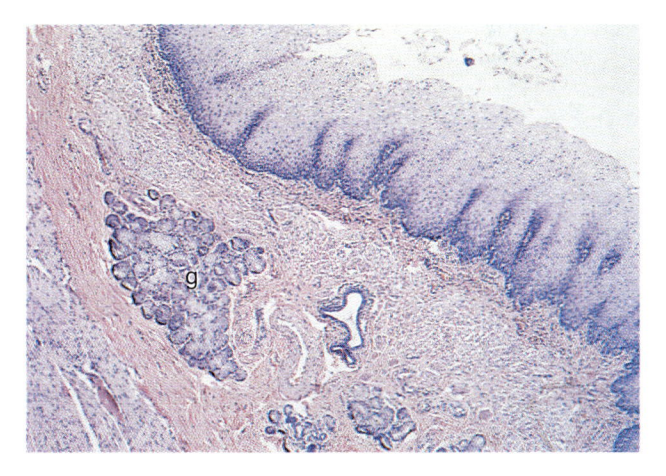

Fig. 15-3. Higher-magnification LM of mucosa and submucosa of esophagus. Esophageal glands (g) are located in submucosa and are involved in production of mucus for lubrication of food during swallowing. (H&E; ×100.)

112 COLOR ATLAS OF HISTOLOGY

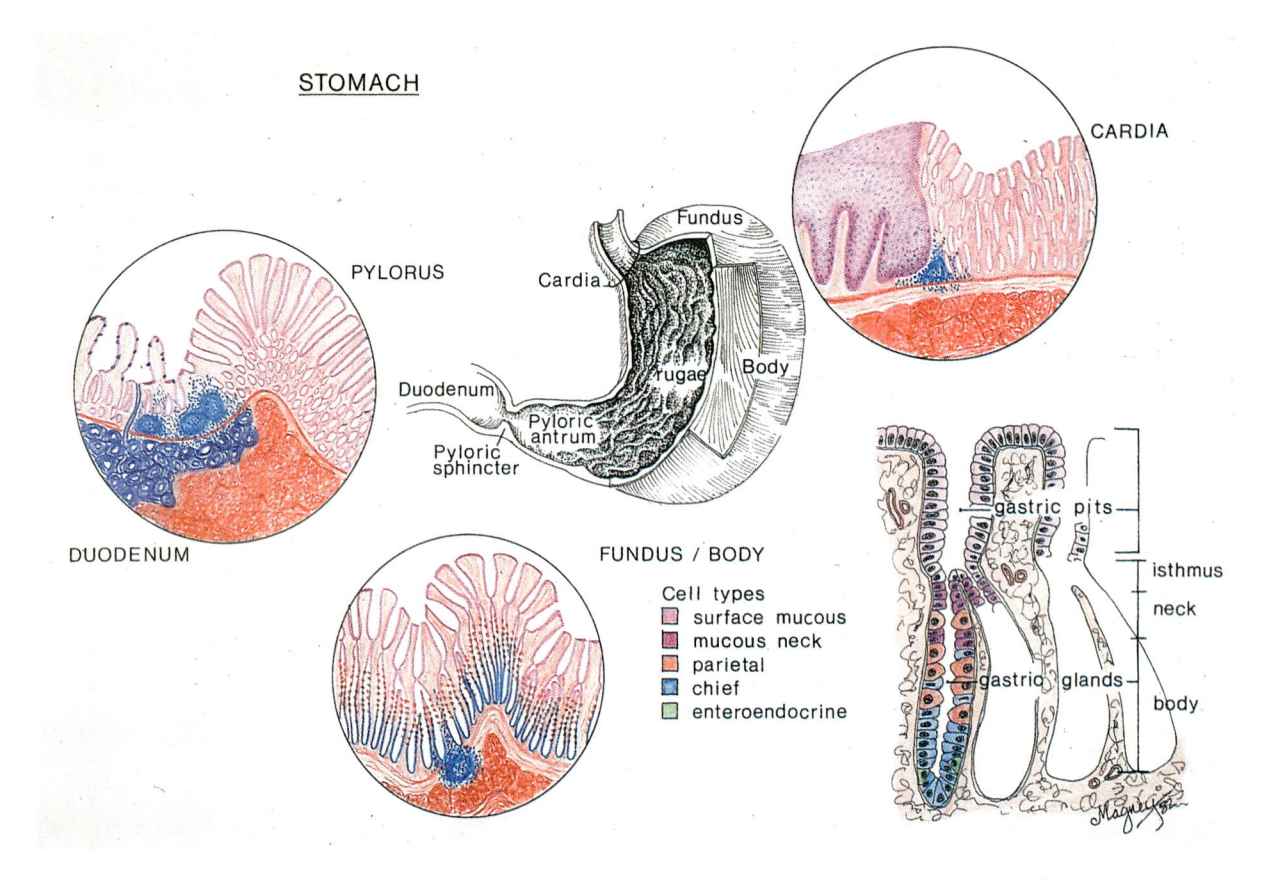

Fig. 15-4. Subdivisions of stomach wall (cardiac, body and fundus, and pyloric regions) and cytologic details of gastric glands in body or fundus of stomach.

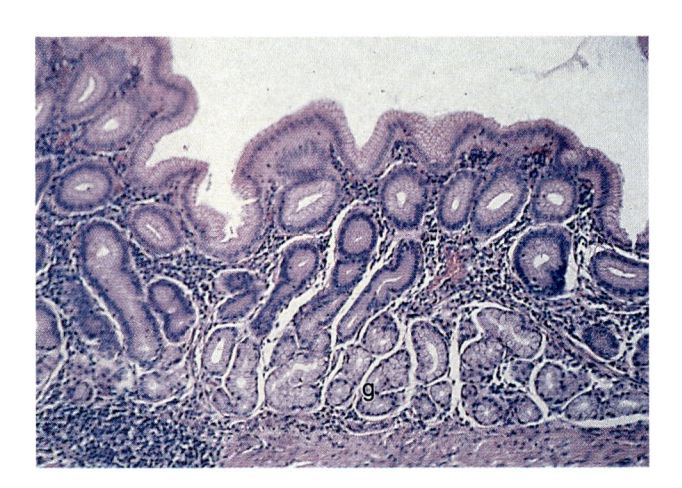

Fig. 15-5. LM illustrating cardiac region of stomach. Observe shallow gastric pits and short cardiac glands *(g)*. (H&E; ×100.)

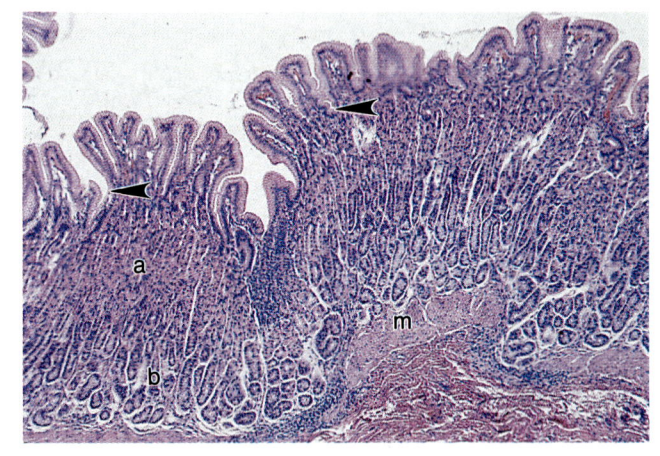

Fig. 15-6. Low-magnification LM of body of stomach, illustrating presence of gastric glands. Observe longer gastric pits *(arrowheads)* and presence of acidophilic *(a)* and basophilic *(b)* regions within gastric glands. Muscularis mucosa *(m)* separates gastric glands from underlying submucosa. (H&E; ×75.)

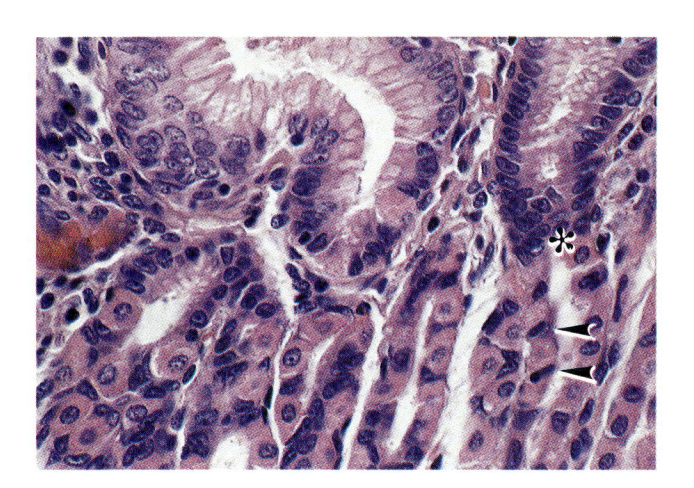

Fig. 15-7. High-magnification LM of bases of gastric pits and their junctions (*) with necks of gastric glands. Surface mucous cells can be seen lining gastric pits, whereas necks of gastric glands consist of acidophilic parietal cells and intervening mucous neck cells *(arrowheads)*. (H&E; ×350.)

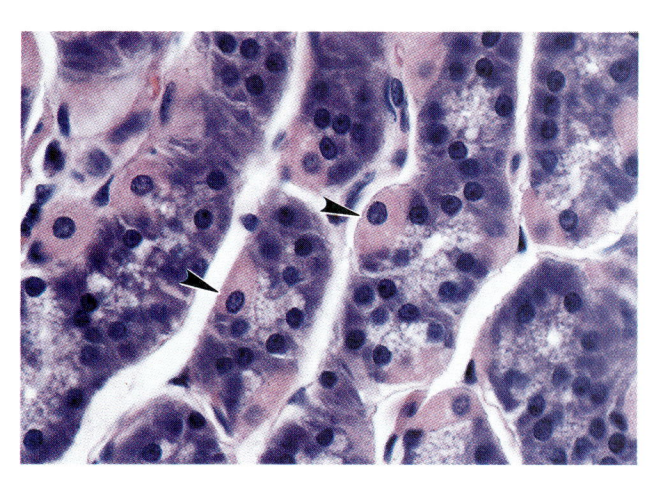

Fig. 15-8. High-magnification LM of body of gastric gland. Acidophilic parietal cells *(arrowheads)* can be seen bulging from basal surface of gastric gland. Narrowed apex of these cells opens to lumen of gland. Smaller, basophilic chief cells that lie between parietal cells also secrete into lumen of gland. (H&E; ×250.)

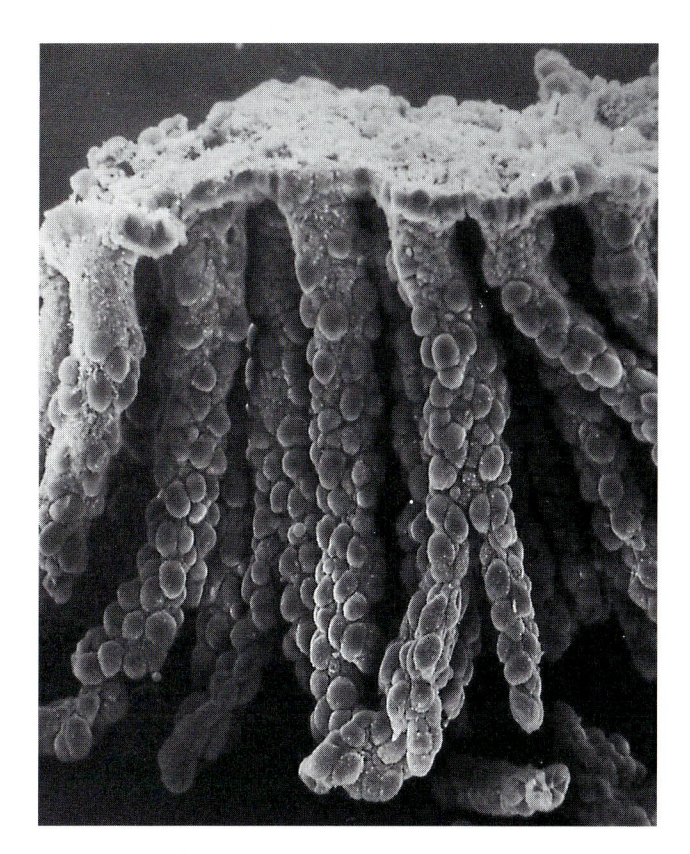

Fig. 15-9. SEM of isolated epithelium from stomach fundus with invaginated gastric glands. Basal surfaces of parietal cells are prominent in glands. (×500.)

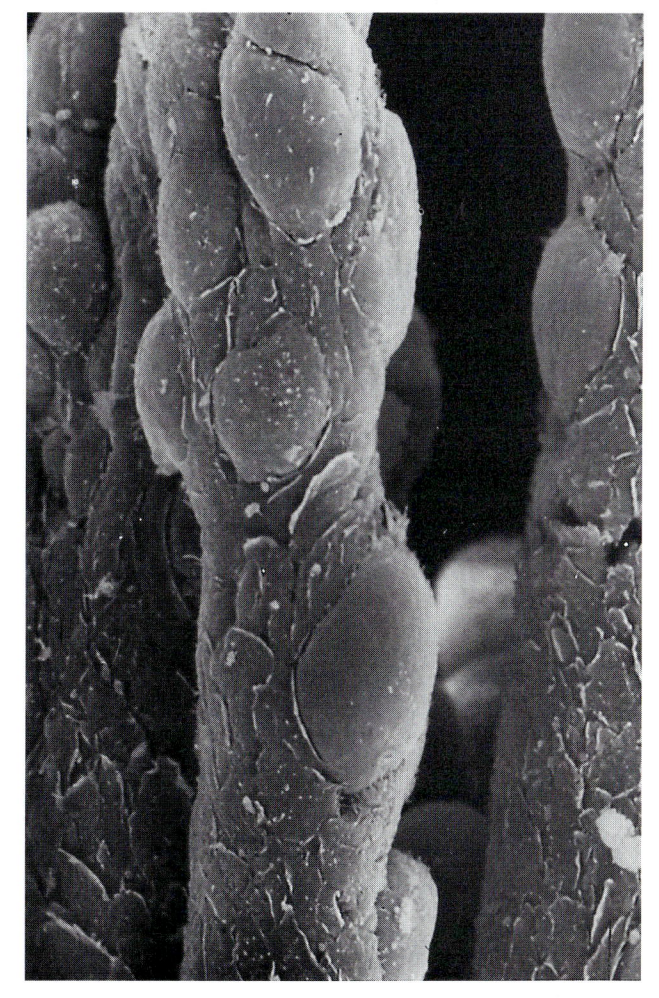

Fig. 15-10. Higher magnification SEM of the basal surface of glandular epithelial cells within fundic stomach. Parietal cells are seen to form prominent dome-shaped bulges on basal surface. (×1,400.)

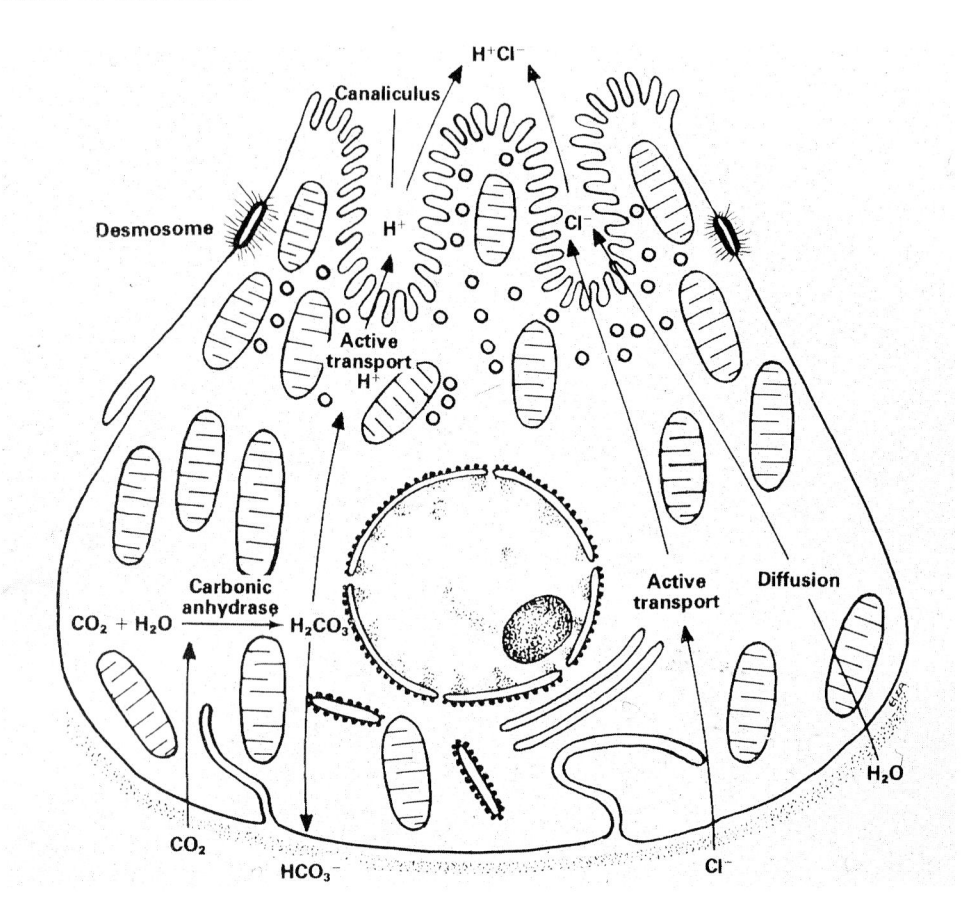

Fig. 15-11. Structure of parietal cell and mechanisms involved in formation of hydrochloric acid.

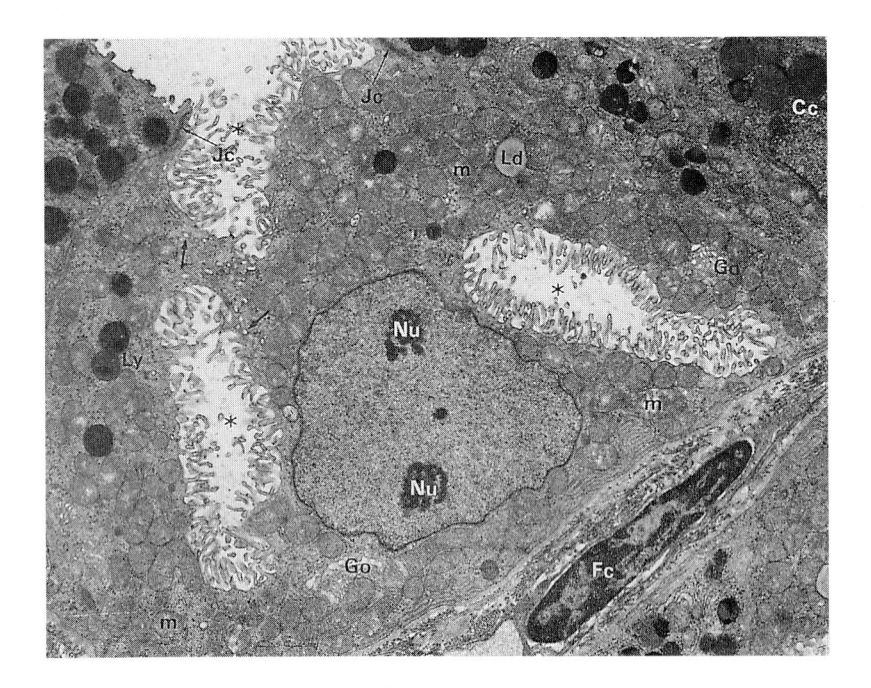

Fig. 15-12. TEM of parietal cell in gastric gland. Observe well-developed intracellular canaliculi. *Ld*, lipid droplet; *Nu*, nucleolus; *Go*, Golgi apparatus; *Fc*, fibroblast; *Cc*, chief cell; *arrows*, canaliculi. ($\times 7,400$.)

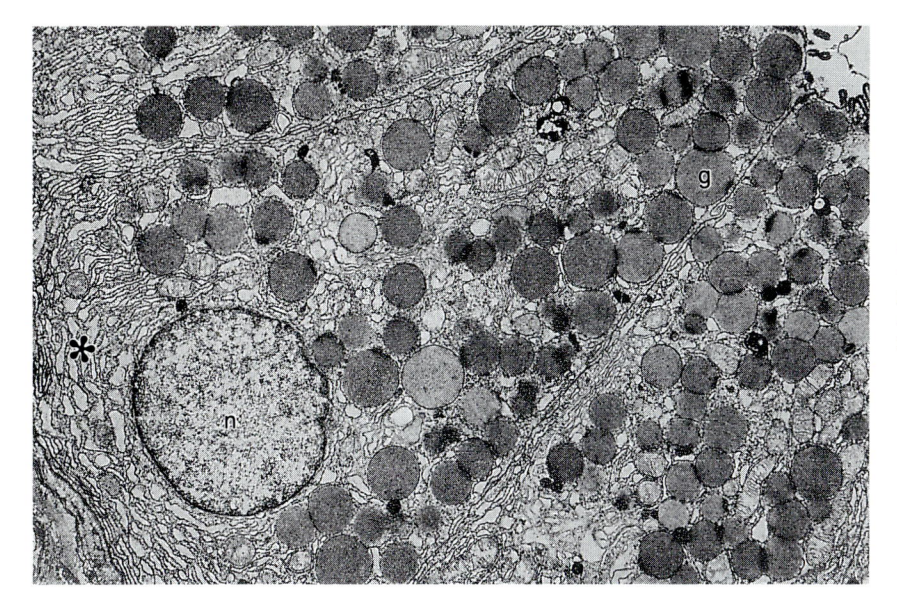

Fig. 15-13. TEM of chief cell showing its exocrine organization. Chief cell of stomach is involved in formation of rennin, pepsinogen, and gastric lipase. *g*, secretion granule; *, RER; *n*, nucleus. (×7,300.)

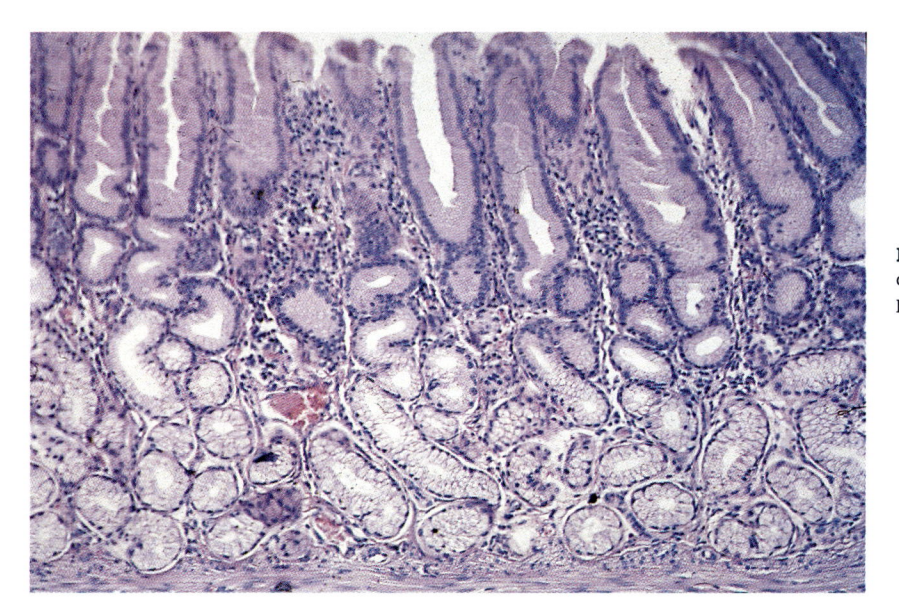

Fig. 15-14. Low-power LM of pyloric mucosa. Note long gastric pits and highly coiled pyloric glands. (H&E; ×200.)

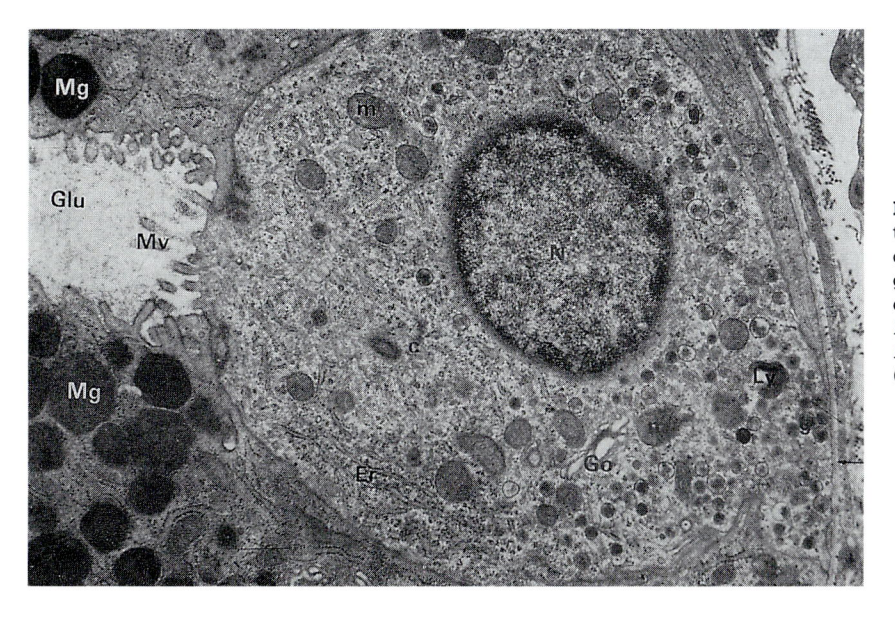

Fig. 15-15. TEM of pyloric gland showing ultrastructure of G cell, or gastrin-producing cell. Observe basal polarization of secretory granules toward connective tissue surface of cell. *Mg*, mucous granule; *Glu*, gland lumen; *Mv*, microvilli; *Go*, Golgi; *m*, mitochondria; *N*, nucleus; *Er*, endoplasmic reticulum. (×5,800.)

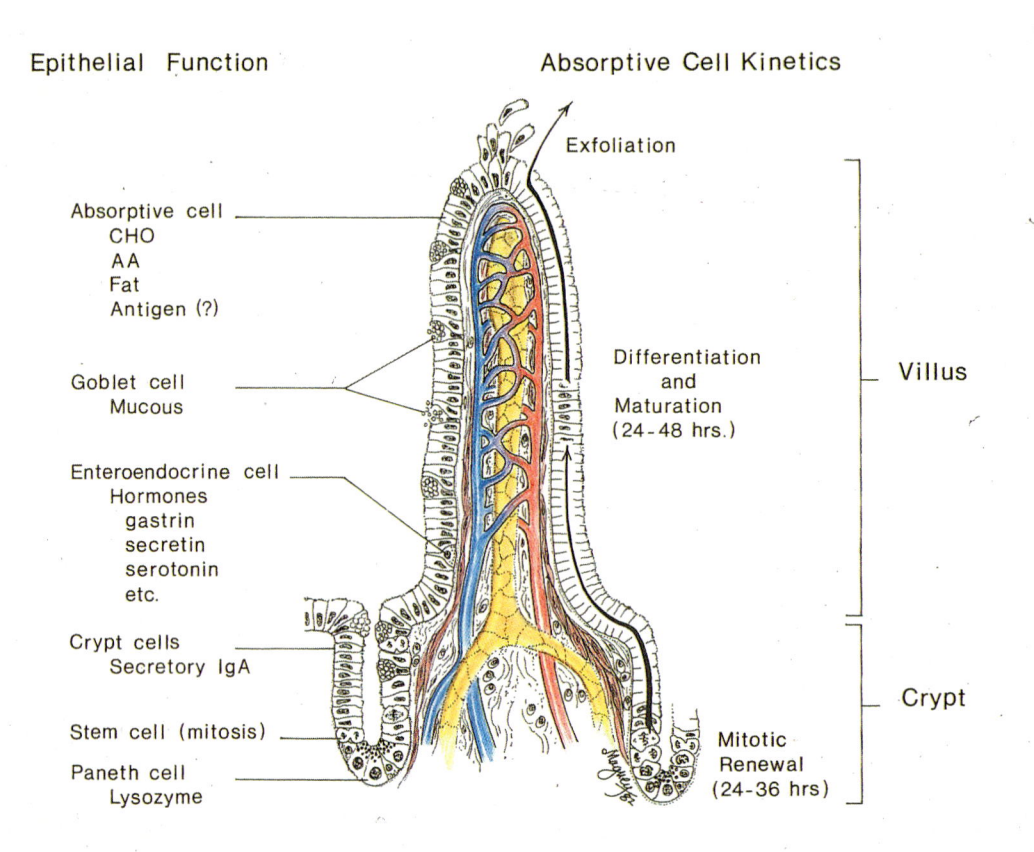

Fig. 15-16. Epithelium of intestinal villus and crypt including several different types of cells with varying functions, such as absorption of nutrients, release of hormones, transport of immunoglobulins, and secretion of mucus and enzymes. Notice also prominent lacteal in core of villus, blood vessels, and smooth muscle. Nerves, not shown in this illustration, supply both villus and crypt.

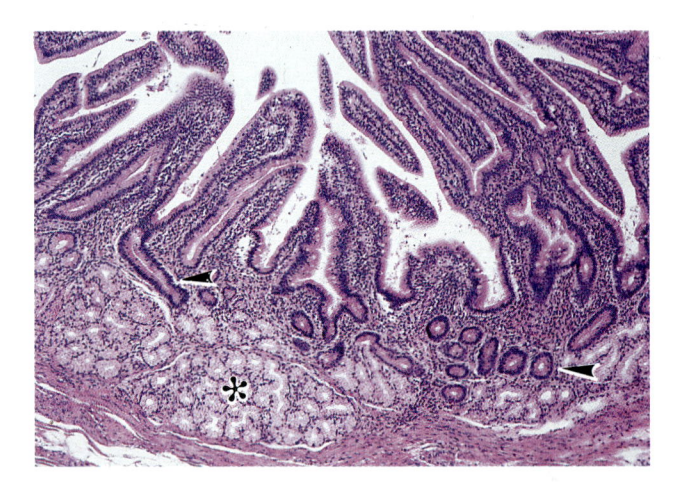

Fig. 15-17. Low-magnification LM of duodenal mucosa. Easily distinguished are numerous fingerlike villi, glandular invaginations called intestinal crypts of Lieberkühn *(arrowheads)*, and beneath muscularis mucosa, mucus-secreting Brunner's glands (*). (H&E; ×75.)

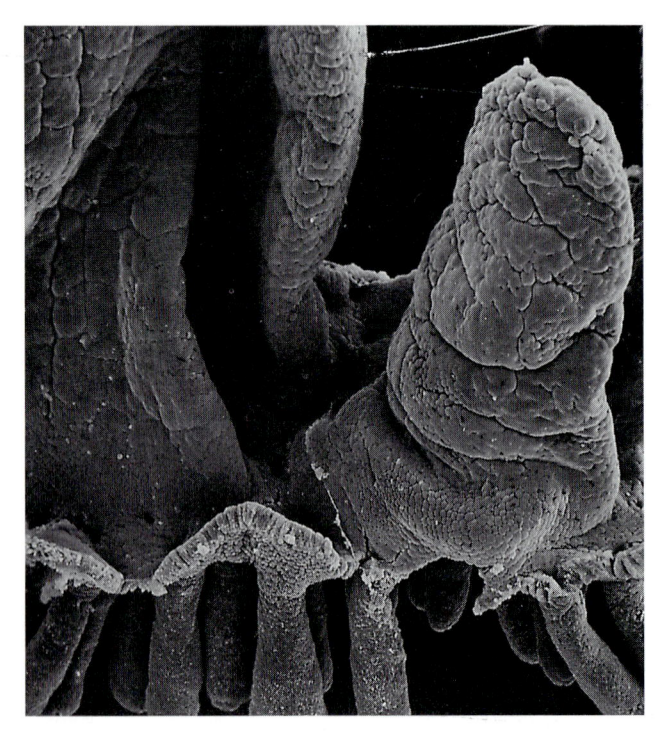

Fig. 15-18. By SEM, furrows that result from smooth muscle contraction are seen on surface of a villus. Examination of intestinal floor reveals openings of intestinal crypts. Outline of apical surface of individual epithelial cells of villus is also evident. (×150.)

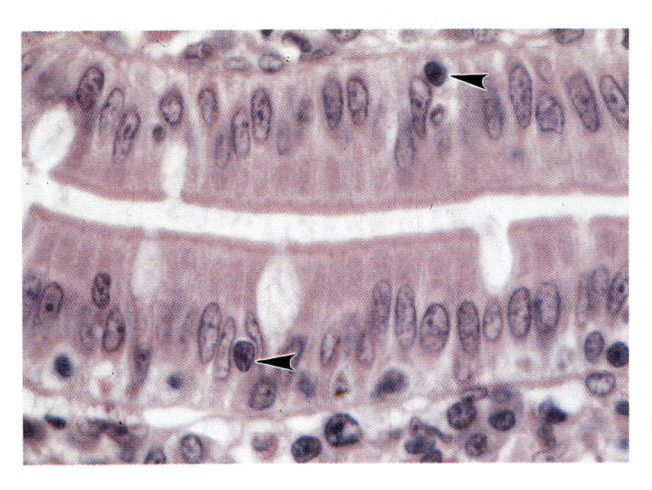

Fig. 15-19. High-magnification LM of epithelium of two adjacent villi. Observe pale-staining goblet cell *(center)*. Several lymphocytes *(arrowheads)* can also be seen traversing epithelium. (H&E; ×1,000.)

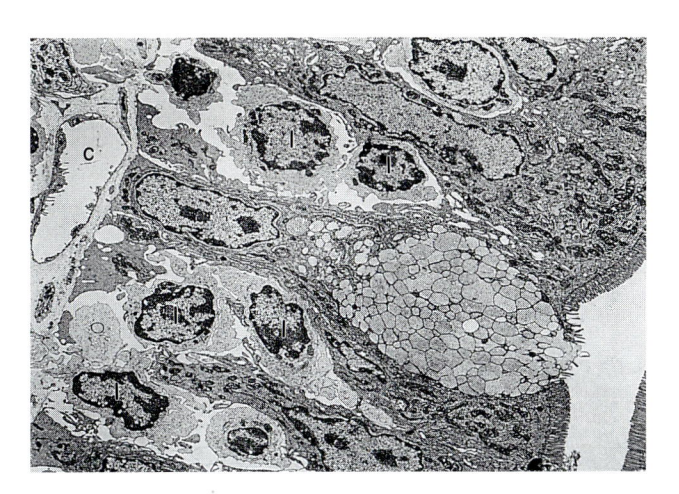

Fig. 15-20. TEM of villus epithelium. Notice goblet cell *(center)* and numerous lymphocytes *(l)* within epithelium. Fenestrated capillary *(c)* is seen in lamina propria at base of goblet cell. (×2,400.)

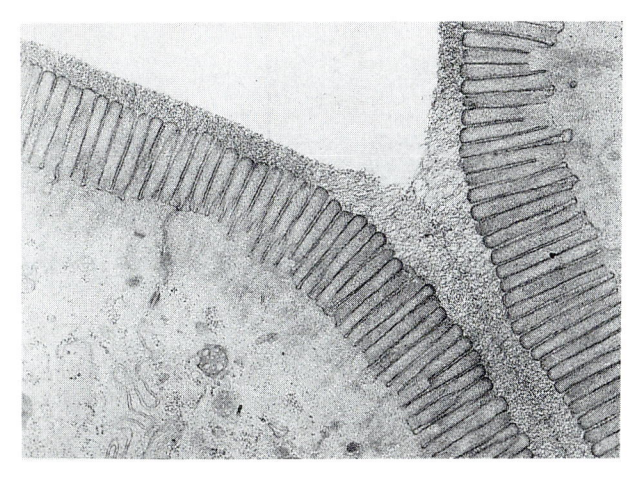

Fig. 15-21. High-magnification TEM of absorptive epithelial cells reveals extensive microvilli on apical surface and presence of glycocalyx, which contains enzymes involved with digestion of disaccharides and small peptides. (×13,600.)

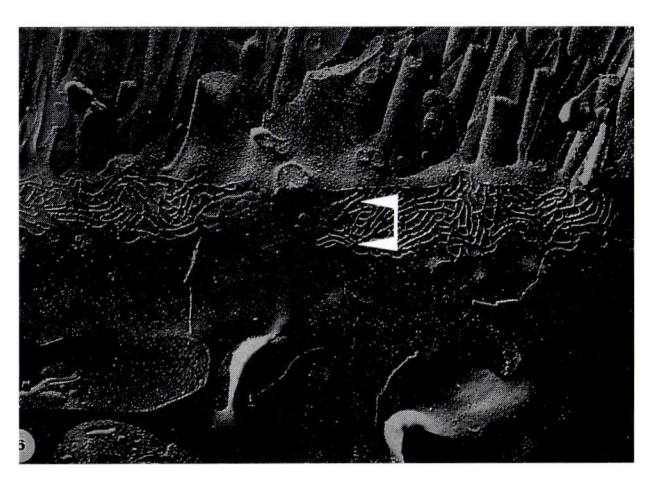

Fig. 15-22. Freeze fracture of junctional complex found near apical surface of absorptive epithelial cells. Extensive zonula occludens *(bracket)* seen in this micrograph illustrates permeability barrier that exists between intestinal lumen and intercellular space beneath junctional complex. (×28,000.)

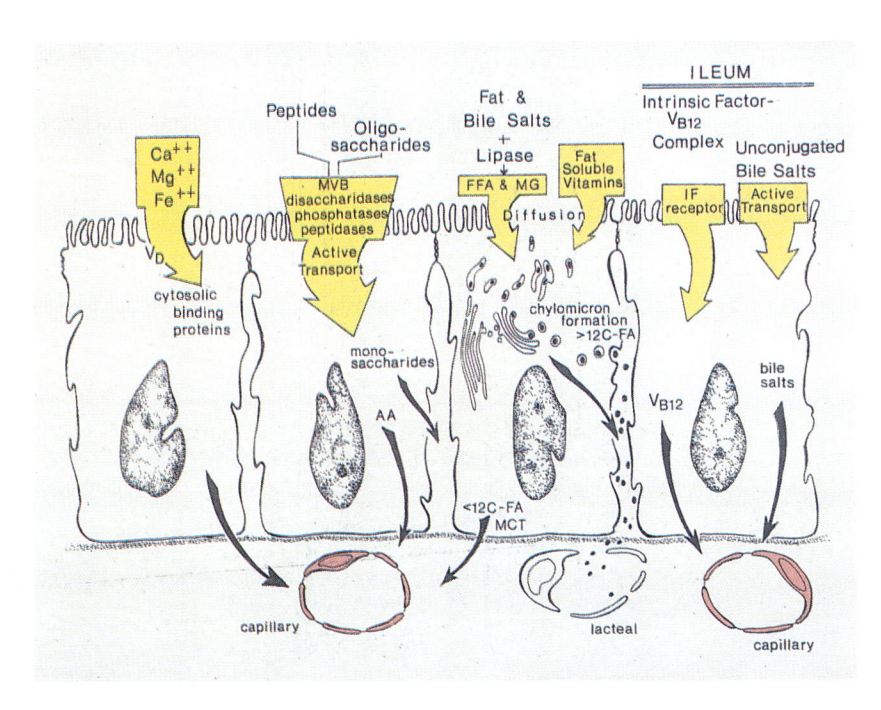

Fig. 15-23. Absorption of nutrients across microvillus border of intestinal epithelial cells. Enzymes (disaccharidases and peptidases) involved in transport of monosaccharides and amino acids are located within glycocalyx of microvillous border. Absorption of most nutrients is completed in upper small intestine; however, absorption of intrinsic factor–vitamin B_{12} complex occurs by specific receptors on absorptive cells in ileum as does reabsorption of bile salts as a part of enterohepatic circulation. Absorption of fat is enhanced by its breakdown into free fatty acids and monoglycerides, which passively diffuse into absorptive cell. Free fatty acids (>12 carbon atoms) and monoglycerides are reesterified in smooth endoplasmic reticulum and then transferred to Golgi where chylomicrons are formed. Chylomicrons are released into extracellular space and enter lacteals in lamina propria. Small fatty acid chains (<12 carbon atoms) can diffuse through epithelium and enter capillaries directly.

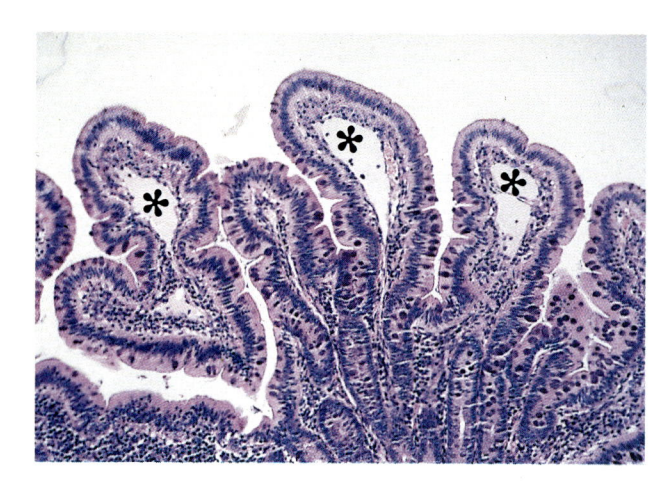

Fig. 15-24. LM of ileal mucosa reveals presence of lacteals (*) within intestinal villi. (H&E; ×100.)

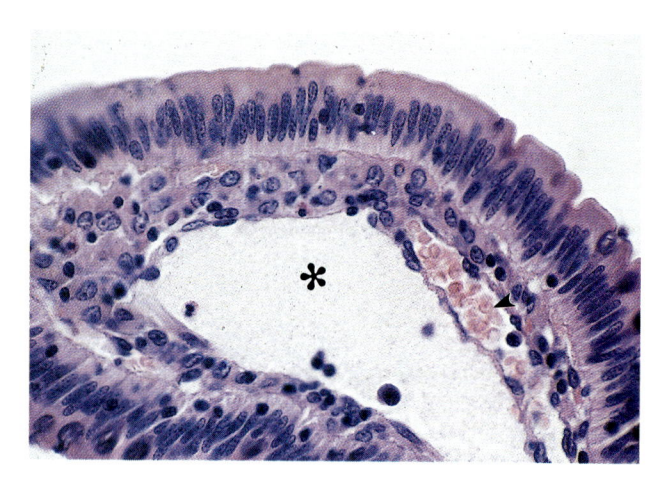

Fig. 15-25. High-magnification LM of intestinal villus showing presence of lacteal (*) within lamina propria. Compare lacteal with small venule *(arrowhead)*. (H&E; ×350.)

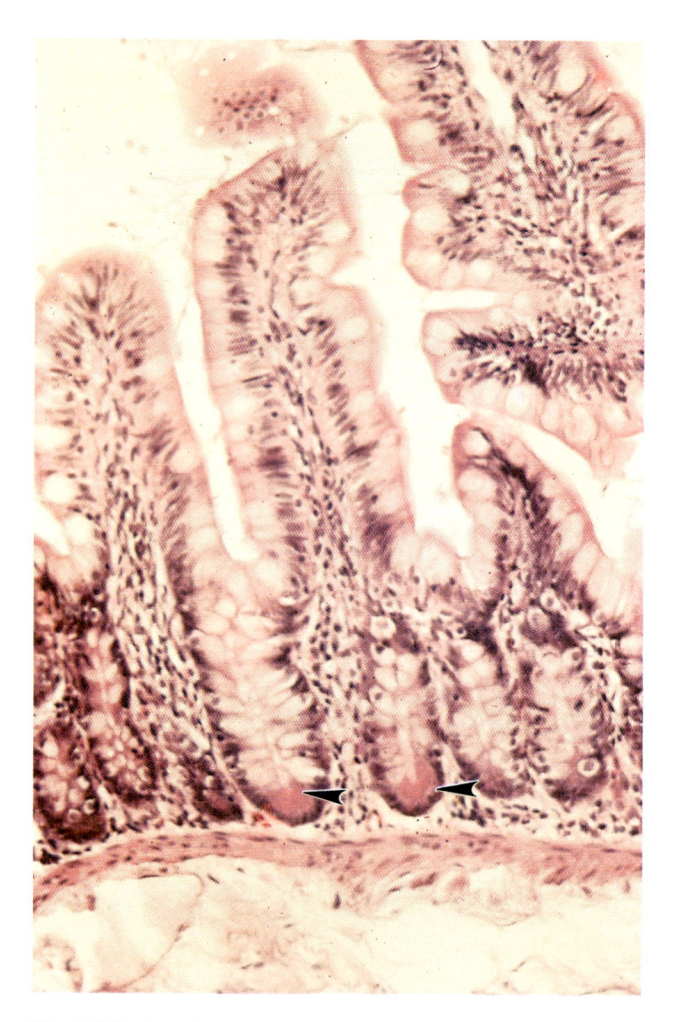

Fig. 15-26. LM of ileal mucosa. Observe large number of goblet cells within epithelium and presence of acidophilic Paneth cells *(arrowheads)* at base of intestinal crypts. Muscularis mucosa lies immediately beneath intestinal crypts. (H&E; ×200.)

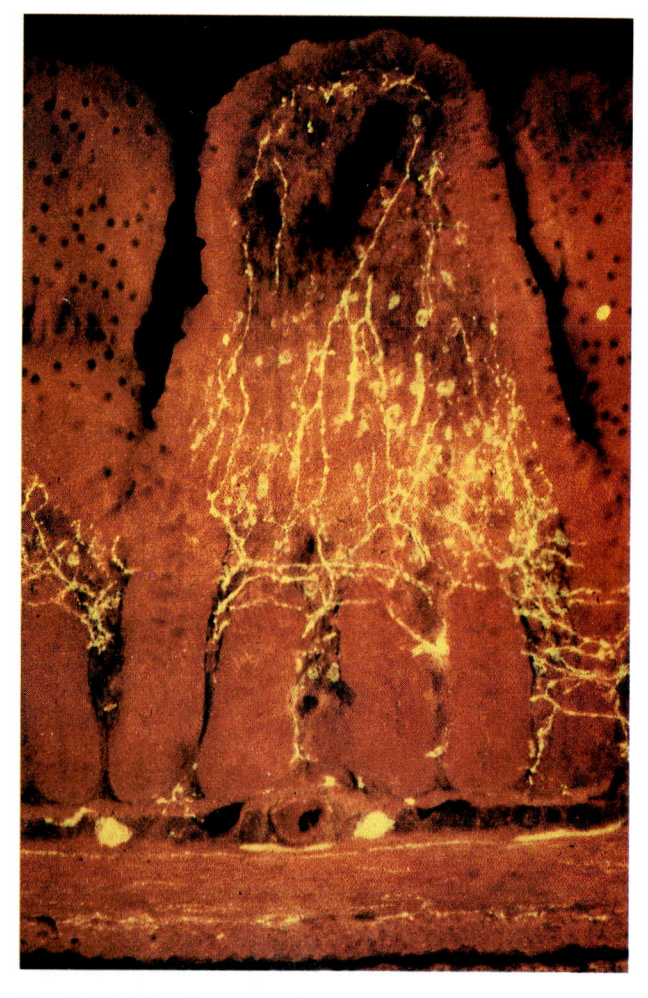

Fig. 15-27. LM of frozen section of ileum immunocytochemically stained for neurotransmitter VIP. Plexus of nerve fibers *(yellow)* surrounds apical portion of crypts and extends up into villus just beneath epithelium, while two autonomic ganglion cells containing VIP are seen in submucosa. (×200.)

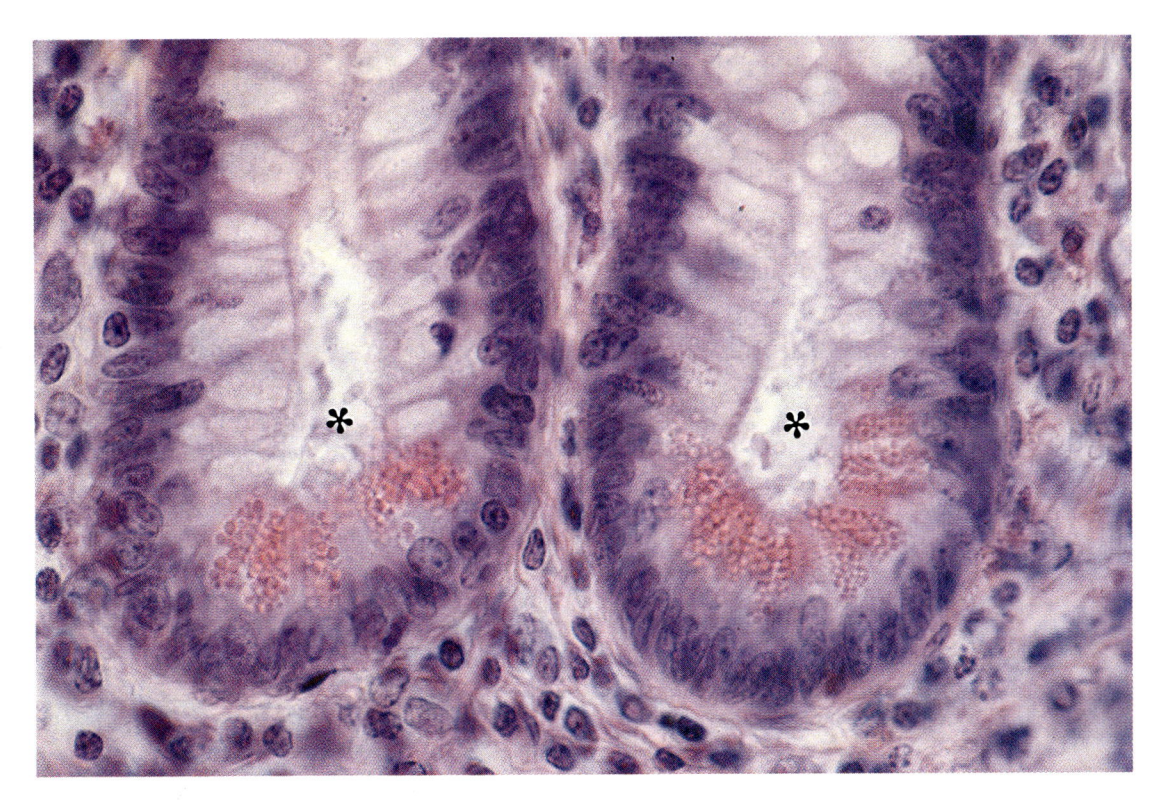

Fig. 15-28. High-magnification LM of bases of intestinal crypts (*) revealing presence of numerous Paneth cells. Acidophilic secretion granules lie in cell apices that abut crypt lumen into which their enzymatic secretion product, lysozyme, is released. (H&E; ×900.)

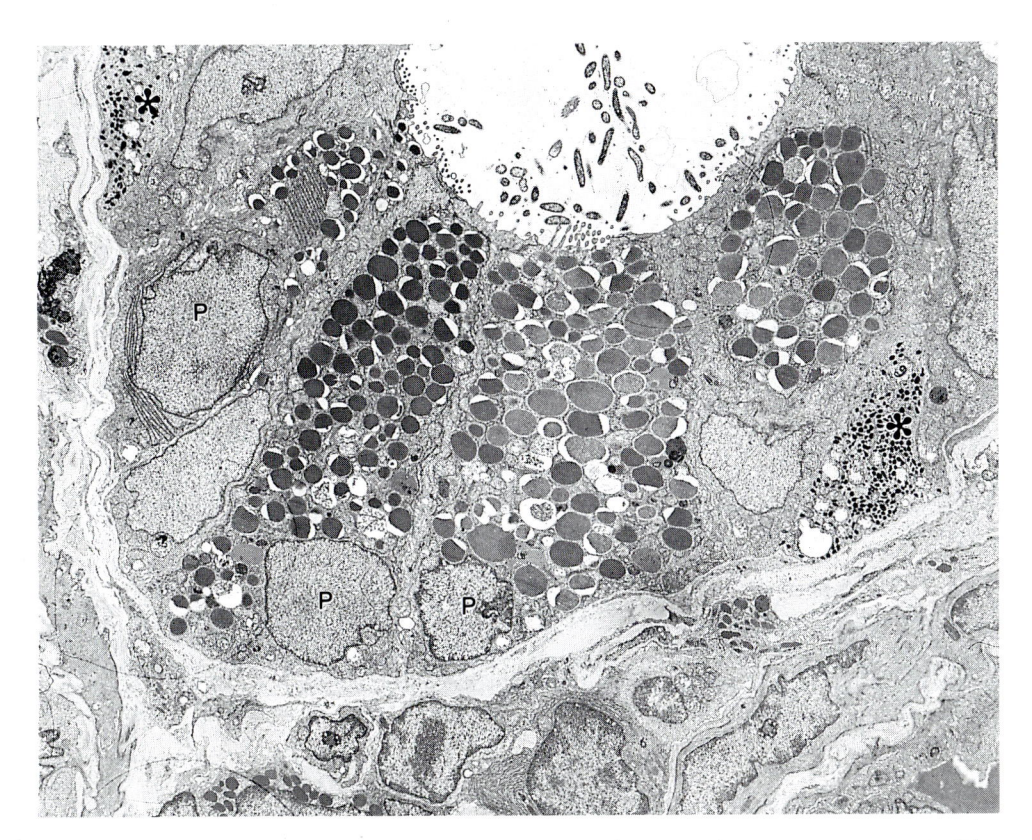

Fig. 15-29. TEM of base of an intestinal crypt (rat ileum) that contains many Paneth cells *(P)*. These serous cells secrete lysozyme, a bactericidal enzyme. Paneth cells also contain an extensive lysosomal apparatus and are capable of endocytosis of microorganisms found within crypt lumen. Two examples of enteroendocrine cells (*) are also visible. (×1,900.)

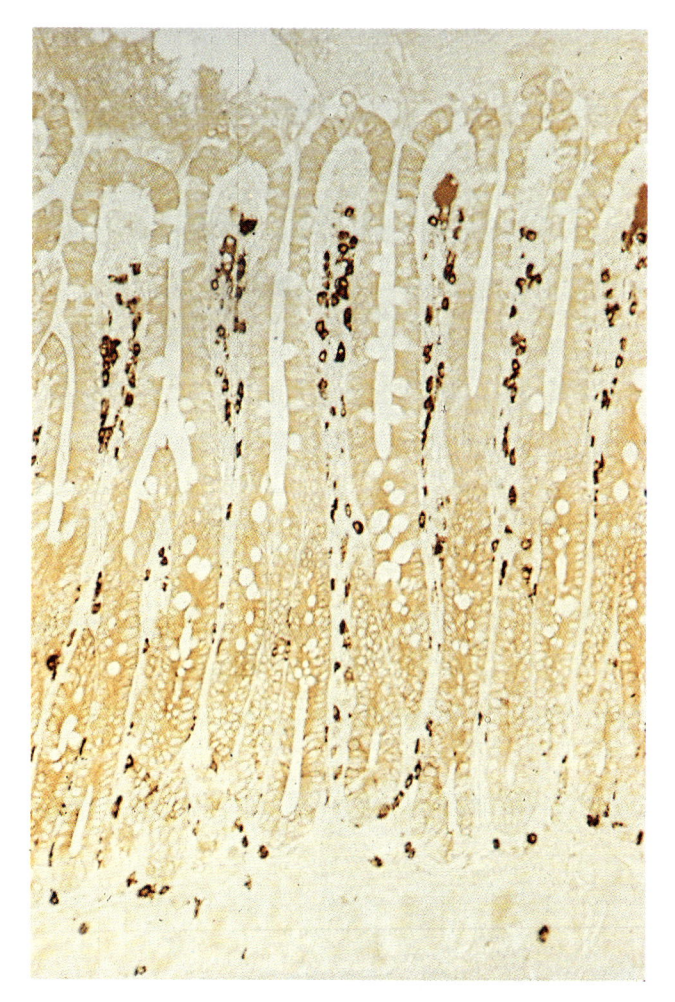

Fig. 15-30. LM of intestine stained immunocytochemically for localization of secretory IgA. Large numbers of dark-staining plasma cells can be seen within lamina propria of intestinal villi and also within submucosa. Apical portions of cells of intestinal crypts of Lieberkühn are also stained for secretory IgA, for these cells are involved in transport of this immunoglobulin from lamina propria into the lumen of intestine. (×150.)

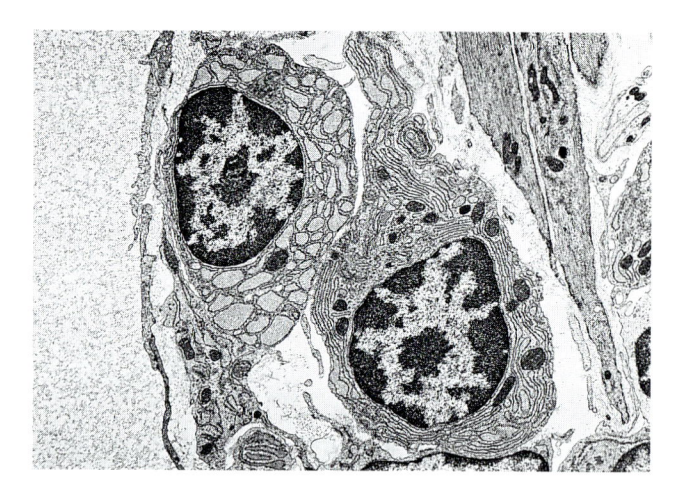

Fig. 15-31. TEM of plasma cells within lamina propria. A lacteal can be seen *(far left)*. Plasma cells within intestine produce secretory IgA within RER, release it into lamina propria, and after binding to secretory component, it is transported across epithelium into intestinal lumen. (×2,800.)

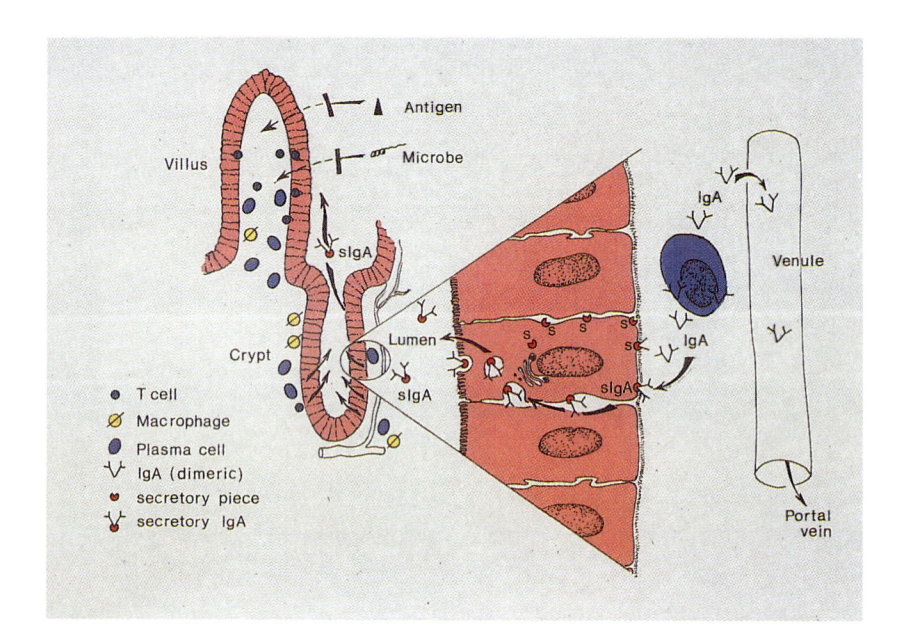

Fig. 15-32. Synthesis, transport, and secretion of secretory IgA in intestinal mucosa.

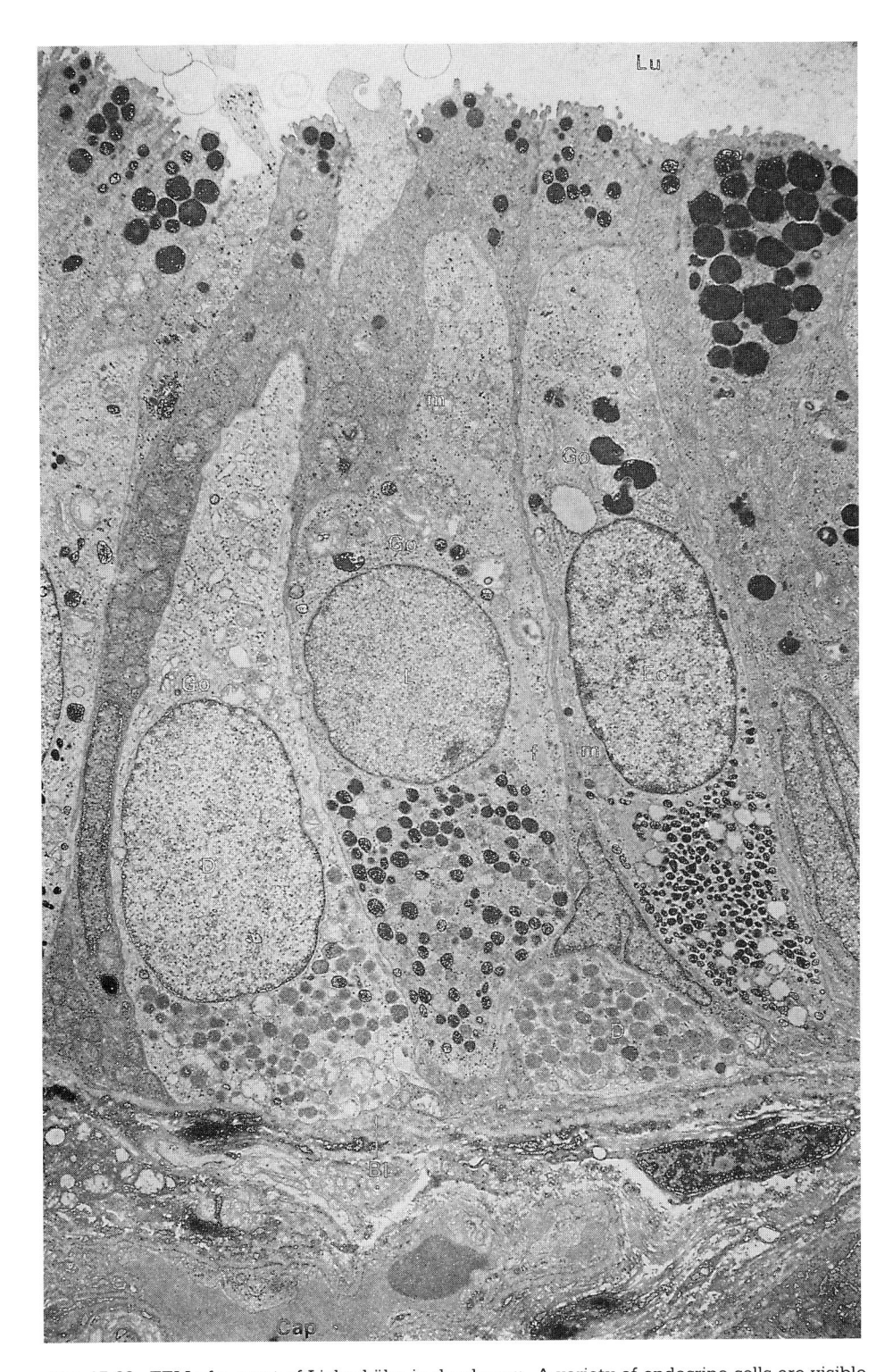

Fig. 15-33. TEM of a crypt of Lieberkühn in duodenum. A variety of endocrine cells are visible in epithelium. Each of these cells is involved in elaboration of a distinct intestinal hormone. Granules are polarized in base of cell, where their secretion will be released into lamina propria. Undifferentiated crypt cells in intestine contain large granules near lumen of gland and may be involved in epithelial transport of secretory IgA. *Lu*, Lumen; *Go*, Golgi complex; *m*, mitochondria; *R*, rough ER; *f*, cytoplasmic filaments; *Bl*, basal lamina; *Ec*, enterochromaffin cell: *D*, type of enteroendocrine cell: *L*, type of enteroendocrine cell. (×4,100.)

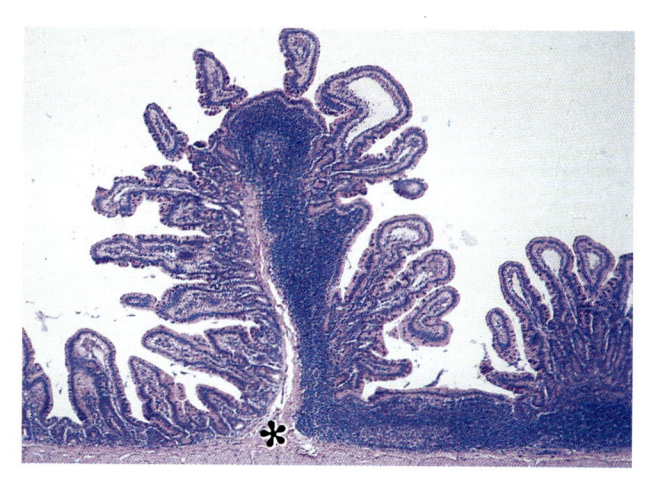

Fig. 15-34. LM illustrating individual folds (plica circulares) in cross section. Submucosa (*) extends up into fold, and extensive amounts of lymphoid tissue can be seen within both submucosa and lamina propria. (H&E; ×50.)

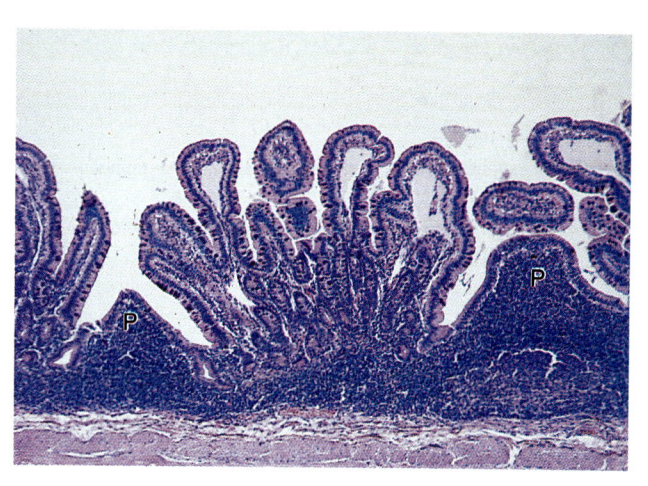

Fig. 15-35. LM of rat ileum illustrating presence of Peyer's patches (P). Because of accumulation of lymphoid tissue beneath epithelium, intestinal villi are absent in region of Peyer's patches. Lacteals can be seen within villi. (H&E; ×50.)

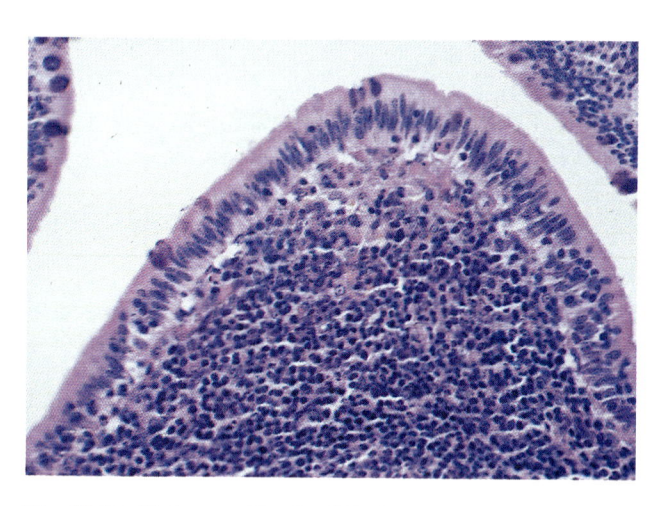

Fig. 15-36. High-magnification LM of intestinal epithelium overlying Peyer's patch. Specialized cells called M cells are present within epithelium but are not easily distinguished by light microscopy. (H&E; ×350.)

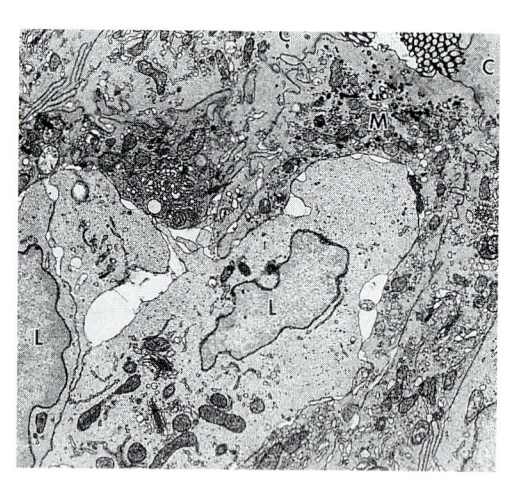

Fig. 15-37. High-magnification TEM of intestinal epithelium overlying Peyer's patch 30 minutes after introduction of horseradish perioxidase (HPO) into intestinal lumen. Reaction product for HPO can be seen (upper right) surrounding microvilli and filling vesicles and tubules within an M cell, suggesting that it may play a role in transporting antigenic material from intestinal lumen to underlying lymphocytes. M, M cell; C, columnar cells; L, lymphocytes; G, Golgi. (×4,500.)

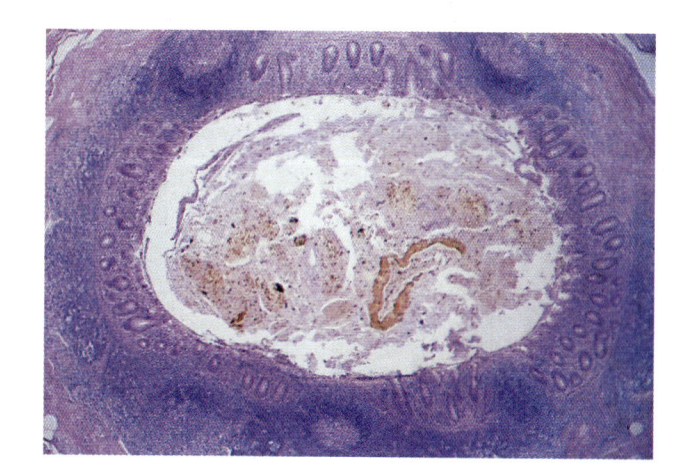

Fig. 15-38. LM of appendix in cross section. Observe detritus within lumen and presence of lymphoid follicles within lamina propria and submucosa. (H&E; ×20.)

DIGESTIVE SYSTEM 123

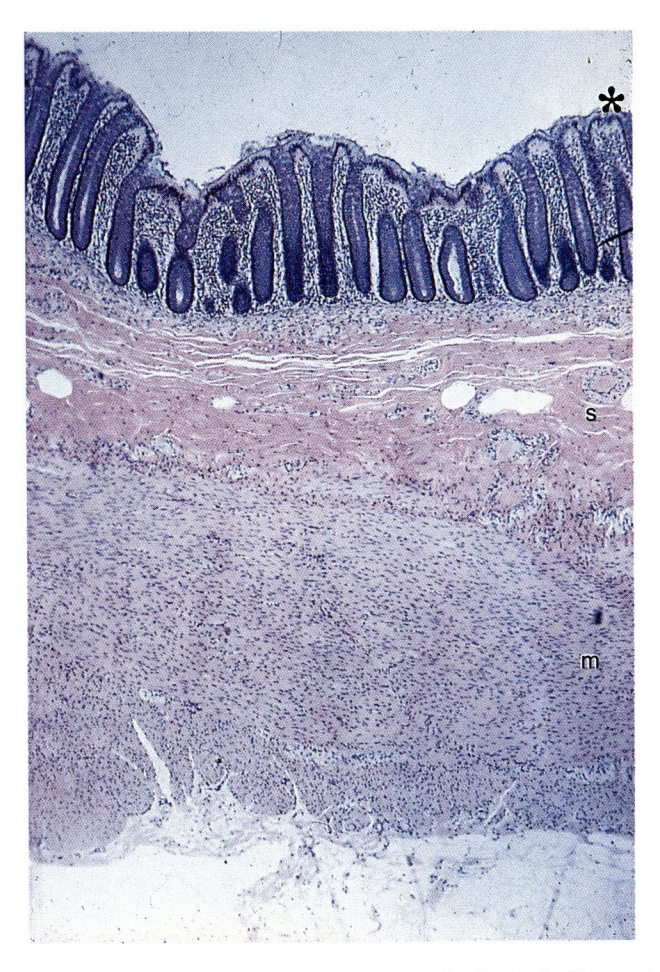

Fig. 15-39. Low-magnification LM of large intestine. Notice lack of villar projections within mucosal surface (*), relatively thick submucosa (s), and thickened muscularis (m) seen in outer wall. (H&E; ×40.)

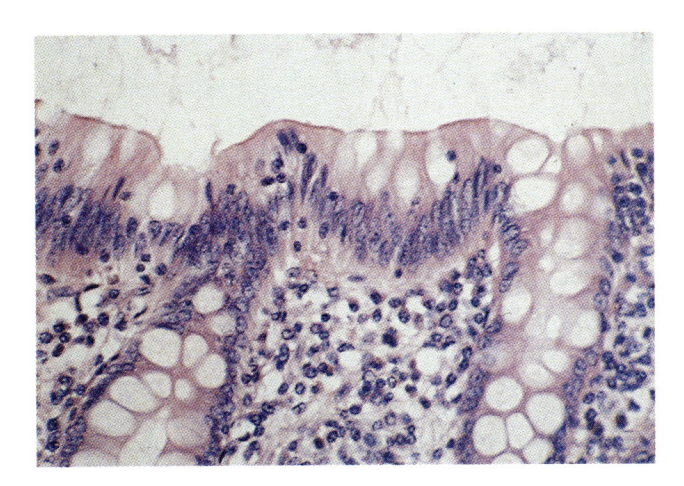

Fig. 15-40. Higher-magnification LM of colonic epithelium. Owing to large number of lymphocytes and other leukocytes in lamina propria and also in epithelium, the gastrointestinal tract is considered to be a site of chronic inflammation. (H&E; ×350.)

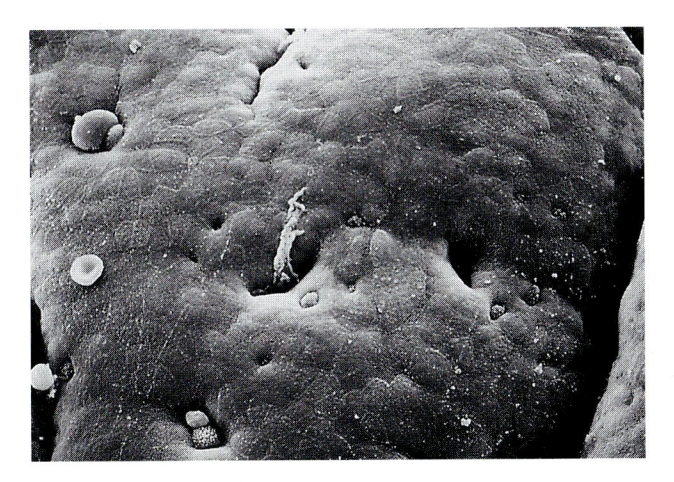

Fig. 15-41. SEM of surface of colonic mucosa. Note openings of crypts of Lieberkühn onto the surface and example of presence of mucous discharge (center) from crypt. Lateral margins of surface epithelial cells are easily distinguished, as are openings of several goblet cells within mucosa. (×500.)

CHAPTER 16

LIVER AND GALLBLADDER

THE LIVER AND gallbladder, like the pancreas, develop in the embryo as an epithelial evagination of the foregut. The liver and gallbladder function as a unit to produce, concentrate, store, and regulate the flow of bile, which is important in the emulsification and absorption of fatty acids.

LIVER

In producing bile the liver acts as an exocrine gland, but, by synthesizing and secreting plasma proteins and glucose into the blood for use elsewhere, it functions as an endocrine gland. The liver can act as a storehouse for nutrients that are received directly from the intestine by way of the portal vein. This complex gland also (1) produces cholesterol, triglycerides, and phospholipids, (2) detoxifies and processes drugs, immunoglobulin complexes, and foreign material ingested with food, (3) produces somatomedin, and (4) converts T4 to T3.

A dense connective tissue capsule (Glisson's capsule) surrounds the liver. The parenchymal cells, **hepatocytes,** are supported by a reticular fiber stroma and are arranged in cords around a **central vein** to form the roughly hexagonal **classic hepatic lobule.** Between adjacent liver lobules, connective tissue **portal canals** transmit **hepatic arteries, portal venules,** and **bile ductules** (known as the **portal triad**), together with lymphatics and nerves. In each lobule, blood flows from vessels in the portal canal through **sinusoids** that run between cords of hepatocytes into a **central vein.** Blood from the portal venule carries carbohydrates, amino acids, and vitamins to liver cells for processing, while hepatic arterial blood supplies oxygen and lipids that have entered the circulatory system by way of the thoracic duct. **Bile,** synthesized by hepatocytes, flows through **bile canaliculi,** in an opposite direction to the blood flow, to enter bile ductules in the portal canal.

Fenestrated liver sinusoids allow for passage of large molecules to and from microvillus-covered hepatocytes that are separated from the endothelium of the sinusoids by the narrow (1 to 2 μm) **space of Disse.** Fixed macrophages **(Kupffer cells)** span sinusoids and phagocytose immune complexes, opsonized bacteria, and particulate matter.

Lobule architecture may be based on endocrine function **(classic lobule),** exocrine function **(portal lobule),** or metabolic function **(liver acinus** or **Rappaport's lobule).** In the **classic lobule,** described above, plasma proteins and glucose are secreted by hepatocytes into sinusoidal blood and leave the liver by way of the central vein, collecting veins, and hepatic veins, which drain into the inferior vena cava. The **portal lobule** is triangular in shape, centered on a bile ductule into which canaliculi from adjacent lobules discharge bile, and defined peripherally by three central veins that form the apices of the lobule. In the oval **liver acinus,** a central axis is formed by terminal vessels derived from adjacent portal triads. Metabolites and oxygen are distributed to hepatocytes in three concentric zones (based on the relative decreasing nutrient concentration available to cells in each zone), which lie between the central axis of the acinus and two peripherally placed central veins into which nutrient-poor blood drains.

Hepatocytes are multifaceted cells arranged in cords between sinusoids. Where hepatocyte surfaces are apposed, **bile canaliculi** (small, extracellular tubular spaces) are formed by the membranes of adjacent cells joined, on either side of the canaliculus, by tight junctions. The cells contain numerous **mitochondria** and **lysosomes,** consistent with complex metabolic activity. **RER** and **Golgi** apparatus are associated with synthesis of plasma proteins and bile, while **SER** is involved with synthesis of cholesterol and phospholipids and the detoxification of drugs.

LIVER AND GALLBLADDER **125**

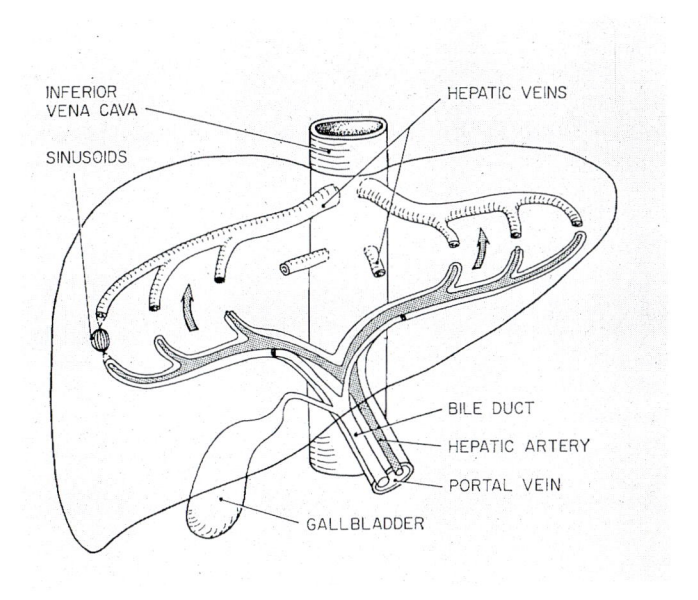

Fig. 16-1. Major vessels entering and leaving liver (hepatic artery, portal vein, and hepatic veins). Relationship of sinusoids to these vessels is shown at left.

GALLBLADDER

The cystic duct, a diverticulum of the hepatic duct system, leads to the **gallbladder,** a small hollow organ lying beneath the inferior surface of the right lobe of the liver. Its function is to concentrate bile by absorbing water from it and to store bile until required for the digestion of fat. The gallbladder mucosa is composed of simple columnar epithelial cells (with microvilli and numerous mitochondria) resting on a lamina propria, and it may be thrown into deep folds or rugae when the gallbladder is empty. Beneath the mucosa lies the muscularis externa, which is hormonally stimulated by cholecystokinin to contract when food is present in the small intestine. Contraction of the gallbladder expels bile into the duct system and then to the small intestine. A relatively thick connective tissue adventitia surrounds the organ and binds it to the liver. Its free surface is covered with (peritoneal) serosa.

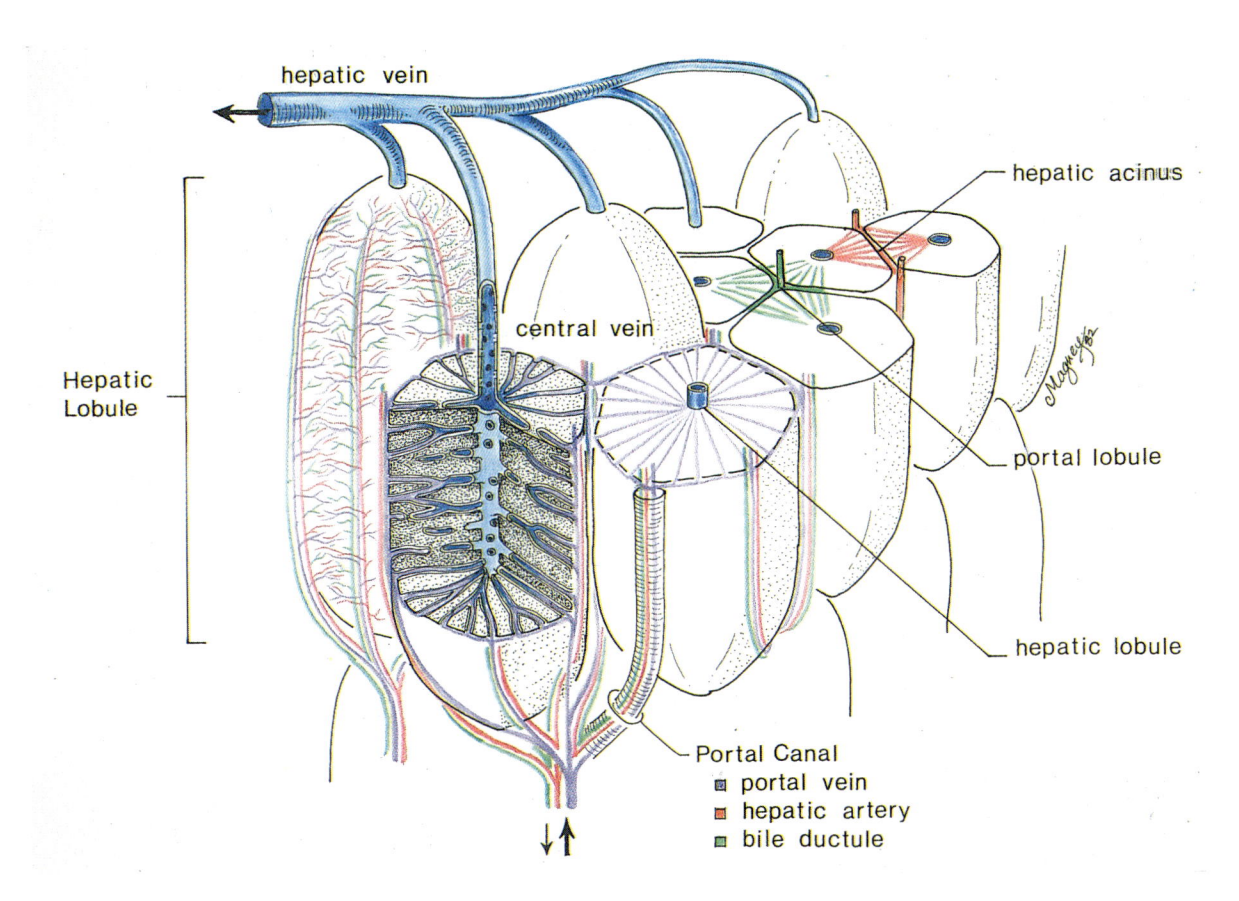

Fig. 16-2. Relationships of liver lobules to marginally located portal canals (containing vessels, lymphatics, nerves, and bile duct) and to centrally located tributaries (central veins) of hepatic vein.

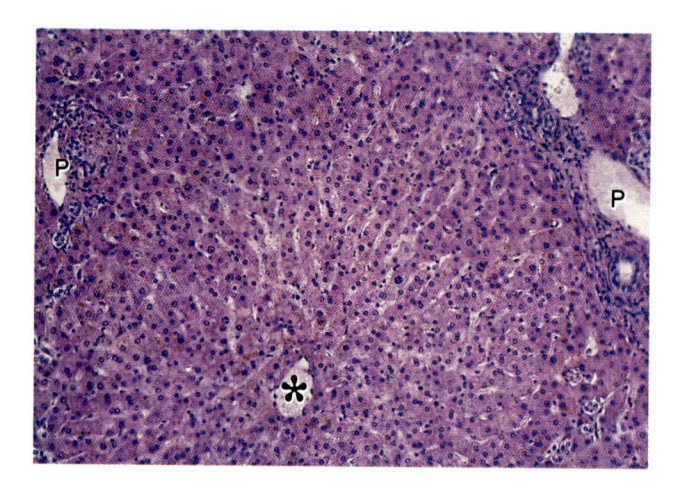

Fig. 16-3. LM of liver showing relationship between central vein (*) and portal canal *(p)*. Observe radial arrangement of cells around central vein. Compare this LM to Fig. 16-2. (H&E; ×100.)

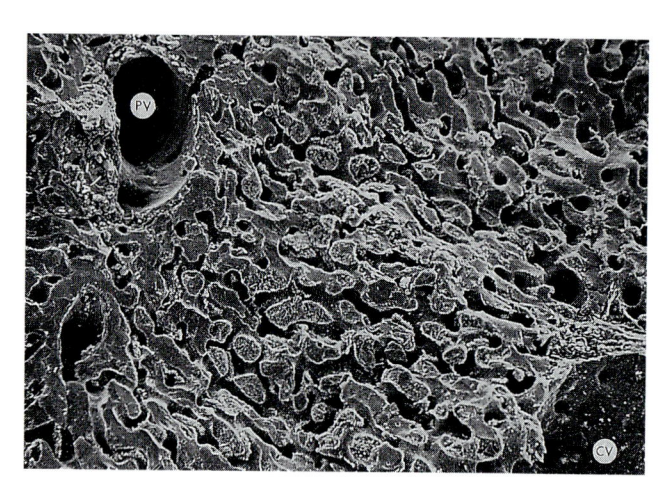

Fig. 16-4. SEM of liver illustrating radial arrangement of cells from central vein toward portal canal. *CV*, Central vein; *PV*, portal vein. Compare to Figs. 16-2 and 16-3. (×150.)

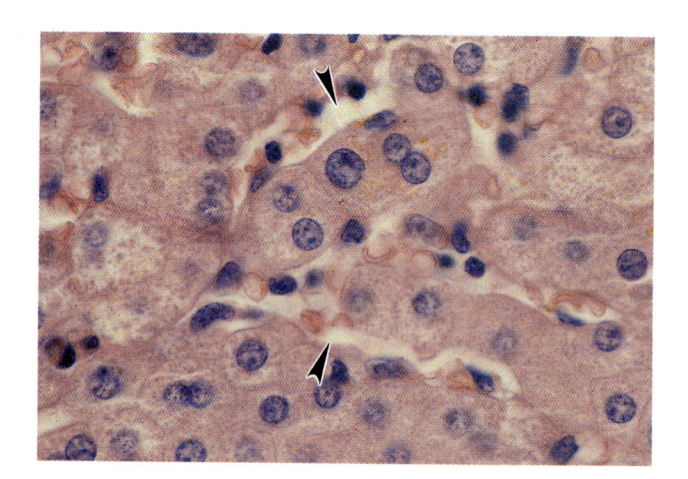

Fig. 16-5. High-magnification LM of liver parenchyma. Note cordlike arrangements of hepatocytes (liver cells) separated by liver sinusoids *(arrowheads)*. (H&E; ×600.)

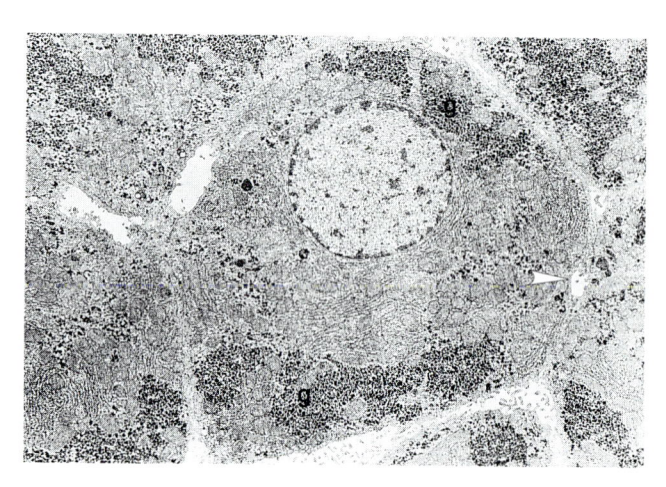

Fig. 16-6. TEM of hepatocytes from a fed rat illustrating accumulation of particulate glycogen *(g)* within cytoplasm. Bile canaliculus *(arrowhead)* can be seen between adjacent hepatocytes. (×2,800.)

LIVER AND GALLBLADDER 127

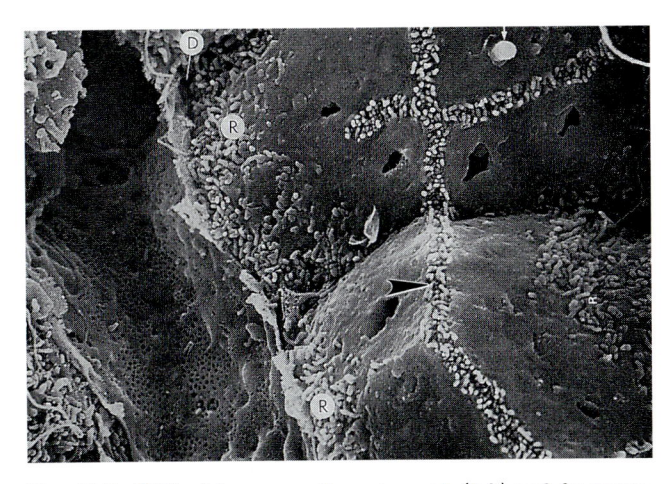

Fig. 16-7. SEM of liver revealing sinusoid *(left)* and fractures showing liver cell surfaces *(right)*. Bile canaliculi *(arrowhead)* seen on surface of hepatocytes contain small microvilli. Luminal surface of sinusoid possesses both fenestrations and large perforations. In space of Disse (D), surface of hepatocyte facing sinusoidal lumen is covered by microvilli (R). (×2,500.)

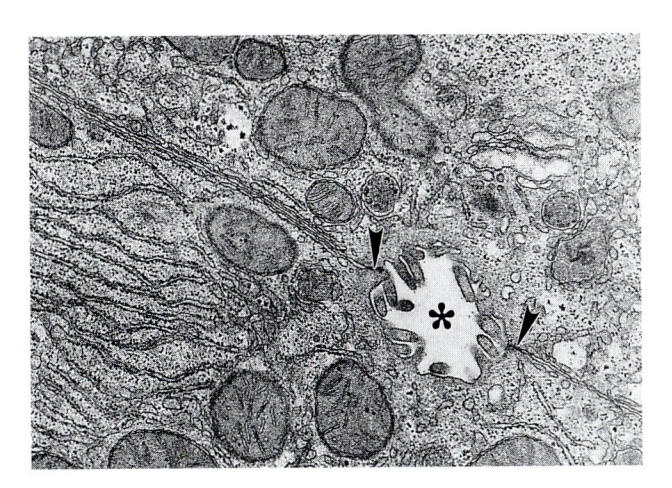

Fig. 16-8. TEM of interface between two hepatocytes revealing bile canaliculus (*). Luminal surface of canaliculus exhibits numerous microvilli and is sealed from lateral intercellular spaces by zonulae occludens *(arrowheads)* between adjacent cells. Observe Golgi apparatus and pericanalicular dense bodies within hepatocytes (×15,000.)

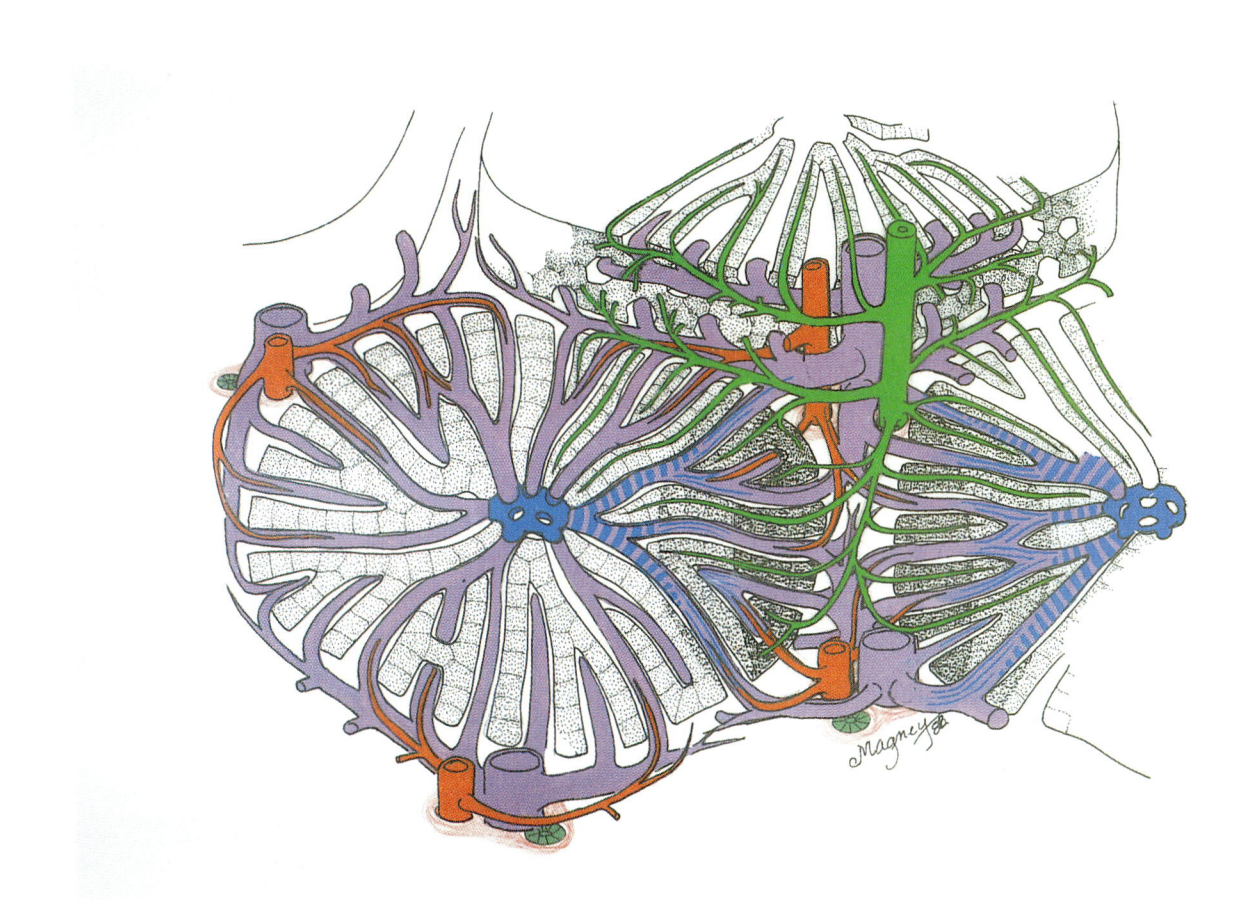

Fig. 16-9. Classic lobule showing flow of blood from portal triads to central vein and flow of bile from canaliculi in liver cords to bile ducts in portal triad.

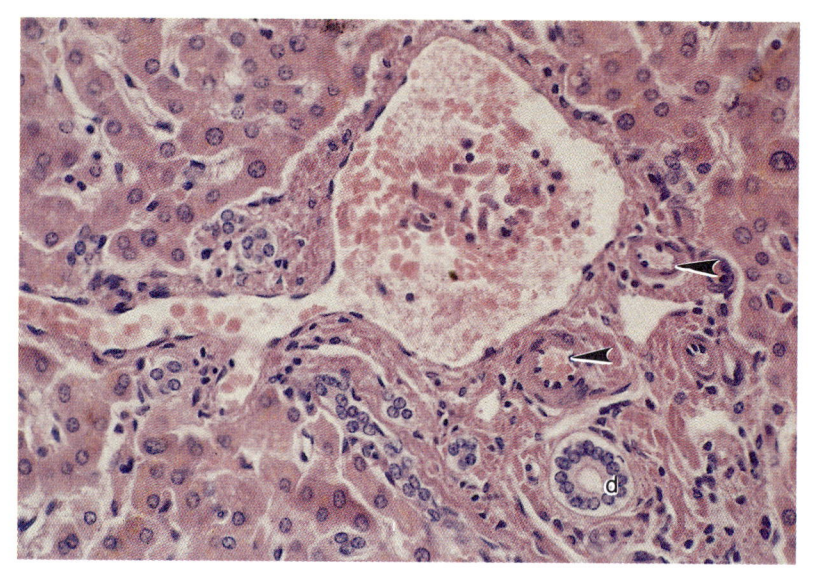

Fig. 16-10. LM of portal triad. Portal vein *(center)* has large branch *(left)* from which several smaller branches extend to supply sinusoids that lie between cords, or plates, of liver cells. Other members of triad are bile ductule *(d)* and branches of hepatic artery *(arrowheads)*. (H&E; ×450.)

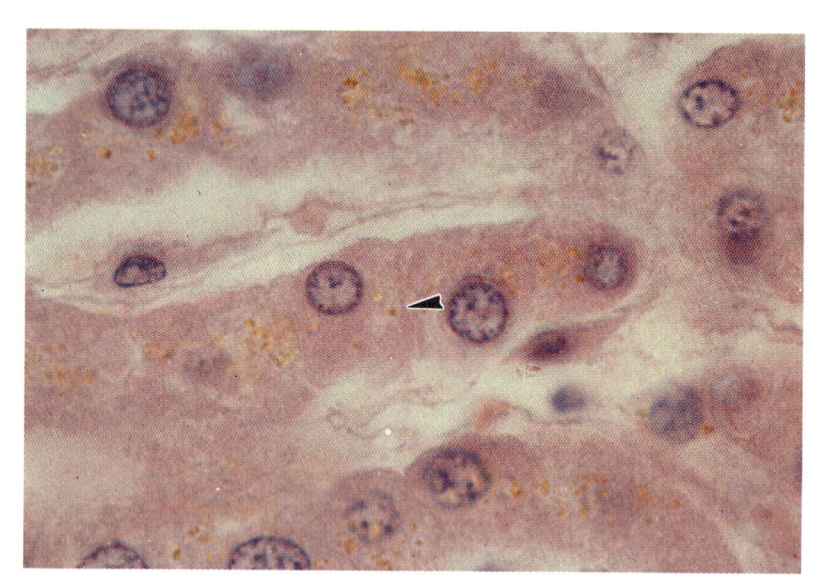

Fig. 16-11. High-magnification LM of liver cords and adjacent sinusoids. Two liver cells *(center)* abut one another and contain a small bile canaliculus *(arrowhead)* at their interface. Gold-brown lipofuscin pigment is seen in most of these cells. (H&E; ×900.)

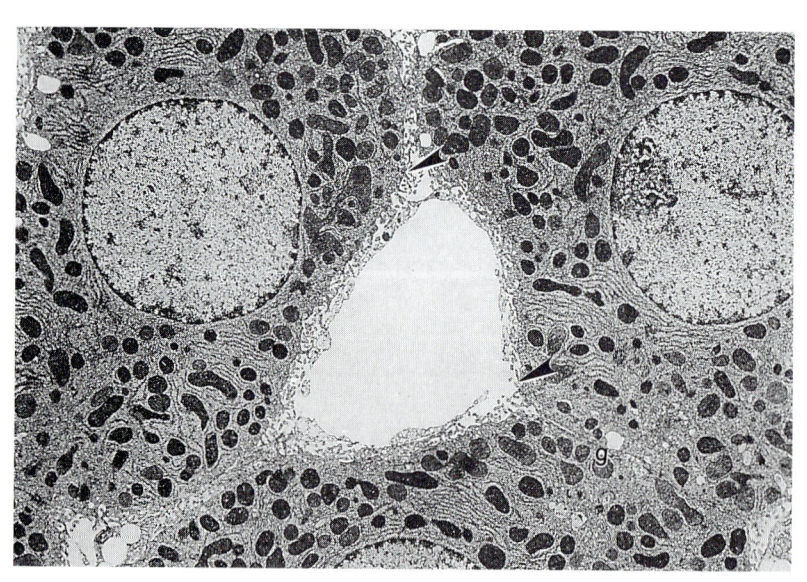

Fig. 16-12. TEM of liver parenchyma showing relationships of hepatocytes to liver sinusoid. Luminal portion of hepatocyte plasmalemma, exposed to sinusoid, possesses microvilli as surface specialization. Where adjacent hepatocytes appose each other, their membranes may be characterized by gap junctions *(g)* and microvilli *(arrowheads)*. Observe numerous mitochondria. (×3,100.)

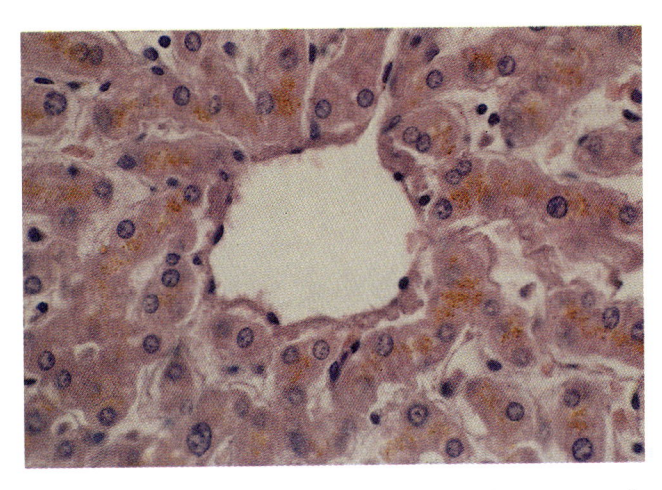

Fig. 16-13. LM of central vein of liver lobule. Hepatocytes adjacent to central vein contain abundant amounts of lipofuscin pigment. Sinusoids can be seen *(top)* emptying into central vein. (H&E; ×500.)

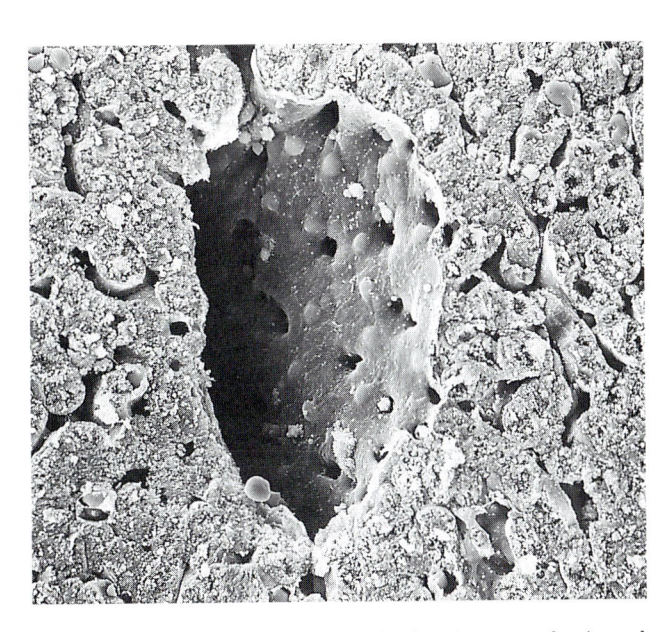

Fig. 16-14. SEM of classic liver lobule showing central vein and openings of sinusoids into lumen. (×500.)

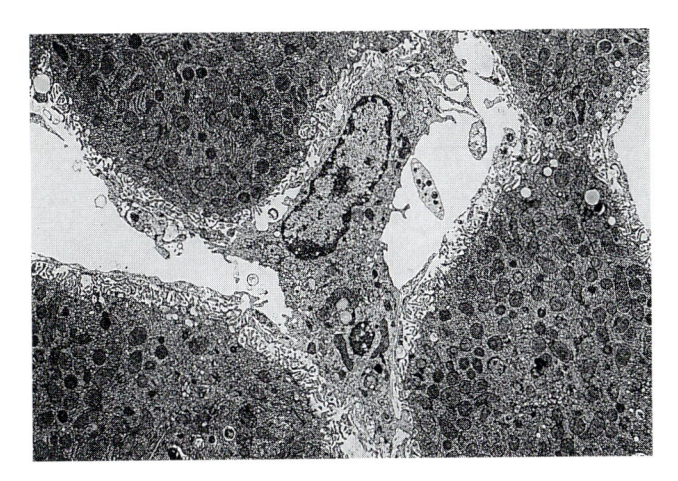

Fig. 16-15. TEM of rat liver showing a Kupffer cell with short cytoplasmic processes spanning sinusoidal lumen. This cell has many endocytic functions, is derived from monocyte precursors in bone marrow, and is part of mononuclear phagocyte system. (×2,500.)

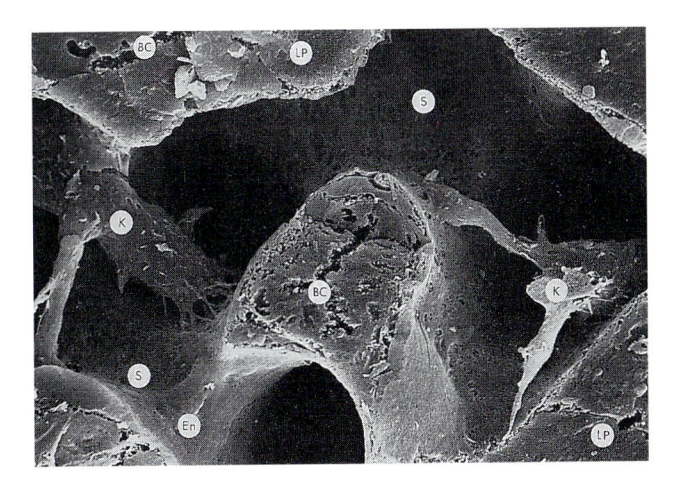

Fig. 16-16. SEM of fracture surface exposing liver sinusoids. Kupffer cells can be seen spanning sinusoidal lumen at left and right. *K*, Kupffer cells; *S*, sinusoidal lumen; *En*, endothelial cell; *BC*, bile canaliculus; *LP*, liver plate. (×1,000.)

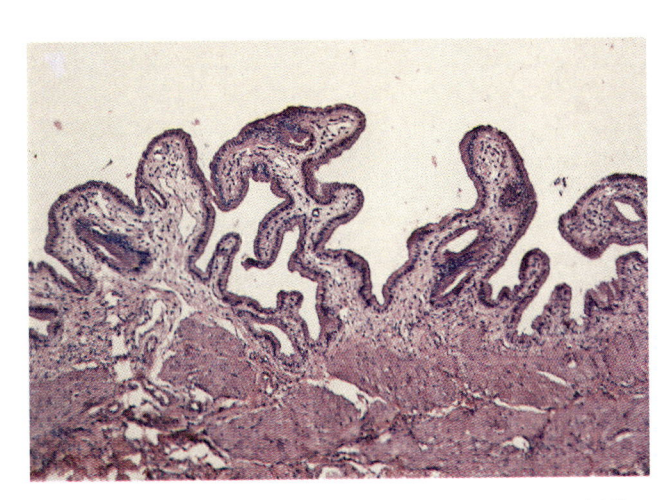

Fig. 16-17. Low-magnification LM showing pronounced folding of gallbladder mucosa. (H&E; ×25.)

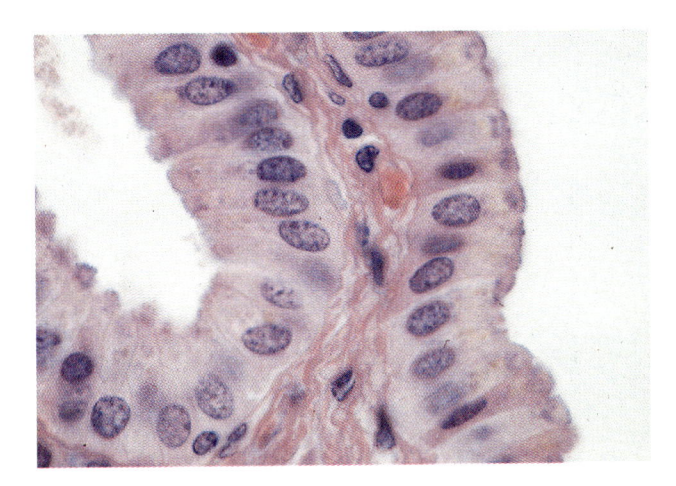

Fig. 16-18. High-magnification LM of gallbladder mucosa. Epithelium consists of simple columnar cells with well-developed microvillous border. Lamina propria is rich in blood vessels and contains connective tissue fibers. (H&E; ×800.)

CHAPTER 17
RESPIRATORY SYSTEM

THE RESPIRATORY SYSTEM can be divided into a **conducting** portion and a **respiratory** region. The function of the conducting portion is to warm or cool air, humidify it, and remove particulate matter from it as it moves into the respiratory region where exchange of gasses between air and blood **(external respiration)** takes place. **Internal respiration** describes gaseous exchange between blood and the cells of the bodily tissues. Lung tissues are supplied oxygenated blood by the **bronchial arteries,** branches of the thoracic aorta. From the right ventricle, **pulmonary arteries** carry deoxygenated blood to the alveolar capillary beds, where carbon dioxide is exchanged for oxygen. Venous blood from both arterial systems returns to the left atrium through **pulmonary veins.**

CONDUCTING PORTION

Organs of the conducting portion of the respiratory system include **nasal cavity, nasopharynx, larynx, trachea,** several **bronchi** of decreasing size, many generations of **bronchioles, and terminal bronchioles.** Characteristics that many of these organs share are **respiratory epithelium** (pseudostratified columnar epithelium with goblet cells and cilia), **seromucous glands** in the lamina propria, **smooth muscle, elastic fibers,** and **cartilage.** Changes along the course of the conducting airways include gradual disappearance of cartilage, glands, and cilia; reduction in the height of the epithelium to simple cuboidal epithelium; and an increase in smooth muscle.

Air passing through the nasal cavity is warmed by a venous plexus immediately beneath the respiratory epithelium lining the cavity. Mucus secreted by goblet cells of the epithelium and glands in the lamina propria moistens the air and traps particulate matter, which is then transported by ciliary action to the pharynx, where it is expectorated or swallowed. Beneath the respiratory epithelium of the nasopharynx, a collection of lymphatic nodules (pharyngeal tonsils) provides a first line of defense to pathogens. Air passes from the nasopharynx through the oropharynx into the **larynx,** the initial segment of the tubular "airway" leading to the lungs.

The walls of the larynx are supported by irregularly shaped hyaline cartilages that keep the airway open. These cartilages provide attachment for **vocal cords** and for skeletal muscle, whose movements regulate volume and pitch of the voice. The larynx is entirely lined with respiratory epithelium except for the true vocal cords (stratified squamous nonkeratinized epithelium), which are subject to abrasion as a result of vibration of the cords as air expelled from the lungs passes between them. The opening between pharynx and larynx is protected by one of the laryngeal cartilages, the **epiglottis,** which prevents food from entering the airway.

The larynx is continuous inferiorly with the **trachea,** a hollow, rigid tube supported by approximately 16 horseshoe-shaped cartilages and closed posteriorly by the trachealis (smooth) muscle. The trachea ends by dividing into right and left **primary bronchi.**

Cartilage supporting the walls of the bronchi is shaped in irregular plates within which smooth muscle encircles the lumen. Primary bronchi enter lung tissue at the hilum and branch dichotomously many times into subdivisions called lobes and lobules. When branching has reduced the diameter of the tube to less than 1 mm, cartilage disappears, the airway wall is supported by smooth muscle and connective tissue, and the airway is called a **bronchiole.**

Bronchioles undergo further branching, during which the epithelium changes to simple columnar and smooth muscle and elastic fibers predominate. The final segment of the conducting portion of the respiratory system is called the **terminal bronchiole.**

RESPIRATORY REGION

Terminal bronchioles give rise to **respiratory bronchioles,** where gaseous exchange first take place in small spherical outpocketings of the bronchiolar wall called **alveoli.** The principal epithelial **(type I)** cell of an alveolus is a simple squamous cell; a **"great alveolar", septal** or **type II** cell is cuboidal and secretes surface tension–reducing **surfactant.** Type I cells rest on a basement membrane fused with that of the endothelial cells of the capillaries surrounding each alveolus. This trilamminar structure is called the **respiratory membrane,** or the **blood-air barrier,** and it is across this membrane that gases diffuse between air and blood.

Respiratory bronchioles, in turn, branch to become **alveolar ducts,** alveolus-studded passageways terminating in rotunda-like spaces called **alveolar sacs** from which clusters of individual alveoli arise. Adjacent alvioli are connected by openings called **alveolar pores,** which serve to equalize intra-alveolar air pressure. **Alveolar macrophages,** also called **dust cells,** are often visible in alveoli. In conjunction with surfactant, mucus, and cilia that beat toward the pharynx, these macrophages provide for the defense of the lung tissues.

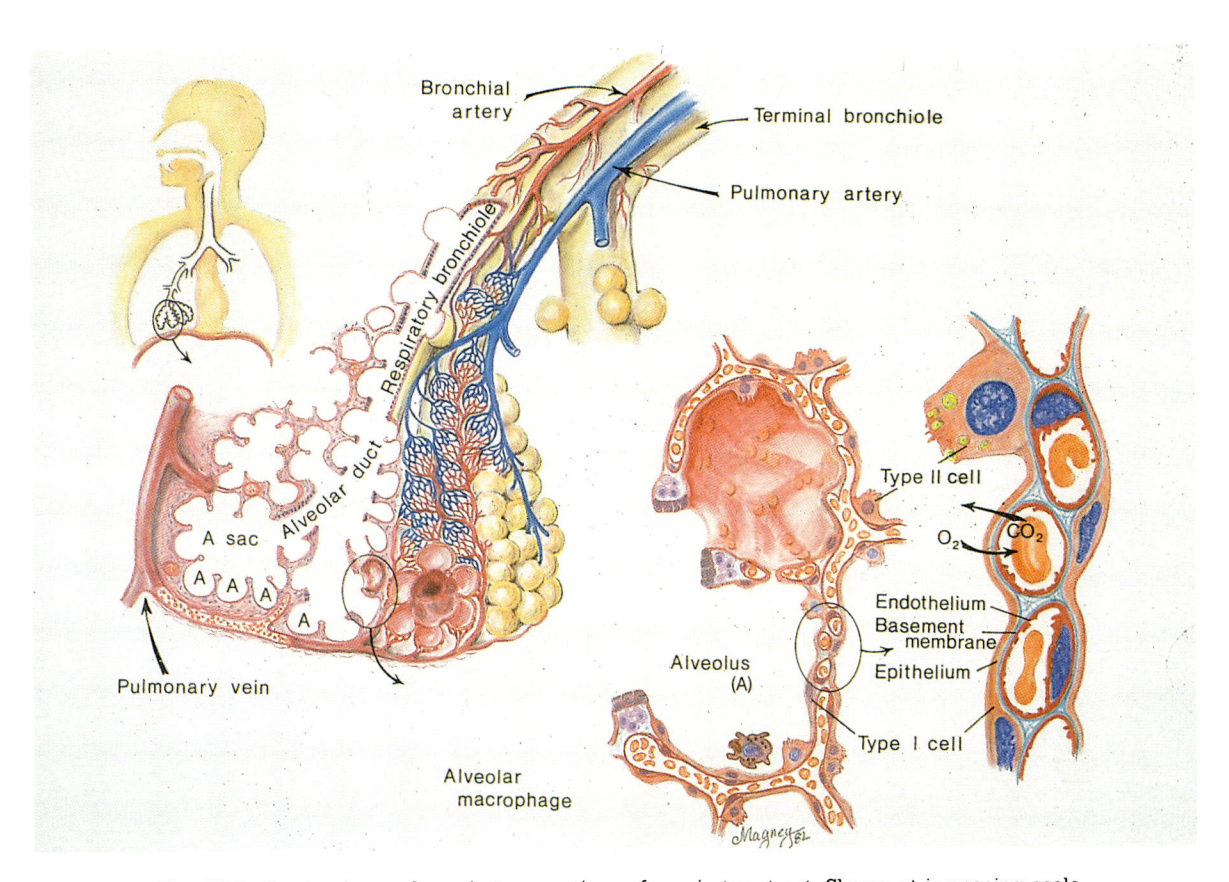

Fig. 17-1. Conducting and respiratory portions of respiratory tract. Shown at increasing scale are respiratory portion of lung, two alveoli depicting surface topography and cross sectional structure of alveolar wall, and microanatomy of cells composing blood-air barrier.

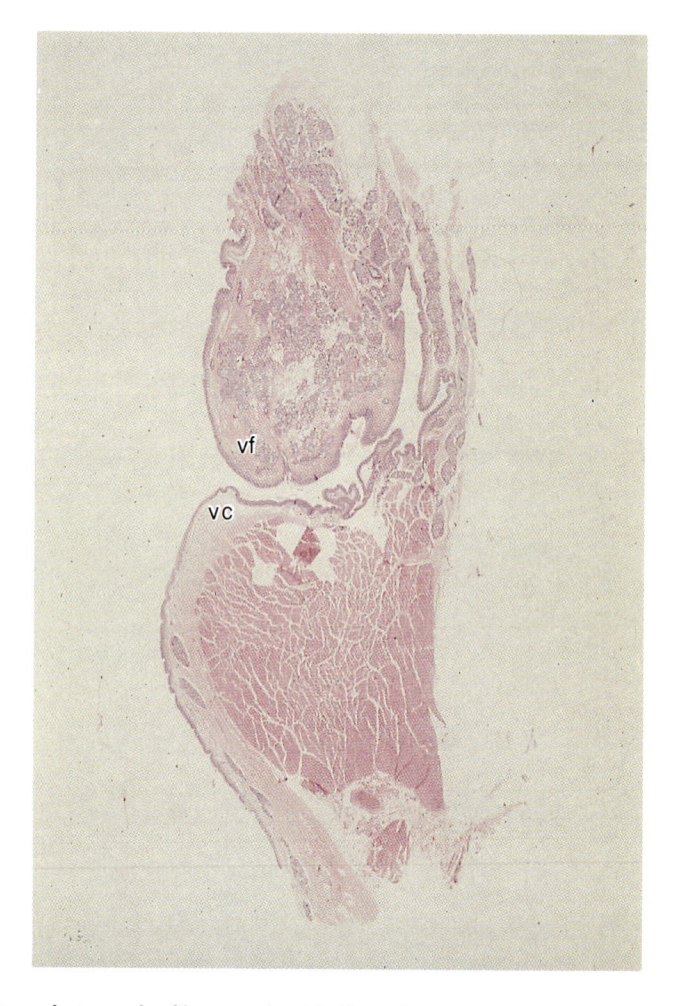

Fig. 17-2. Macrophotograph of laryngeal epithelium showing both vestibular folds *(vf)* or false vocal cords and true vocal cords *(vc)*. Between them, opening of laryngeal saccule can be seen. Many seromucous glands are present within vestibular fold; within vocal cord fibroelastic connective tissue underlies epithelium. Vocalis muscle, part of thyroarytenoid, is deep to fibroelastic connective tissue. (H&E; ×6.)

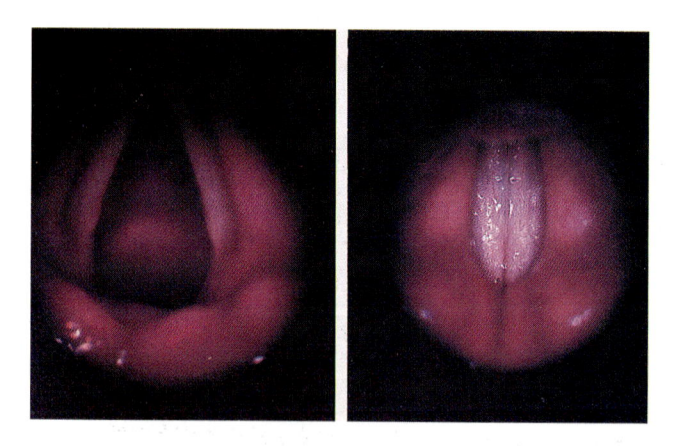

Fig. 17-3. Endoscopic views of vocal cords within larynx. By changes in position of laryngeal cartilages, rima glottidis, or opening, between vocal cords can be adjusted. Relaxed vocal cords *(left)* are wide open at rest, i.e., when we breathe but do not speak. At right, vocal cords are closed and appear white. During speech stretched vocal cords form a narrow opening through which air is forced, causing them to vibrate.

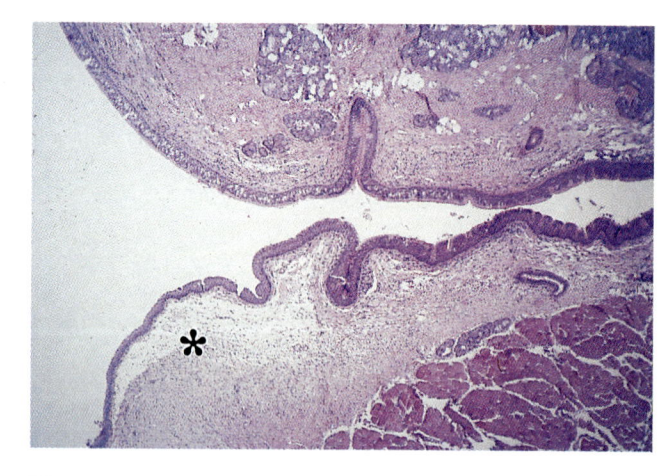

Fig. 17-4. LM of vestibular fold and true vocal cord. Observe glands within former and fibroelastic connective tissue (*) within latter. True vocal cord is lined with stratified squamous epithelium; vestibular fold with pseudostratified columnar epithelium. (H&E; ×125.)

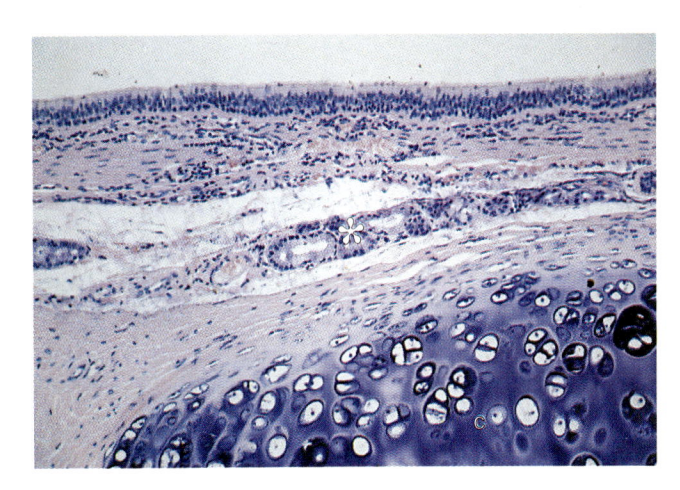

Fig. 17-5. LM of tracheal wall. Observe pseudostratified columnar epithelium characteristic of respiratory tract, underlying fibroelastic tissue, small seromucous glands (*), and portion of cartilaginous ring (c). (H&E; ×200.)

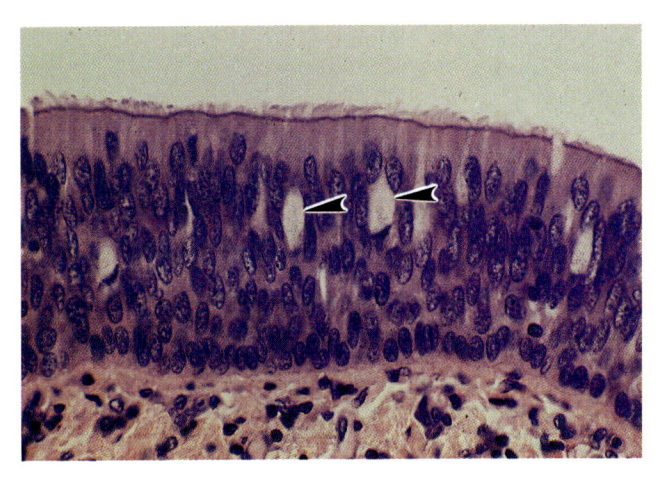

Fig. 17-6. High-magnification LM of pseudostratified columnar epithelium of trachea. Cell types include mucous cells (arrowheads), ciliated cells, basal cells involved in mitotic renewal of epithelium, endocrine cells, and nonciliated cells with extensive microvillous border. Basement membrane separates epithelium from underlying lamina propria. (H&E; ×500.)

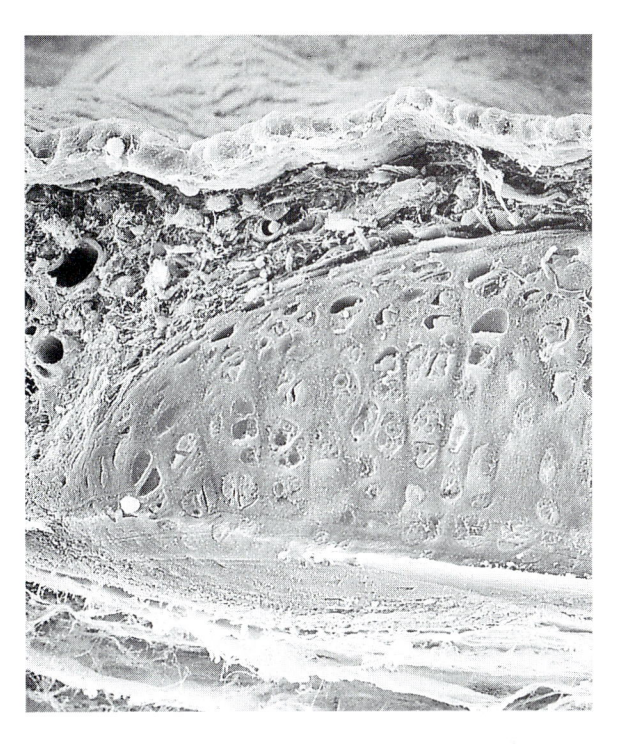

Fig. 17-7. SEM of fractured tracheal wall. Compare with Fig. 17-5, observing location of pseudostratified columnar epithelium, underlying fibroelastic tissue, and portion of cartilaginous ring. (×300.)

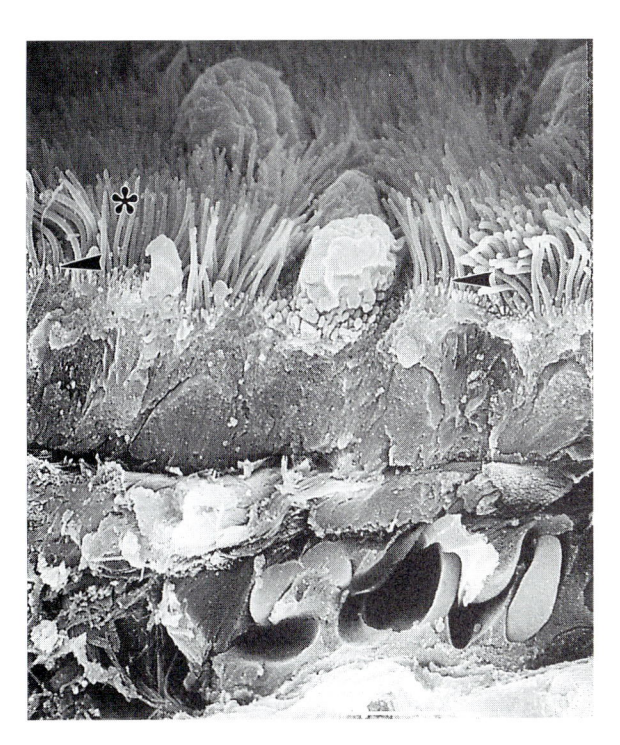

Fig. 17-8. SEM of tracheal epithelium. Dome-shaped cells indicate sites of secretory activity. Note appearance of cilia (*) and microvilli (arrowheads) in surrounding cells and presence of capillaries within lamina propria. (×3,000.)

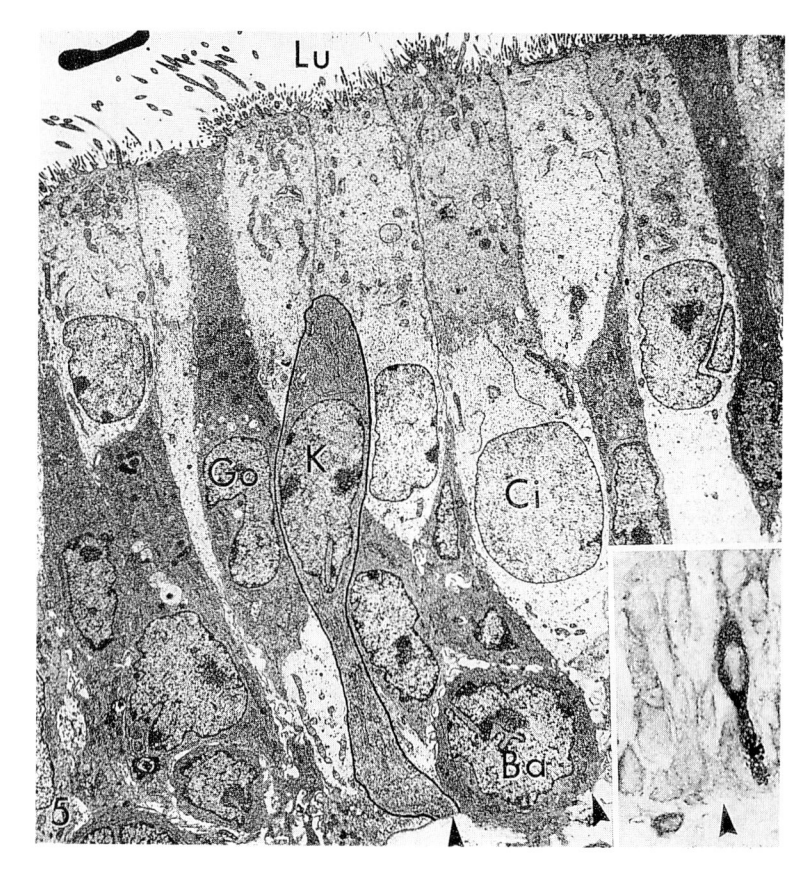

Fig. 17-9. TEM of tracheal epithelium. Ciliated cells *(Ci)*, basal cells *(Ba)*, endocrine cells *(K)*, and cells possessing microvillous border can be distinguished. Inset LM *(lower right)* illustrates staining for hormones within endocrine cell, outlined in black in center of field. *Lu,* lumen; *Go,* goblet cell. (×1,800.)

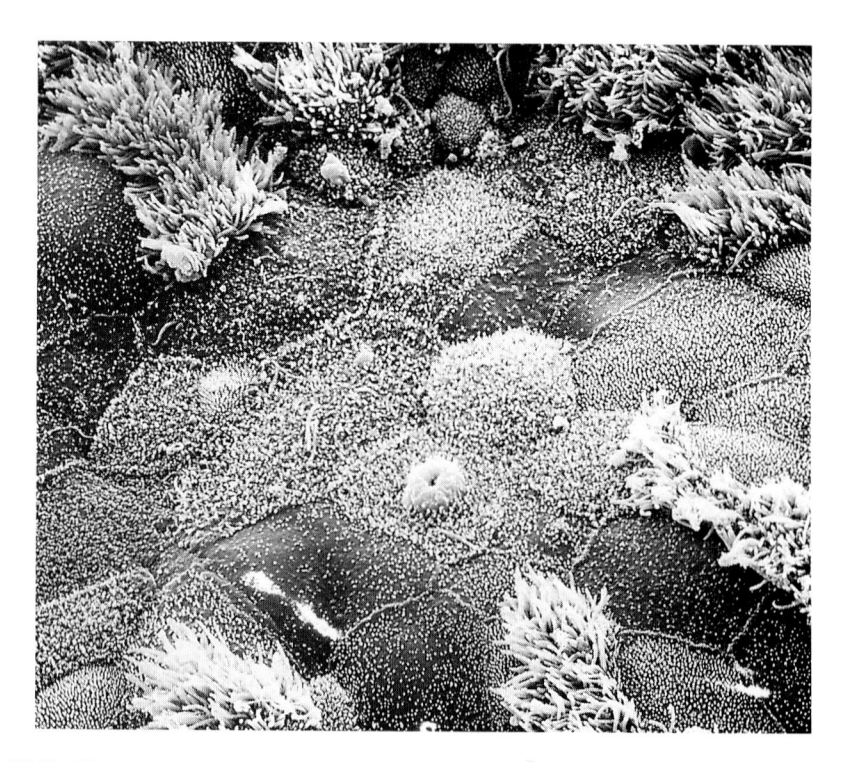

Fig. 17-10. Higher-magnification SEM of epithelial surface of trachea. Observe presence of ciliated cells and cells possessing microvilli. Presence of craterlike structures in surface of some cells suggests possible secretory activity. Higher density of microvilli occurs near lateral margin of cells, thereby outlining their borders. (×2,000.)

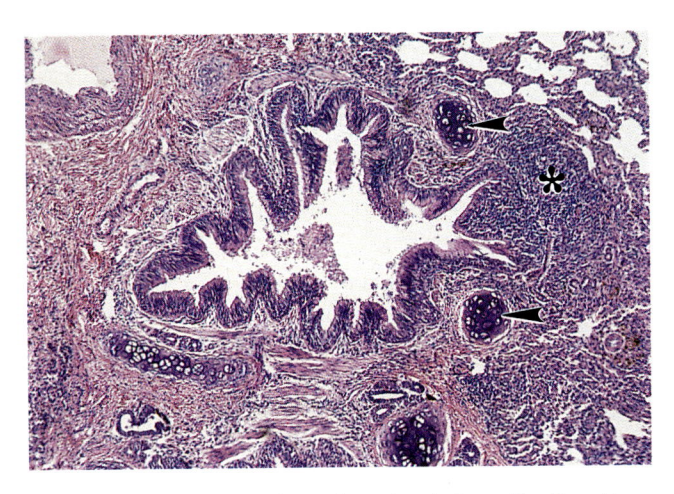

Fig. 17-11. LM of cartilaginous bronchus in lung. Small portions of hyaline cartilage *(arrowheads)* can be seen beneath mucosal surface. Substantial amounts of lymphoid tissue (*) are also present. (H&E; ×20.)

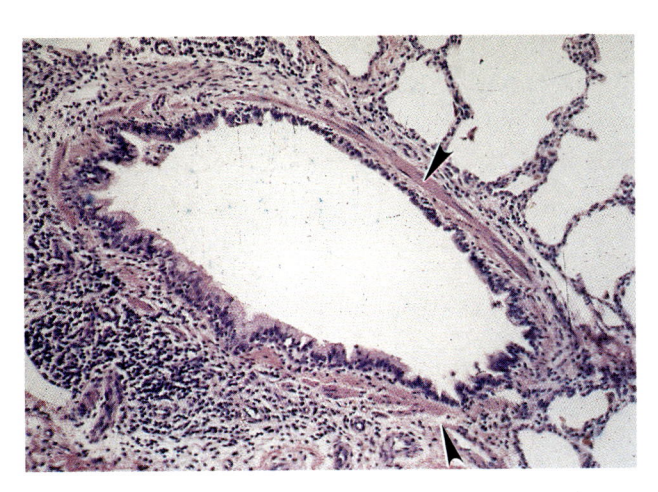

Fig. 17-12. LM of bronchiole in lung. Smooth muscle *(arrowheads)* within wall plays important role in regulating diameter of bronchiole (H&E; ×100.)

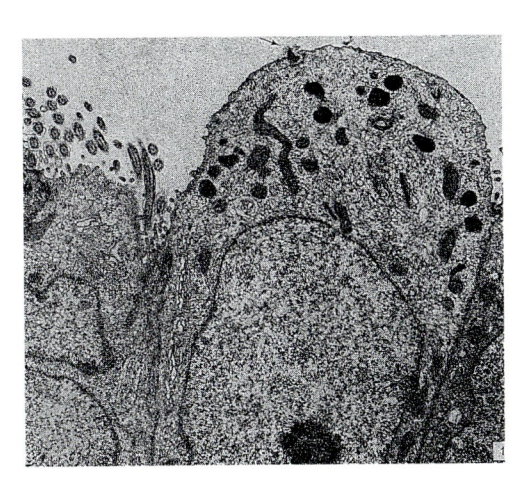

Fig. 17-13. TEM of bronchiolar epithelium showing protrusion of Clara cell into lumen. Note ciliated cell at left. (×12,000.)

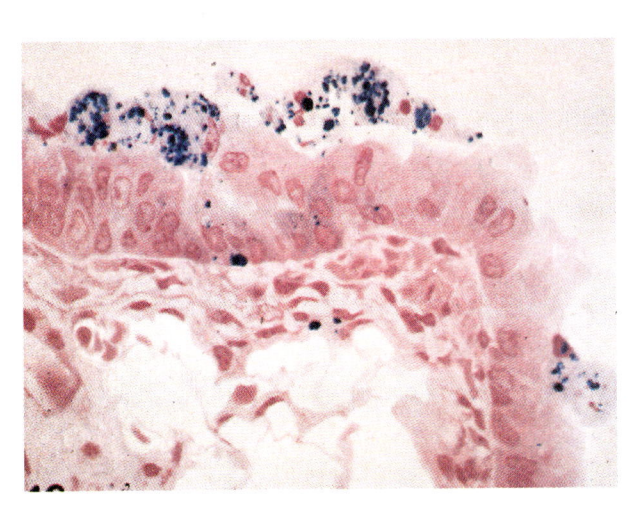

Fig. 17-14. LM of bronchiolar epithelium illustrating presence of clusters of macrophages on luminal surface of epithelium. (colloidal iron and Ponceau counterstain; ×500.)

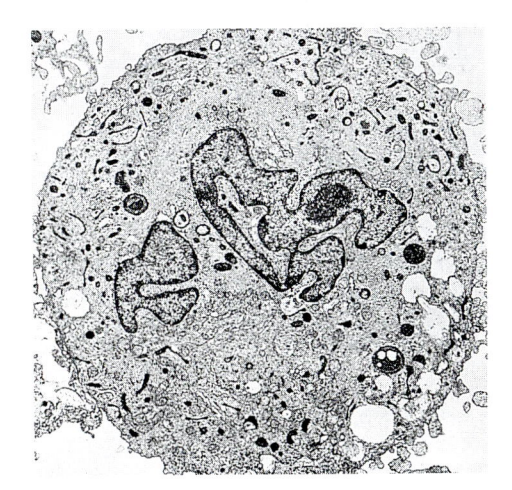

Fig. 17-15. TEM of alveolar macrophage washed from lungs of normal, nonsmoking subject. (×4,500.)

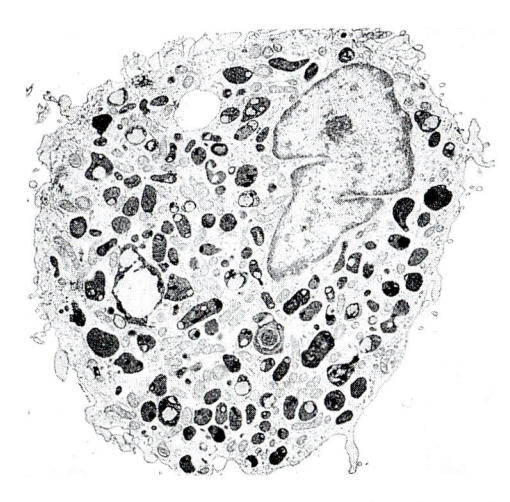

Fig. 17-16. TEM of alveolar macrophage from lungs of normal, tobacco-smoking subject. Note large number of residual bodies with myelin figures. (×4,500.)

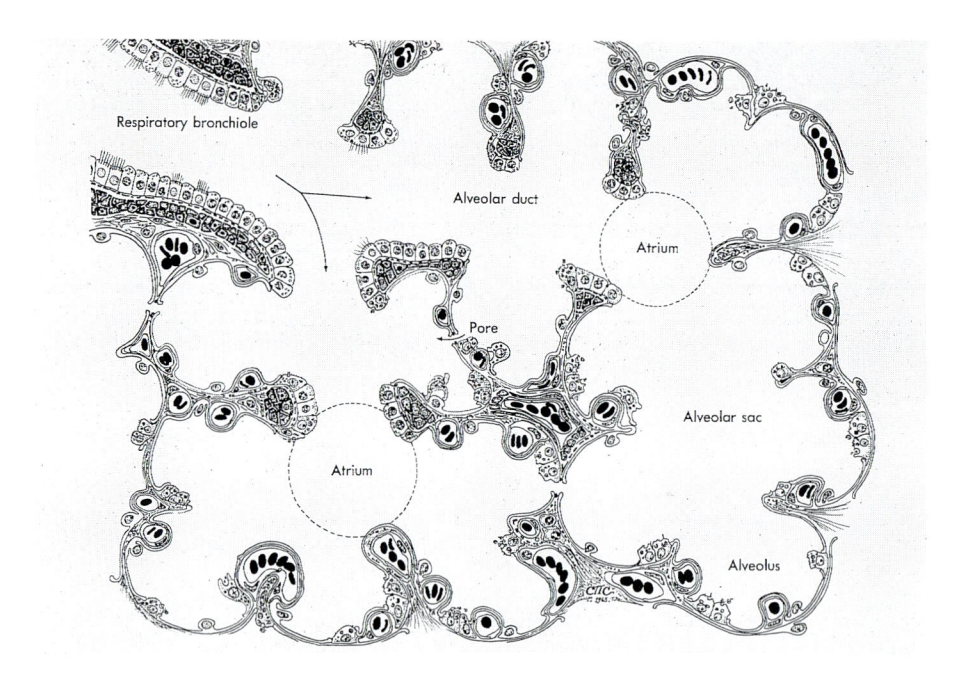

Fig. 17-17. Respiratory subdivisions in lung showing continuity of airway from respiratory bronchiole through alveolar duct to alveolar sac and alveoli. Gaseous exchange can occur in alveoli associated with respiratory bronchiole *(upper right)*. Alveolar duct has multiple openings to alveoli or alveolar sacs and terminates in space called atrium, which serves as common entrance into multiple avleolar sacs *(circular areas)*. Capillaries containing red blood cells can be seen immediately beneath epithelial lining of alveololi, and smooth muscle cells are present in thickened rim surrounding opening to individual alveoli.

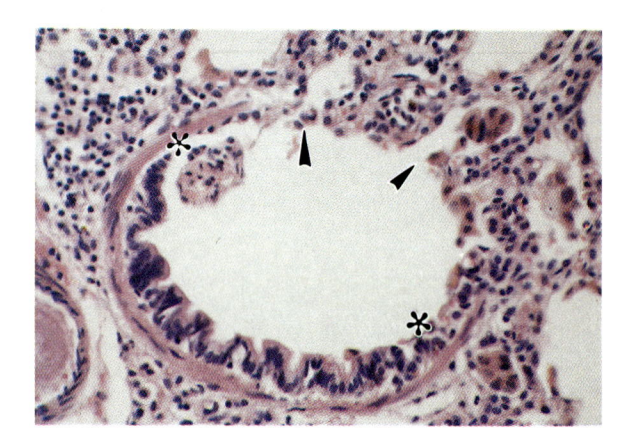

Fig. 17-18. LM of respiratory bronchiole in lung. Observe changes (*) in epithelium in transition from terminal bronchiole to respiratory bronchiole. Note openings *(arrowheads)* of alveoli. (H&E; ×200.)

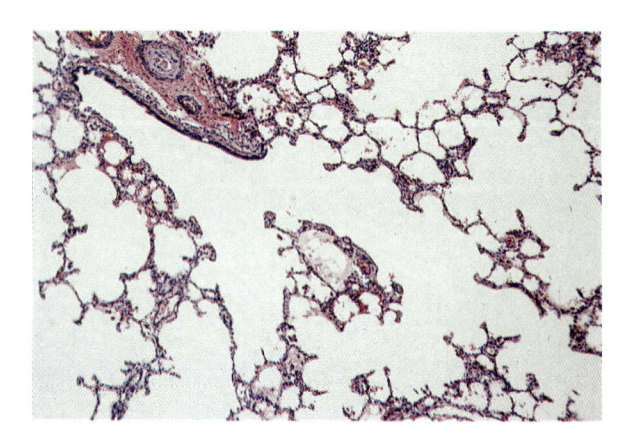

Fig. 17-19. Low-magnification LM of lung. Compare with Fig. 17-17 and find examples corresponding to respiratory bronchiole, alveolar duct, atrium, alveolar sac, and alveoli. (H&E; ×20.)

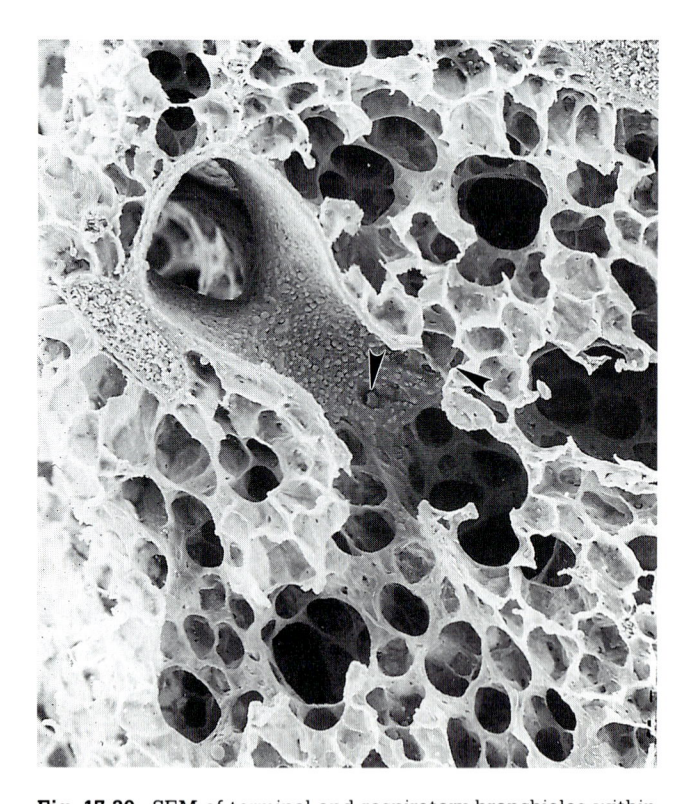

Fig. 17-20. SEM of terminal and respiratory bronchioles within rat lung. Terminal and respiratory bronchioles can be differentiated by openings of alveoli *(arrowheads)* into latter. (×140.)

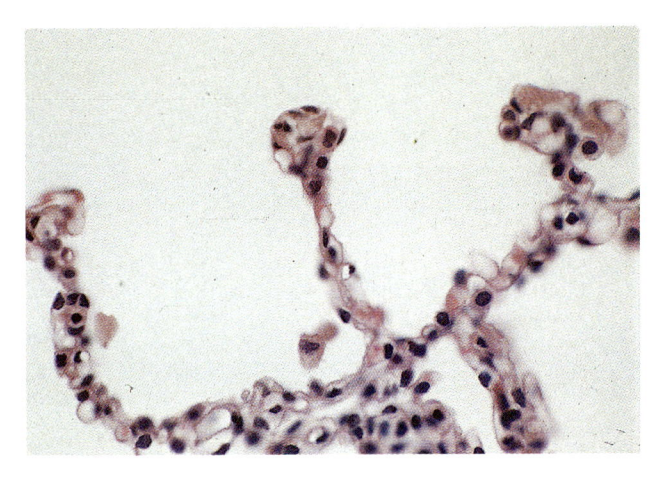

Fig. 17-21. LM of two adjacent alveoli in lung. Locate capillaries by identifying red blood cells within them. Blood-air barrier consists of alveolar epithelium, capillary endothelium, and their fused basement membranes. (H&E; ×300.)

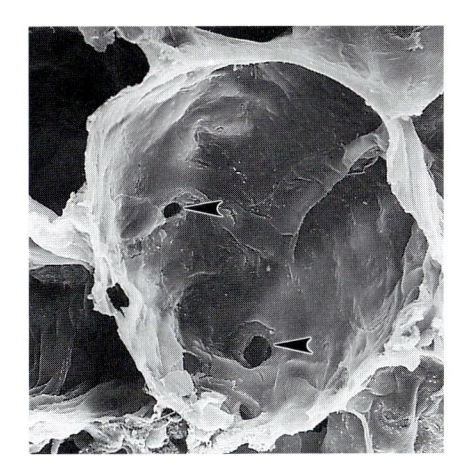

Fig. 17-22. SEM of alveolus in rat lung. Capillary loops can be seen in relief beneath epithelium lining alveolus. Openings of alveolar pores *(arrowheads)* are also visible. (×500.)

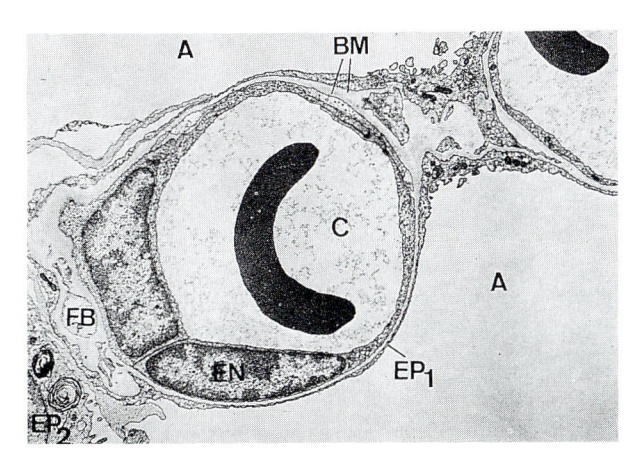

Fig. 17-23. TEM of interalveolar wall. Note thickness of wall and route that gas molecules must traverse to move from red blood cell to alveolar space and vice versa. *A*, alveolar space; *BM*, basement membrane; *C*, capillary lumen; *EP1*, type I epithelial cell; *EP2*, type II epithelial cell; *FB*, fibroblast. (×4,000.)

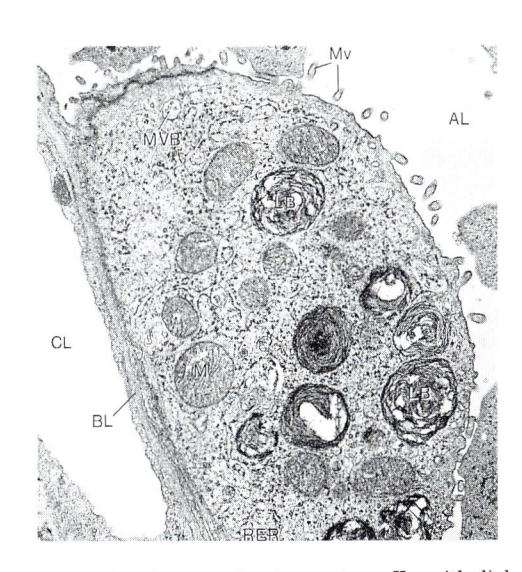

Fig. 17-24. TEM of great alveolar, or type II, epithelial cell in rat lung. Type II cell is larger than adjacent type I cells and possesses large numbers of lamellar bodies containing surfactant. *AL*, alveolar lumen; *Mv*, microvilli; *MVB*, multivesicular body; *LB*, lamellar body; *CL*, capillary lumen; *BL*, fused basement membrane of endothelial cell and type II cell; *M*, mitochondria. (×8,100.)

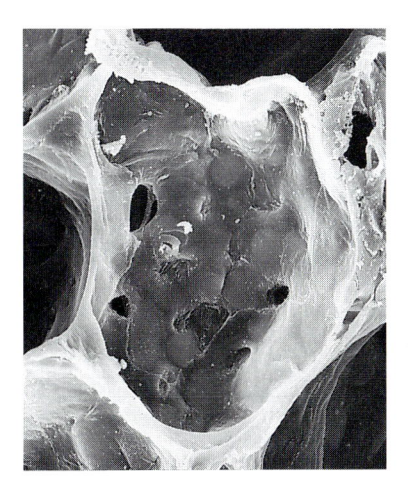

Fig. 17-25. SEM of alveolus in rat lung. Note presence of alveolar pores in wall of alveolus that permit equilibration of air pressure within adjacent alveoli. (×500.)

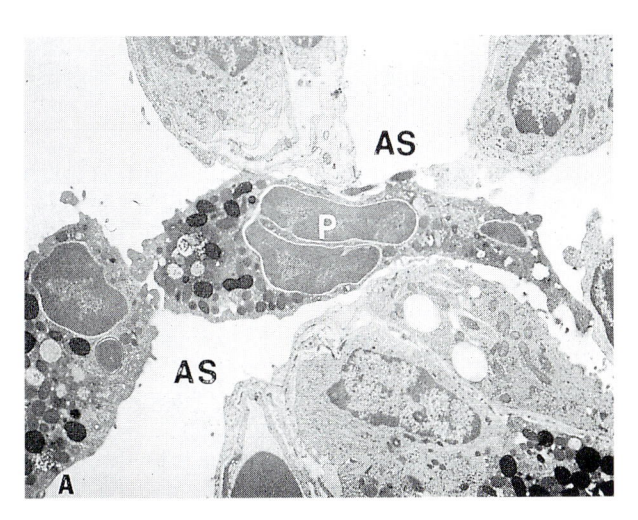

Fig. 17-26. TEM of alveolar pore between adjacent alveoli. Leukocytes *(P)* are seen passing from one alveolar space *(AS)* into an adjacent alveolar space. (×2,500.)

CHAPTER 18

URINARY SYSTEM

THE **KIDNEY** IS a bean-shaped organ with a lateral convex border and a medial concave border called the hilum through which vessels, nerves, lymphatics, and the ureter enter or leave the organ. The kidney regulates the volume and composition of body fluids and secretes substances into the blood that influence blood pressure and erythropoiesis. The end product of kidney function is **urine,** which leaves the kidney and enters a series of tubular organs, the **urinary tract,** consisting of **renal pelvis, ureters, urinary bladder,** and **urethra.** Blood is supplied to each kidney by a direct branch of the abdominal aorta, the **renal artery,** and it is drained by a **renal vein** into the inferior vena cava.

KIDNEY

A thin capsule of collagen fibers and a scanty interstitial reticular fiber stroma support epithelial cells arranged in **uriniferous tubules** that make up the parenchma of the kidney. The distribution of uriniferous tubules gives a characteristic pattern to the hemisected kidney, dividing it into **cortex** and **medulla.** Six to 17 cone-shaped **medullary pyramids** are arranged around a central cavity called the **renal sinus.** The apex **(papilla)** of each pyramid inserts into a **minor calyx,** a cup-shaped initial segment of the urinary tract lying within the renal sinus. Several minor calyces join to form a **major calyx,** and two or three major calyces coalesce into the **renal pelvis.** The base of each medullary pyramid is oriented toward the capsule and is separated from it by **cortex,** which also extends inward between the pyramids as **renal columns of Bertin.** A lobe is composed of a medullary pyramid and its overlying and surrounding cortex.

Uriniferous tubules are tightly packed within cortex and medulla, separated only by small amounts of stroma. Each uriniferous tubule is subdivided into the **nephron,** where urine is formed, and the **collecting duct,** which drains urine through the papilla into a minor calyx. A nephron consists of a **renal corpuscle** confluent with a **renal tubule.** The renal corpuscle is formed by a blind end of the tubule reflected onto a tuft of capillaries, the **glomerulus. Visceral epithelium** is modified tubular epithelium in contact with the capillary endothelium. It is separated by the **urinary space** from the **parietal epithelium,** which forms **Bowman's capsule.**

At the **urinary pole** of the renal corpuscle, Bowman's capsule narrows to become the first (proximal) part of the renal tubule. The glomerulus is supplied with blood by an **afferent arteriole** and is drained by an **efferent arteriole.** These vessels enter and leave the renal corpuscle at its **vascular pole,** opposite the urinary pole. Glomerular capillaries are arranged into **lobules** with central (axial) regions where anastomoses occur and peripheral regions that border on the urinary space.

The renal artery divides into **segmental arteries** at the hilum, and each supplies a discrete portion of the kidney. These branch into **interlobar arteries** that run between medullary pyramids to the corticomedullary interface, where they arch over the base of the pyramid as **arcuate arteries.** Each arcuate artery gives off a number of **interlobular arteries,** which, as they course toward the kidney capsule, define the periphery of a unit of parenchyma called a **lobule. Afferent arterioles** branch from the interlobular artery, and each supplies a glomerular capillary bed where filtration of blood takes place, with the filtrate passing into the urinary space and the renal tubule.

Efferent arterioles draining the glomerulus are part of an arterial portal system. They immediately branch into a second capillary plexus surrounding the convoluted renal tubules. If the renal corpuscle is close to the renal capsule (superficial), the efferent arteriole provides a **peritubular** capillary plexus around cortical tubules; if the corpuscle lies deep in the cortex (juxtamedullary), the second capillary bed enters the medulla parallel with the renal tubule and is called the **vasa rectae.** Both capillary beds then drain into arcuate veins, interlobar veins, and renal vein.

Within the renal corpuscle are fenestrated **endothelial cells** of the capillaries, contractile **mesangial cells** and **matrix** supporting axial regions of the glomerulus,

podocytes (modified visceral epithelial cells), and simple squamous parietal epithelial cells that form Bowman's capsule. Hydrostatic pressure forces water and ions through a **filtration barrier** consisting of fenestrated endothelium, a fused **glomerular basement membrane (GBM),** and **filtration slits** between the foot processes of **podocytes** into the urinary space. The filtrate then passes into the renal tubule where it is modified by reabsorption and secretion to become urine.

As is true in the renal corpuscle, epithelium of the renal tubule varies, depending on function. The first segment of the tubule, the **proximal convoluted tubule (PCT)**, is composed of cuboidal or columnar cells with a thick microvillous **brush border,** and abundant mitochondria within basolateral interdigitations. The PCT reabsorbs approximately 80% of water and sodium chloride, and normally all of the sugar and protein in the glomerular filtrate. The proximal tubule straightens and descends into the medulla where it narrows abruptly to become the **descending thin limb** of the **loop of Henle,** bends back on itself, and becomes the **ascending thin limb** of the loop of Henle. Thin limbs have narrowed lumina and simple squamous epithelium. The ascending thin limb widens into the **medullary ascending thick** limb and enters the cortex as the **cortical ascending thick** limb or **distal tubule (DT),** to return to the renal corpuscle of its origin. The **loop of Henle** establishes a hypertonic medullary interstitium by active and passive transport of sodium chloride and urea from the tubule into the medullary interstitium.

At the renal corpuscle, cells of the DT called the **macula densa,** together with modified secretory smooth muscle cells of the afferent arteriole **(juxtaglomerular cells)** and extraglomerular mesangial cells, form the **juxtaglomerular apparatus (JGA),** which is important in blood pressure regulation. Beyond the JGA the tubule becomes known as the **distal convoluted tubule (DCT)** and exhibits simple cuboidal epithelium with basal folds within which lie numerous mitochondria. In the presence of **aldosterone,** the distal portion of the DCT reabsorbs salt from the filtrate. A connecting segment joins DCT to a **collecting duct,** which carries the filtrate through cortex and medulla toward the papilla. The medullary portion of the collecting duct, in response to **antidiuretic hormone,** concentrates the filtrate by allowing reabsorption of water by the hypertonic medullary interstitium. **Collecting duct** epithelium is cuboidal in the cortex but increases to tall columnar as it passes into the medulla.

The collecting ducts open on the papilla at the **area cribrosa** and empty their contents into the minor calyx. Collecting ducts surrounded by straight profiles of proximal and distal tubules produce **medullary rays** in the cortex. A **cortical lobule** is centered on the medullary ray, which is surrounded by the **cortical labyrinth,** made up of proximal and distal convoluted tubules, renal corpuscles, and, at the periphery, interlobular arteries.

URINARY TRACT

The **urinary tract** consists of intrarenal minor and major calyces and the renal pelvis, which lie within the renal sinus supported by adipose tissue. Although the renal pelvis may lie entirely within the renal sinus, an extrarenal portion usually narrows at the inferior pole of the kidney to become the **ureter.** Descending along the dorsal body wall in an extraperitoneal position, a ureter from each kidney enters the **urinary bladder,** where urine is stored. All of these organs are lined with **transitional epithelium** capable of expansion as urine fills the lumen. The apical membranes of transitional epithelial cells are composed of mosaic-like plaques that may be endocytosed into discoidal vesicles by folding at their margins to reduce the surface area of cells in the relaxed bladder. The exocytosis of diskoidal vesicles adds additional membrane surface area to cells undergoing stretching to accommodate urine being stored in the bladder. The walls of calyces, renal pelves, ureters, and bladder contain increasing quantities of smooth muscle, which contracts (peristalsis) to propel urine from the kidneys to the bladder for storage. When a critical volume is reached, contraction of large bundles of smooth muscle in the bladder wall expels urine from the body through the **urethra.**

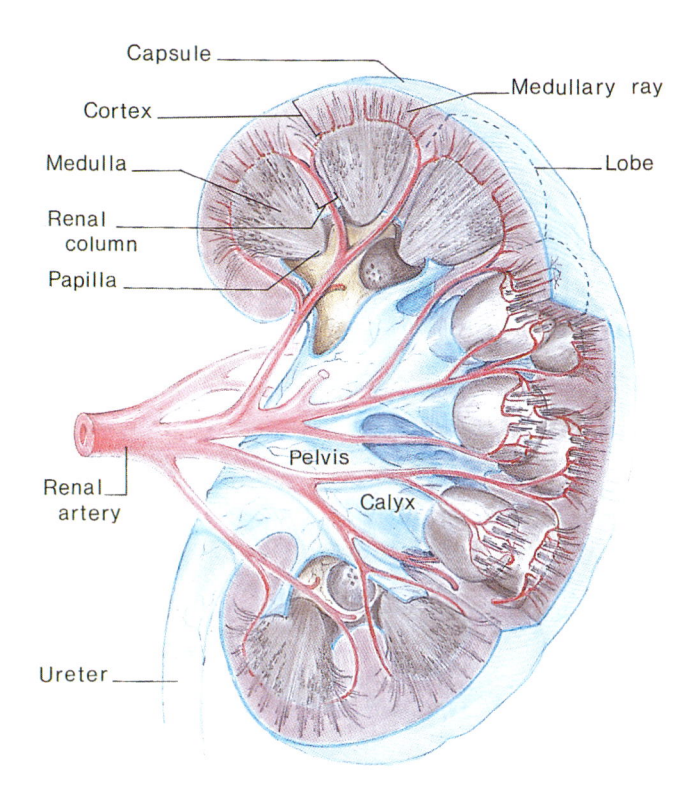

Fig. 18-1. Hemisection of kidney showing relationships of renal pelvis and calyces to arterial supply of renal cortex and medulla.

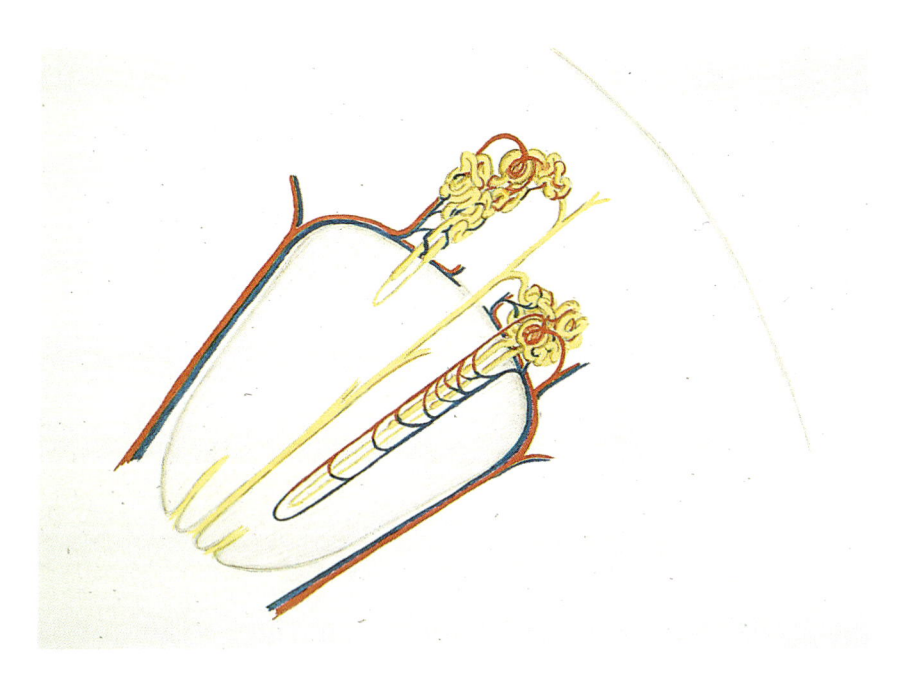

Fig. 18-2. Arteries and veins in renal cortex and medulla. Afferent arterioles *(AA)* derived from interlobular arteries supply cortical and juxtamedullary nephrons. Note peritubular capillary plexus surrounding convoluted tubules and origin of vasa rectae. *LH*, Loop of Henle; *CCD*, collecting duct in the cortex; *MCD*, collecting duct in medulla.

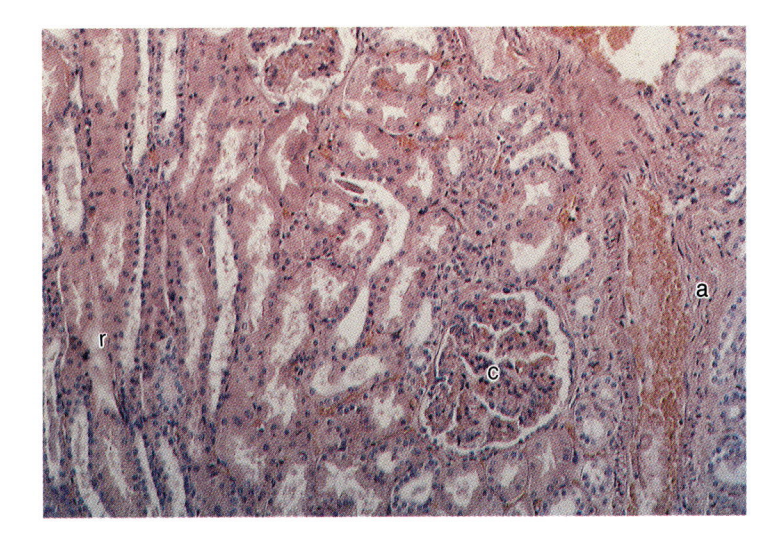

Fig. 18-3. LM of kidney cortex showing interlobular artery (a), renal corpuscle (c) surrounded by convoluted tubules, and a medullary ray (r). (H&E; ×200.)

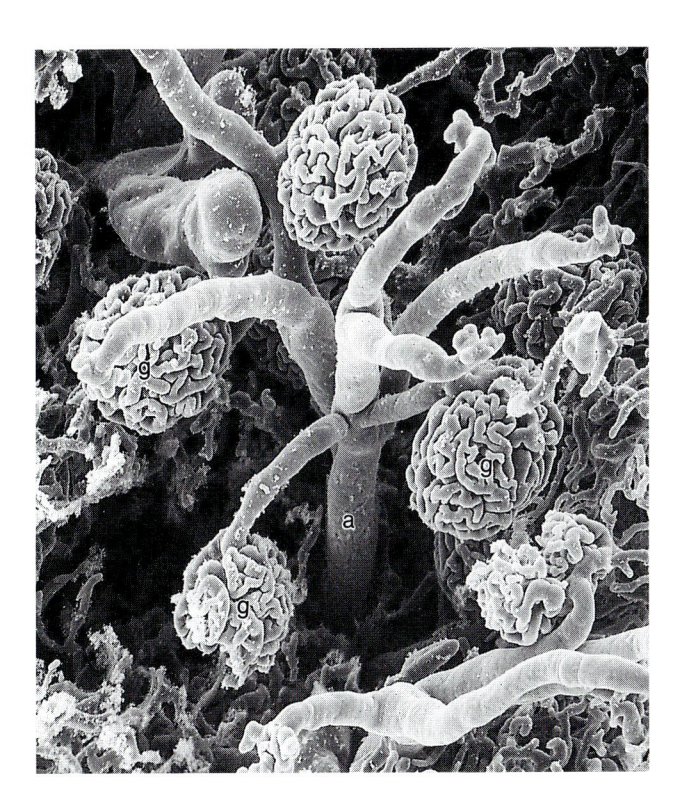

Fig. 18-4. SEM of latex-injected vessels in rat kidney cortex. An interlobular artery (a) and its branches, which are afferent arterioles, supply glomeruli (g) with blood. (×50.)

Fig. 18-5. LM of renal corpuscle showing both vascular and urinary poles. Parietal layer of simple squamous epithelium forms outer wall of Bowman's capsule, while visceral layer (composed of podocytes) surrounds glomerulus (capillary tuft). (H&E; ×350.)

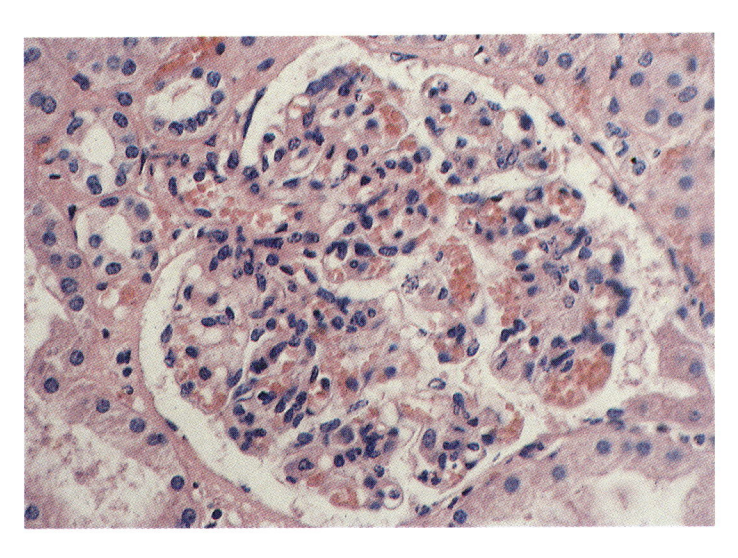

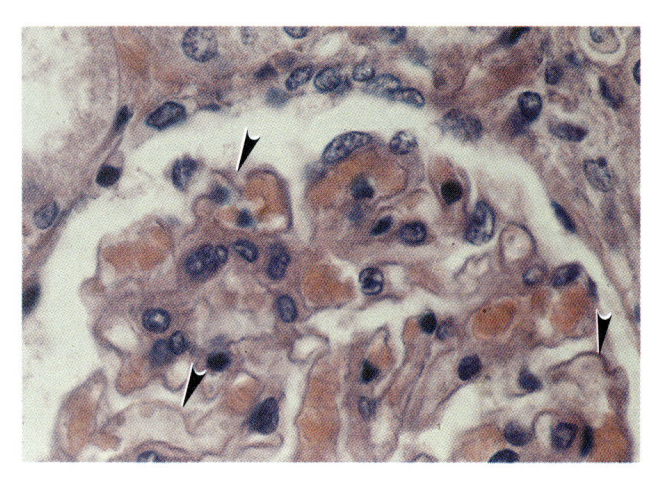

Fig. 18-6. LM of renal corpuscle in kidney. Urinary space separates parietal layer of Bowman's capsule from visceral epithelium (or podocytes). In glomerular tuft arrowheads identify basement membrane between podocytes and endothelial cells and RBCs within capillaries. (H&E; ×1,000.)

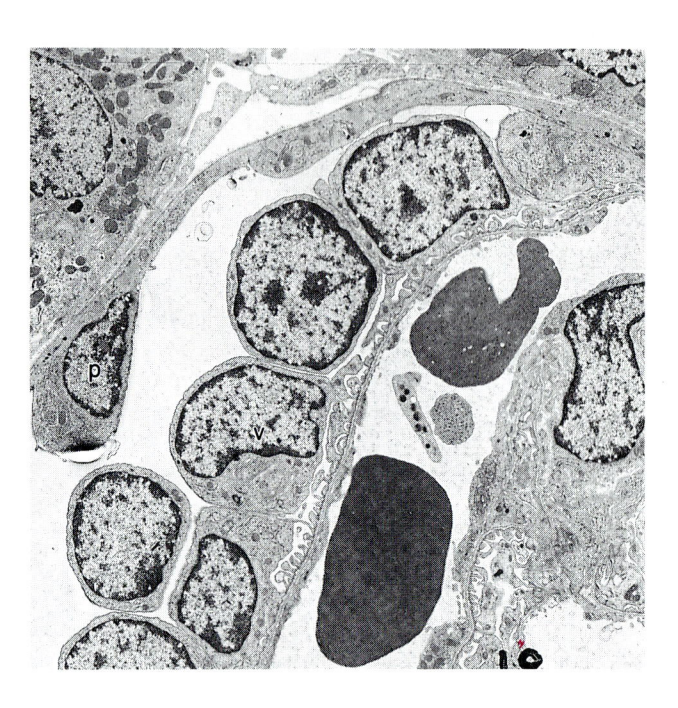

Fig. 18-7. TEM of immature renal corpuscle showing both parietal (p) and visceral (v) epithelial layers. Contrast morphology of these two epithelial cell types, and observe that podocytes rest on glomerular basement membrane. Several blood cells and a platelet can be seen within capillary lumen. (×5,000.)

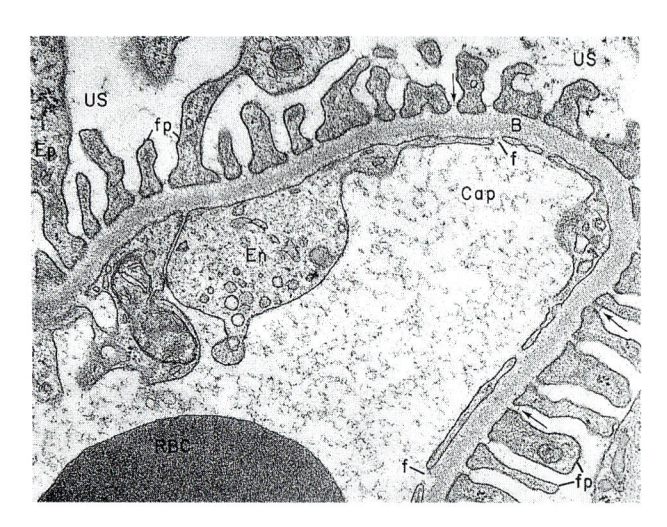

Fig. 18-8. TEM of glomerular capillary and surrounding visceral epithelial cells, or podocytes. Unlike other fenestrated capillaries, fenestrae within glomerular capillaries lack diaphragms. Basal laminae of endothelial cell and podocyte are fused. Foot processes of adjacent podocytes abut basal lamina and are interconnected by slit diaphragms such as those seen at arrow. *US*, urinary space; *Ep*, epithelial cell or podocyte; *fp*, foot process; *B*, fused basal laminae of endothelial cell and podocyte; *f*, fenestrae; *En*, endothelial cell; *Cap*, capillary lumen; *RBC*, red blood cell. (×20,800.)

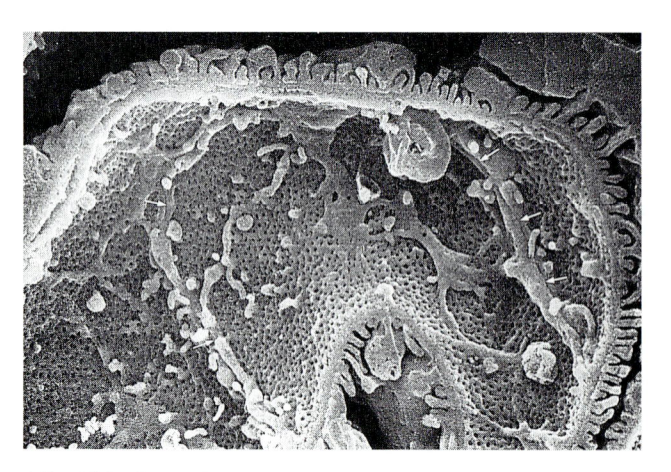

Fig. 18-9. SEM of luminal surface of glomerular capillary. Compare morphology by SEM to that seen by TEM. Note appearance of fenestrae within endothelial cell, and foot processes of podocyte. (×6,000.) Arrows indicate cytoplasmic ridges on luminal surface of endothelial cell.

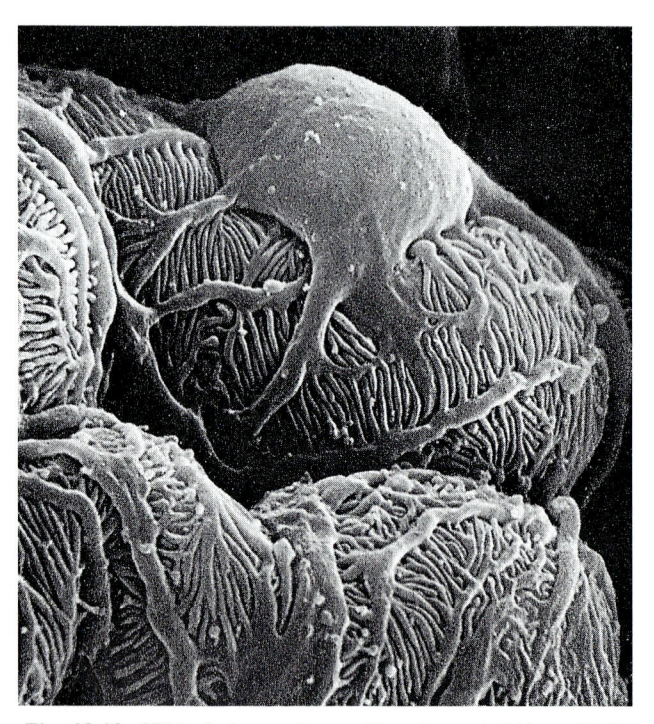

Fig. 18-10. SEM of glomerular capillary loops in kidney. Podocyte extends both primary and secondary rami, which envelop, as foot processes, external surfaces of capillaries. (×6,200.)

	Heparin sulfate
	Type IV collagen
	Laminin
	Sialic acid on glycocalyx
LRE	Lamina rara externa
LD	Lamina densa
LRI	Lamina rara interna

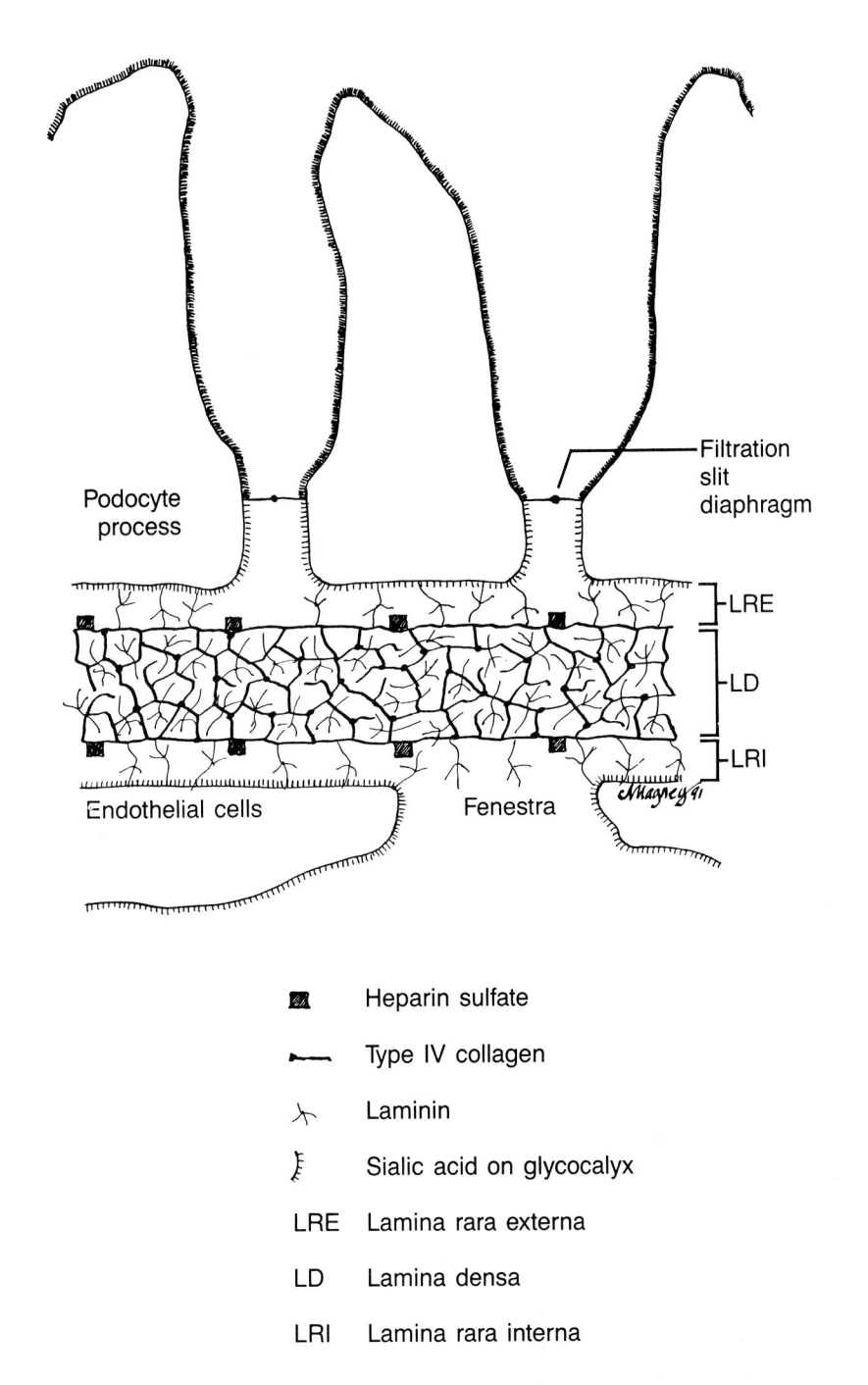

Fig. 18-11. Structure and composition of glomerular filtration barrier. Glomerular barrier functions through both size and charge selection. Fenestrae of endothelial cell, meshwork of basal lamina, and slit diaphragms of podocyte processes contribute to size barrier. Charge selection is accomplished mainly by heparin sulfate proteoglycan in basal lamina, as well as by sialic acid in glycocalyx of endothelial cell and podocyte.

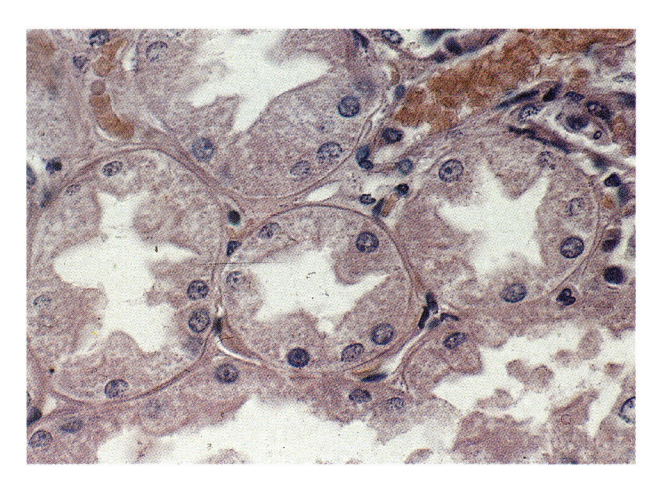

Fig. 18-12. High-magnification LM of kidney cortex showing proximal convoluted tubules in cross section and portion of proximal straight tubule in longitudinal section. (H&E; ×1,000.)

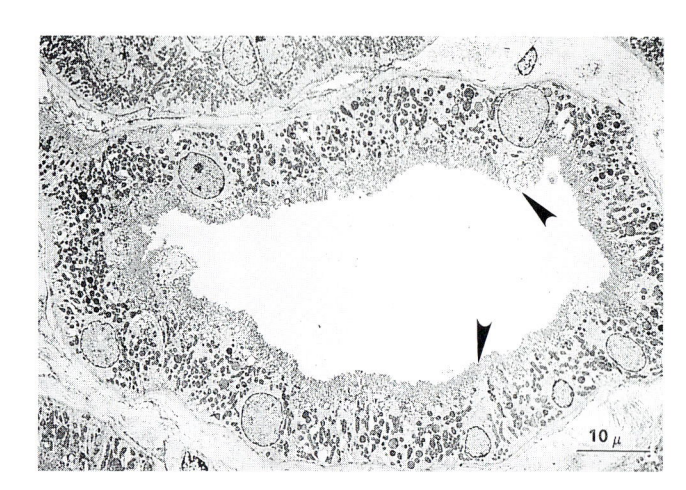

Fig. 18-13. TEM of cross section of proximal convoluted tubule from kidney fixed by perfusion. Unlike fixation for LM, tubule lumen appears round and not collapsed. Extensive microvillus border *(arrowhead)* is also known as "brush border" by LM. (×1,100.)

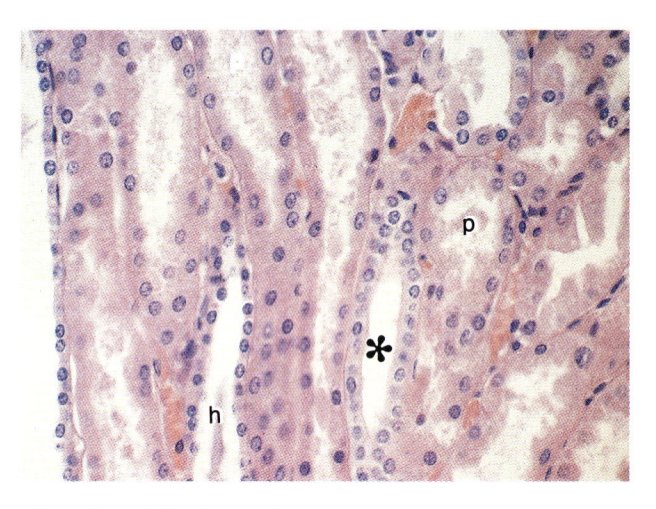

Fig. 18-14. LM of medullary ray containing examples of collecting duct (*), straight portions of proximal tubule *(p)*, and ascending thick segment of loop of Henle *(h)*. (H&E; ×350.)

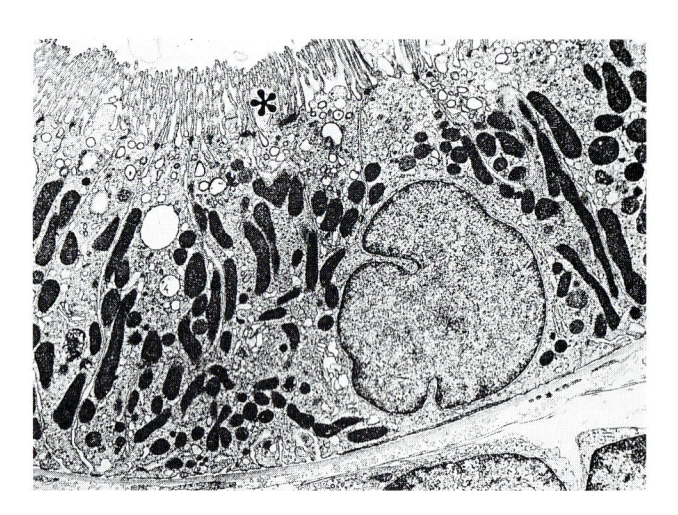

Fig. 18-15. High-magnification TEM of proximal convoluted tubule cell. This cell type is characterized by prominent microvilli (*), numerous dense mitochondria, lysosomal bodies, and extensive infolding of lateral and basal membranes of cell. (×4,200.)

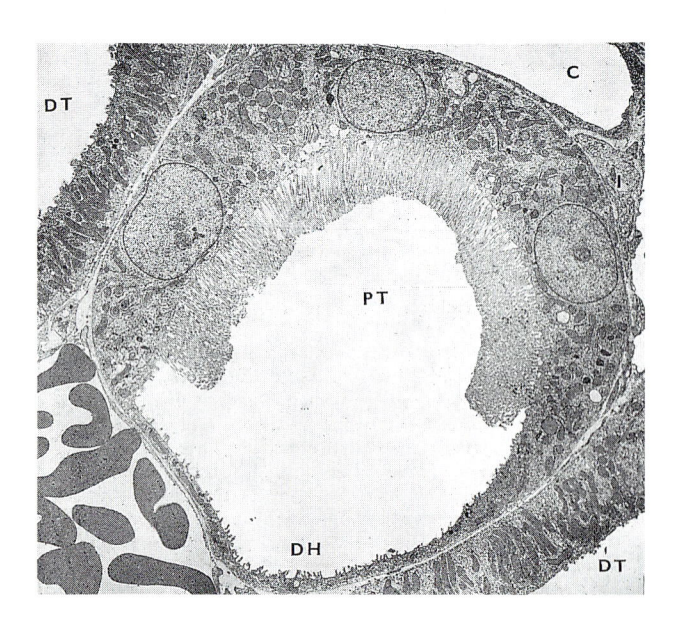

Fig. 18-16. TEM of proximal straight tubule at its junction with thin segment (or descending limb) of loop of Henle. Observe dramatic change in epithelial morphology. *C*, Capillary; *DH*, descending limb of loop of Henle; *DT*, distal tubule. (×2,100.)

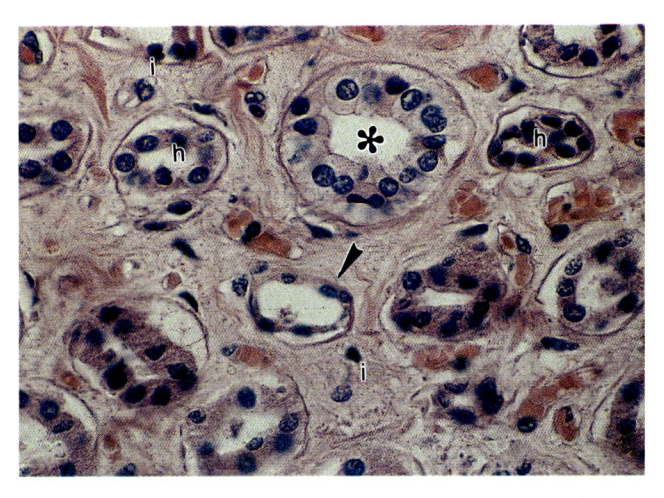

Fig. 18-17. LM of kidney medulla. A collecting duct (*), thin limbs *(arrowhead)* of loop of Henle, capillaries, and ascending thick limbs of loop of Henle *(h)* are easily distinguished. Also note presence of interstitial cells *(i)* within connective tissue between adjacent tubules and capillaries. (H&E; ×1,000.)

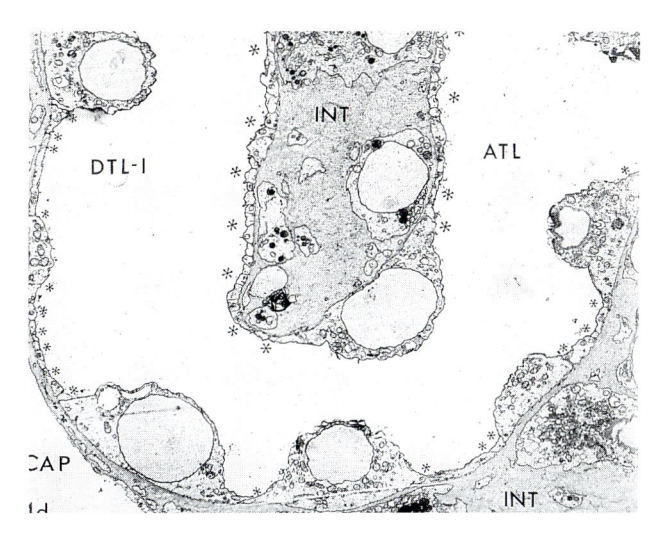

Fig. 18-18. TEM of loop of Henle showing transition between descending thin limb and ascending thin limb of loop of Henle. Interstitial cells lie between limbs. *CAP*, capillary; *INT*, interstitium; *DTL-1*, descending thin limb; *ATL*, ascending thin limb. (×1,600.)

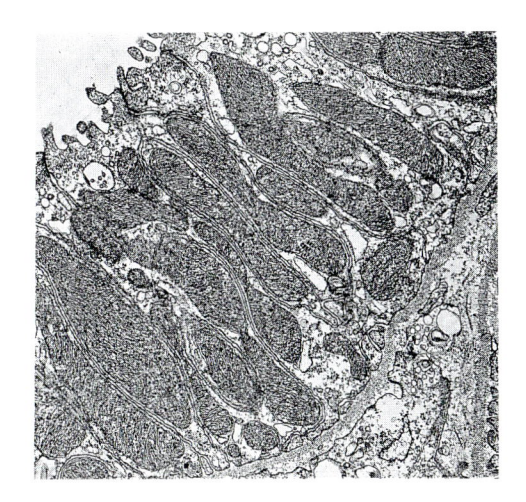

Fig. 18-19. TEM of ascending thick limb of loop of Henle from rat kidney. Compare short, sparse microvilli to prominent microvillous border of proximal tubule (Fig. 18-13). Numerous mitochondria provide energy for active transport of ions from filtrate within tubule into medullary interstitium. (×8,500.)

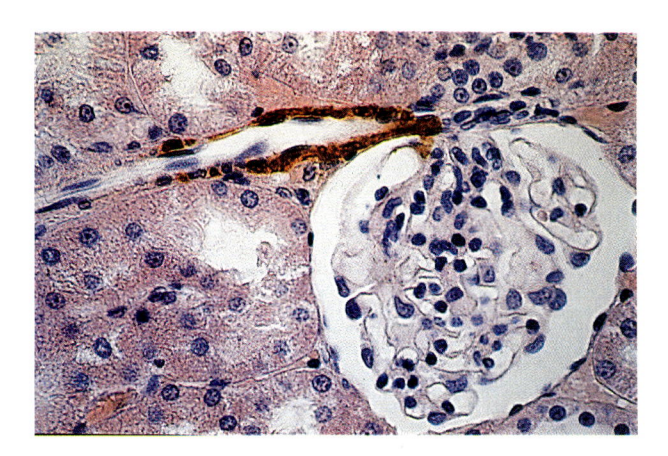

Fig. 18-20. LM illustrating immunocytochemical localization of enzyme renin within smooth muscle cells of afferent arteriole at vascular pole of renal corpuscle. (H&E; ×300.)

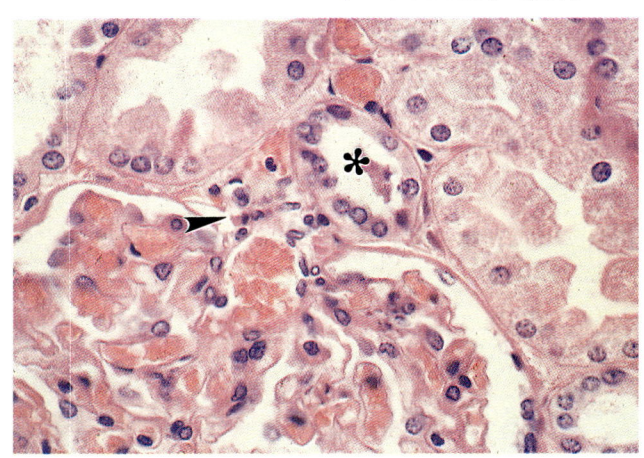

Fig. 18-21. LM showing vascular pole of renal corpuscle at higher magnification. Distal tubule adjacent to renal corpuscle consists of numerous small nucleated cells, polarized toward corpuscle, and is known as macula densa (*). These distal tubule cells together with modified smooth muscle of afferent arteriole, also known as juxtaglomerular cells, and extraglomerular mesangial cells *(arrowhead)*, form the juxtaglomerular apparatus. (H&E; ×350.)

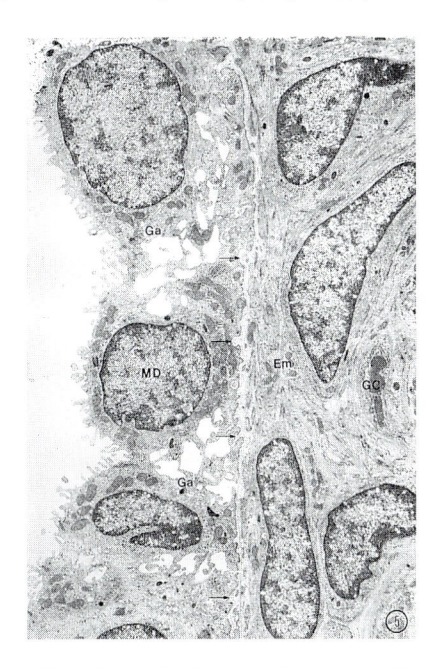

Fig. 18-22. TEM of macula densa and adjacent JG cells of afferent arteriole. Large, irregular, dense granules within cytoplasm of arteriolar smooth muscle cells *(right)* contain renin. Lumen of distal tubule and macula densa forming part of tubule wall are on left. *EM*, extraglomerular mesangium; *Ga*, Golgi apparatus; *GC*, granule complex; *MD*, macula densa. (×2,400.)

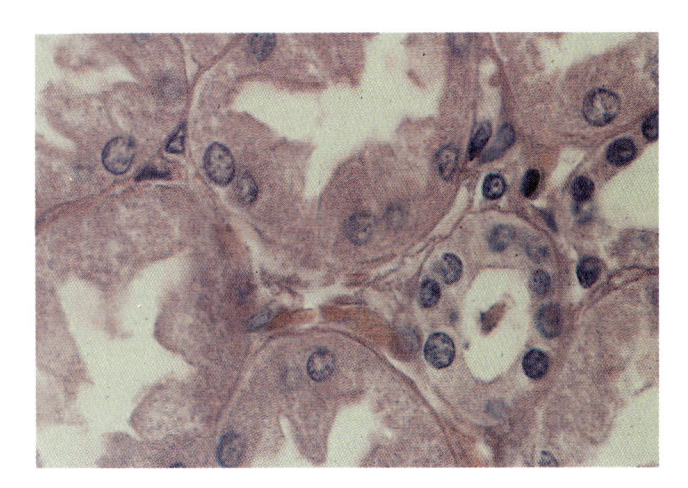

Fig. 18-23. LM depicting several proximal convoluted tubules and a distal convoluted tubule *(right)*. Notice in these tubules differences in height of epithelia, variation in microvillous border, and shape of lumen. (H&E; ×1,200.)

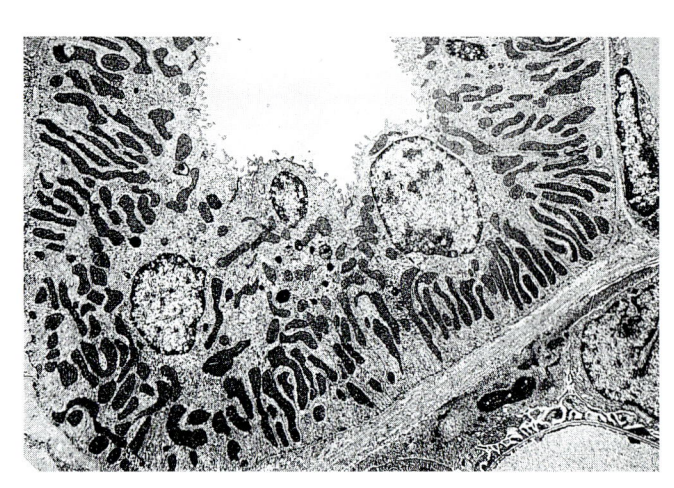

Fig. 18-24. TEM of distal convoluted tubule. Observe lack of well-developed microvillous border and presence of numerous mitochondria within folds in basal cytoplasm. (×3,200.)

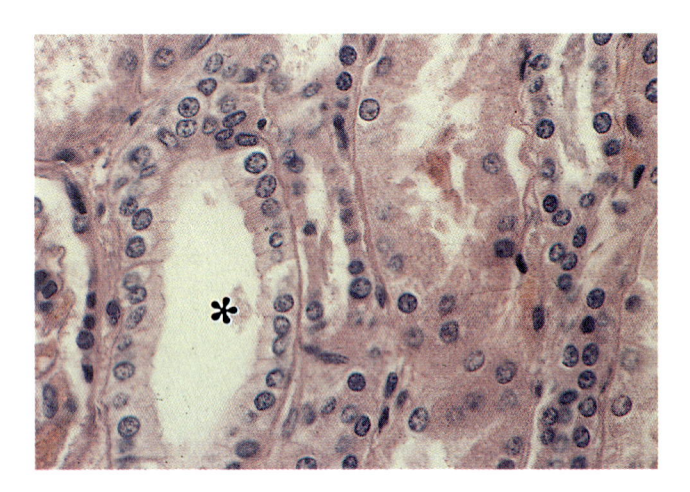

Fig. 18-25. LM of collecting duct (*) found within medullary ray in kidney cortex. Observe columnar shape of cells and large diameter of duct lumen. (H&E; ×800.)

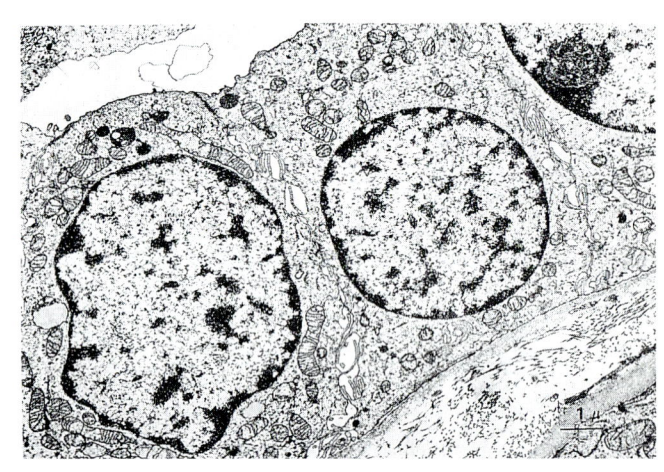

Fig. 18-26. TEM of cells in collecting duct. These cells lack well-developed microvillous border and contain few mitochondria as compared with cells of distal tubule, ascending thick limb of loop of Henle, or proximal convoluted tubule. (×6,100.)

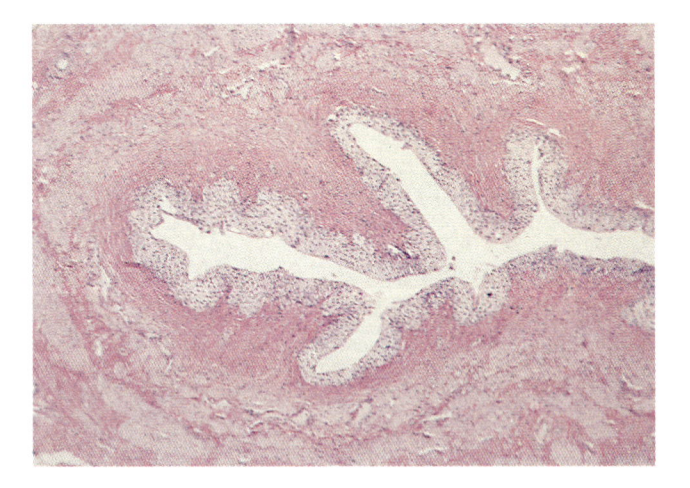

Fig. 18-27. LM showing wall of ureter in cross section. Transitional epithelium lines slitlike, star-shaped lumen and overlies thin lamina propria. Muscularis portion of ureter wall consists of smooth muscle cells arranged in alternating longitudinal, circular, and longitudinal arrays. (H&E; ×50.)

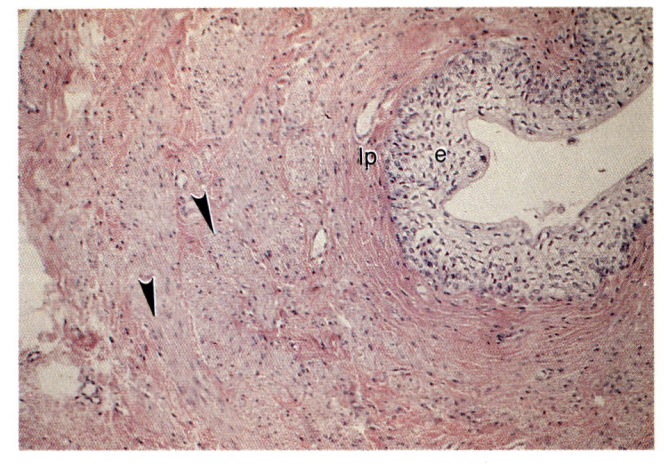

Fig. 18-28. Higher magnification LM of ureter. From lumen outward, observe transitional epithelium *(e)*, delicate layer of connective tissue comprising lamina propria *(lp)*, and alternating layers *(arrows)* of smooth muscle cells in muscularis. (H&E; ×150.)

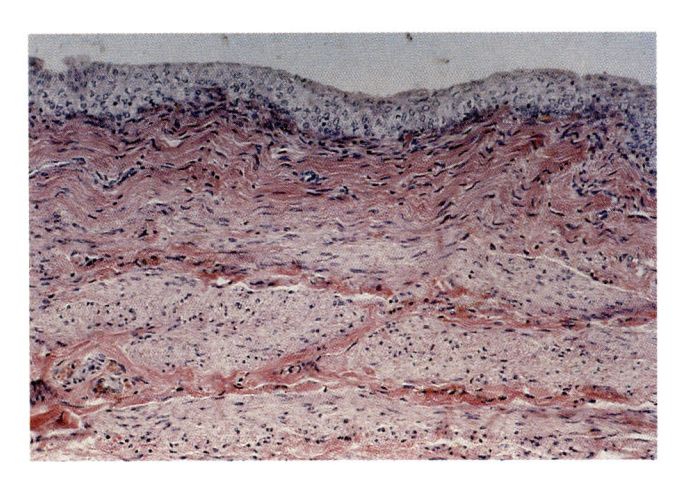

Fig. 18-29. Low-magnification LM of urinary bladder. Large bundles of smooth muscle are found within thick wall of bladder. These are usually arranged at oblique angles to one another, in sharp contrast to well-organized circular and longitudinal arrays found within gastrointestinal tract. (H&E; ×150.)

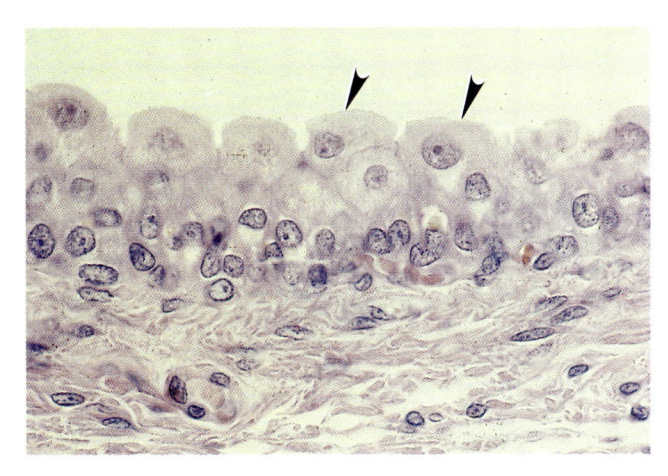

Fig. 18-30. Higher-magnification LM of transitional epithelium lining urinary bladder. This tissue was fixed in relaxed state so that large umbrella cells *(arrowheads)* adjacent to lumen can be seen overlying basal cells within epithelium. (H&E; ×1,200.)

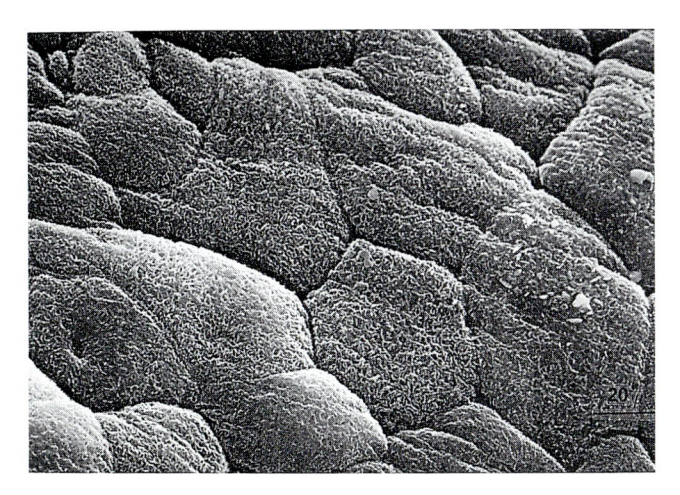

Fig. 18-31. SEM of urinary bladder showing luminal surfaces of umbrella cells. (×2,500.)

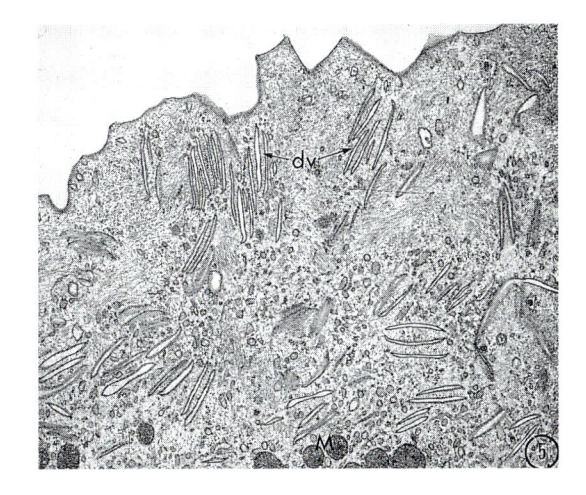

Fig. 18-32. TEM of apical cytoplasm of umbrella cell in transitional epithelium. Many discoidal vesicles are present within apical cytoplasm and represent a form of membrane storage. Upon stimulation these vesicles fuse with the plasma membrane, thereby increasing surface area of umbrella cell. *dv*, disc-shaped vesicles; *M*, mitochondria. (×12,000.)

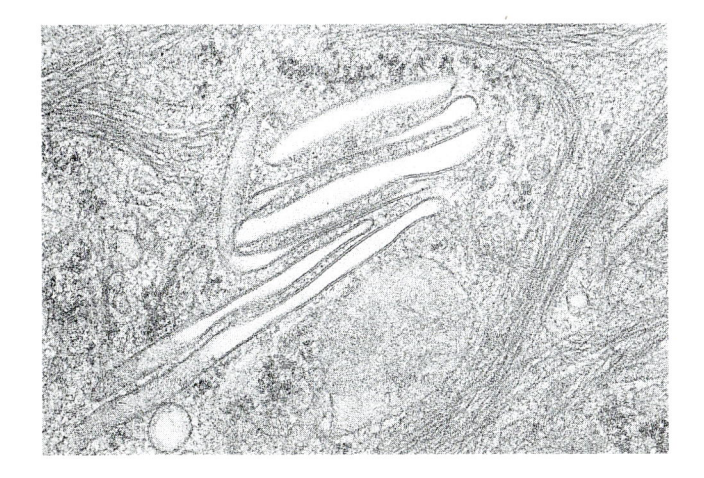

Fig. 18-33. High-magnification TEM showing stack of discoidal vesicles and proximity of actin filaments to cytoplasmic surface of vesicle membrane. In bladder, luminal surface area of epithelium is regulated by removal (endocytosis) or insertion (exocytosis) of discoidal vesicles by an actin-mediated contractile system. (×64,000.)

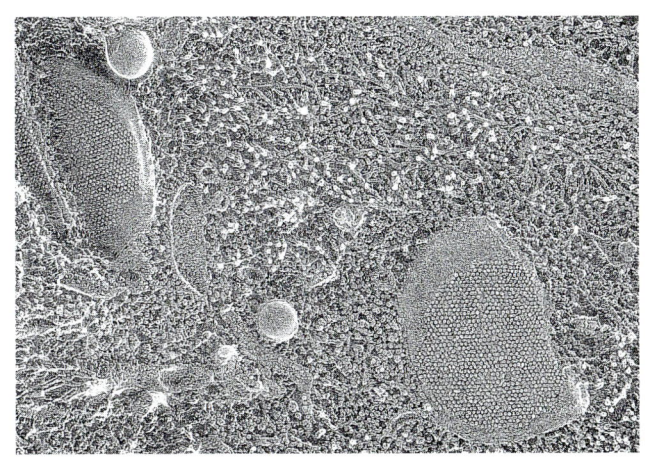

Fig. 18-34. TEM of umbrella cell prepared by quick-freeze, deep-etch method. Discoidal vesicles are easily recognized amidst cytoplasmic filaments. Central portion of cytoplasmic surface of vesicle membrane consists of hexagonal arrays of closely packed particles. (×48,000.)

CHAPTER 19

MALE REPRODUCTIVE TRACT

THE MALE REPRODUCTIVE tract has four parts, each of which contributes to the function of the entire system.
1. The **testes** are double glands in that their exocrine product are germ cells, **spermatozoa,** which are delivered to the female through a duct system. The endocrine product of the testis, **testosterone,** sustains spermatogenesis and promotes and maintains the secondary sexual characteristics of the male.
2. **Conducting tubules** and **ducts** are responsible for maturation of the spermatozoa, their storage within the system, and transport from the testes through the duct system until discharge from the body.
3. **Accessory glands** produce and store secretions that form a transport medium known as semen.
4. A copulatory organ, the **penis,** is responsible for placement of the spermatozoa within the female reproductive system.

TESTES

The testes develop in the abdominal cavity and normally descend into the **scrotum** at birth. Testicular arteries and veins are direct branchs and tributaries of the abdominal aorta and inferior vena cava, respectively, reflecting the abdominal origin of the testes. These male glands are suspended outside the body in the scrotum because spermatozoa will not develop at body temperature. Arterial blood to the testis is cooled by a countercurrent mechanism involving the **pampiniform plexus** of veins. The **spermatic cord,** a fibromuscular structure, transmits these blood vessels and part of the male duct system, the **vas deferens,** between the pelvic cavity and the scrotum.

Each testis is surrounded by a thick fibroelastic capsule, the **tunica albuginea. Septulae testes** are connective tissue partitions that radiate from the mediastinum to the capsule and incompletely divide the testes into approximately 250 pyramidal compartments, each of which contains coiled **seminiferous tubules** embedded in loose connective tissue. Located in the interstitial space between tubules are neural and vascular elements together with the **interstitial cells of Leydig,** which secrete testosterone. The **seminiferous epithelium** contains germinative cells (spermatogonia, spermatocytes, and spermatozoa) and **Sertoli cells** that abut the basement membrane. Tight junctions between adjacent Sertoli cells form the **blood-testis barrier** and divide the epithelium into a **basal compartment,** housing primitive germ cells called spermatogonia, and an **adluminal compartment,** where maturing spermatogonia develop under hormonal stimulation before being released into the lumen of the seminiferous tubule. The developing germ cells undergo reduction division during the process of **spermatogenesis** and pass through several stages of development to become **spermatogonia.**

CONDUCTING TUBULES AND DUCTS

Tubuli rectae connect seminiferous tubules of each lobule to the **rete testis,** an anastomosing network of channels within the mediastinum. These tubules convey spermatogonia to the **efferent ductules,** through which they leave the testes and enter the **epididymis,** a long coiled duct that is continuous distally with the **vas deferens.** The epididymis is lined with a pseudostratified secretory epithelium with long, nonmotile microvilli called **stereocilia.** Maturation of spermatogonia is completed within the epididymis, and spermatogonia are stored in this tubular organ until ejaculation. The vas deferens is a thick-walled muscular tube that passes through the spermatic cord to reach the pelvis, where it ends posterior to the urinary bladder as a distal dilation called the **ampulla.** At this point, the ampulla is joined by the **seminal vesicle** to form the **ejaculatory duct,** which empties into the prostatic urethra. Secretions of the seminal vesicle and prostate gland together with spermatozoa comprise semen, which passes through the penile urethra to be discharged from the body.

ACCESSORY GLANDS

A **seminal vesicle** is formed by a diverticulum of the vas deferens that is coiled and folded so that a section through the organ appears honey-combed. The seminal vesicle is testosterone dependent, and it produces a fluid rich in fructose that is important in nourishing the spermatozoa.

The **prostate gland,** located immediately inferior to the urinary bladder, contains an aggregation of tubuloalveolar glands within a fibrous stroma. The prostate is also testosterone dependent and produces a milky, slightly acidic fluid that makes up the bulk of semen and serves to reduce the acidity of both urethra and the female copulatory organ, the vagina.

PENIS

The penis is the male copulatory organ and houses the urethra, through which spermatogonia are delivered to the female. It is composed of three cylindrical erectile bodies bound together with dense connective tissue (tunica albuginea) and covered with thin skin. There are two dorsal **corpora cavernosa** and one **corpus spongiosum,** enlarged distally as the glans penis, through which the urethra passes. The corpora contain a spongy network of endothelial-lined spaces (sinusoids) that, when engorged with blood, compress venules against the tunica albuginea, preventing the blood from draining and causing the penis to become erect. Detumescence follows ejaculation; the arterial blood supply to the penis is reduced and sinusoids are slowly drained by the venules.

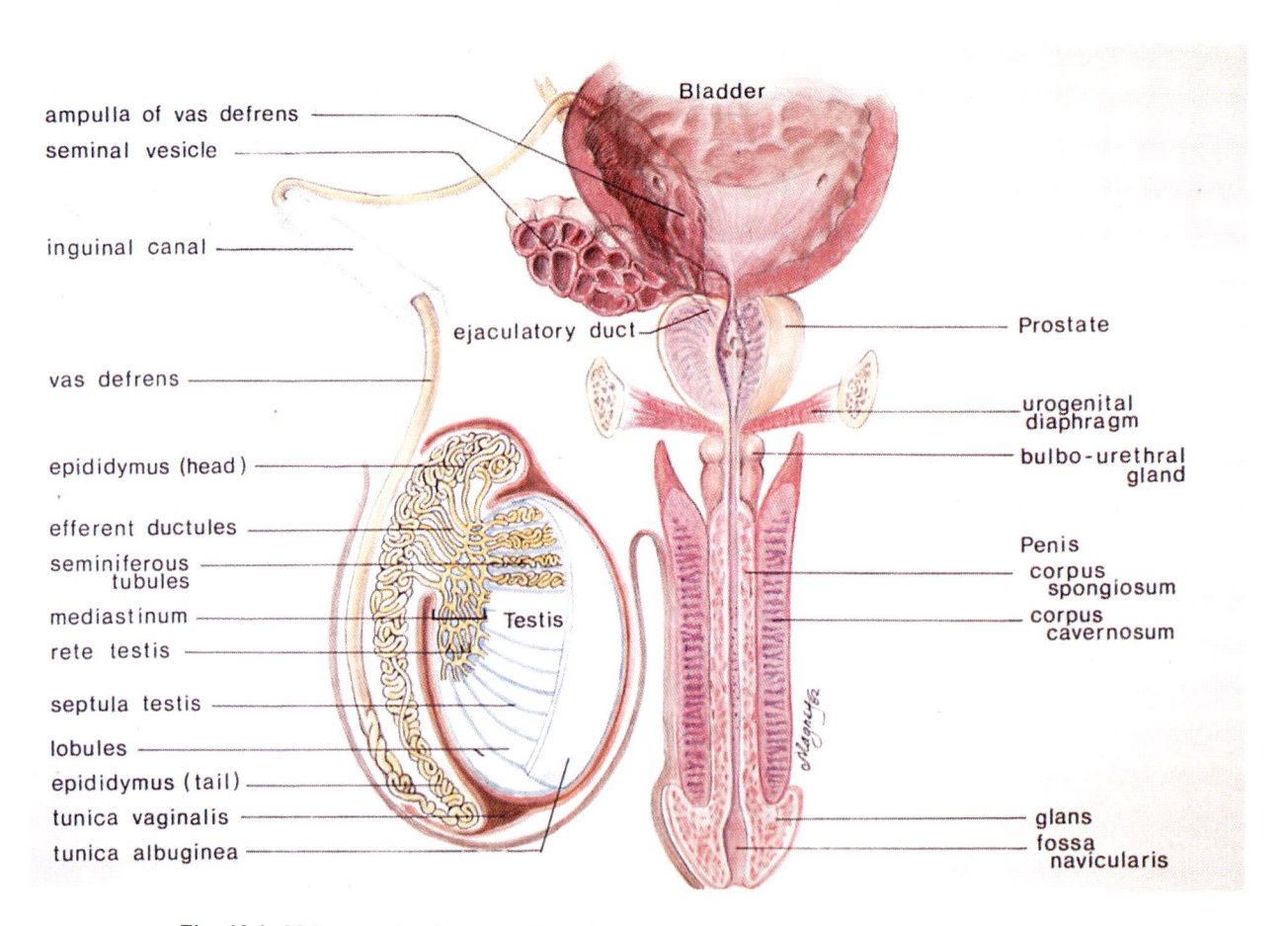

Fig. 19-1. Male reproductive tract. Organization and relationships of testis, accessory male reproductive organs, and penis are illustrated.

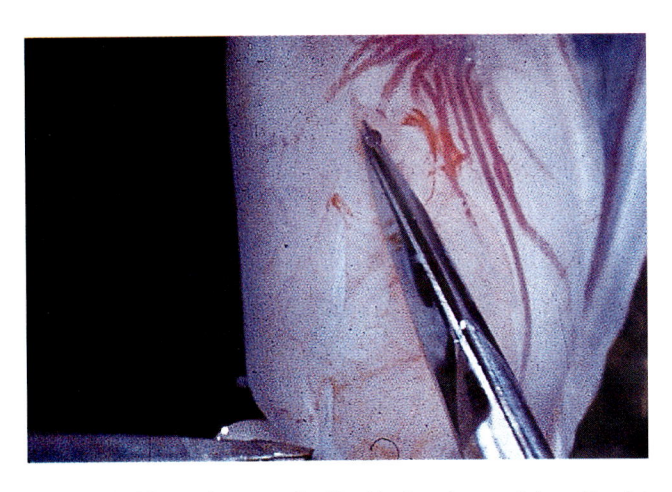

Fig. 19-2. Macrophotograph of testis showing excision of tunica albuginea and underlying seminiferous tubules.

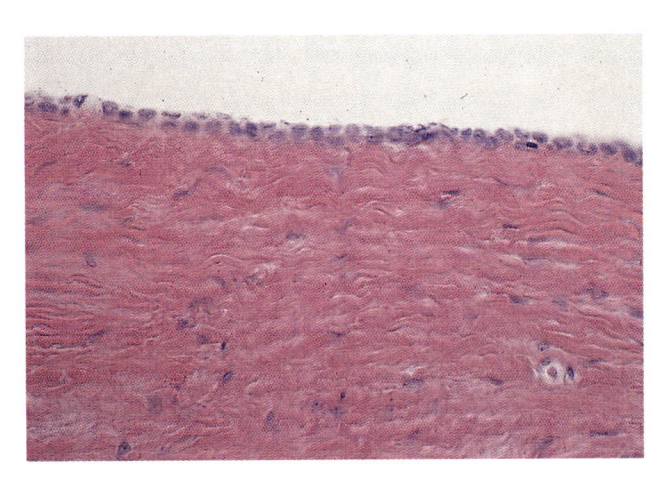

Fig. 19-3. LM of tunica albuginea and overlying epithelium in testis. Observe thick collagenous nature of this capsulelike stroma. (H&E; ×300.)

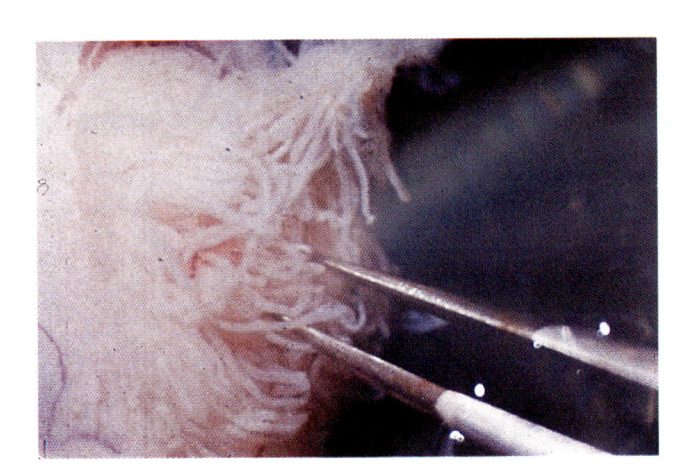

Fig. 19-4. Macrophotograph showing arrangement of seminiferous tubules within testis. Tunica albuginea has been removed to reveal seminiferous tubules. Compare with Figs. 19-2 and 19-5.

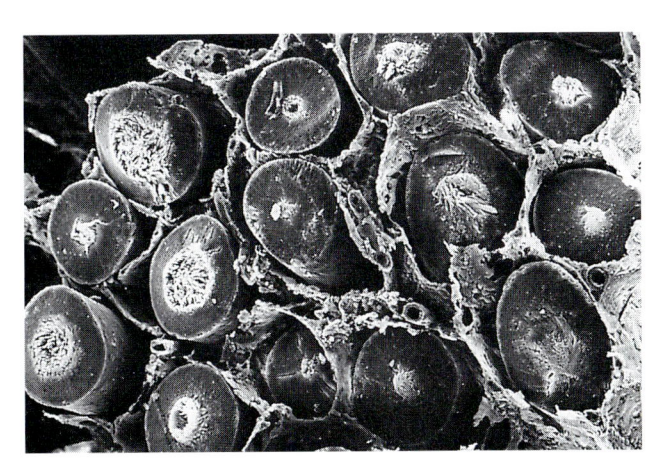

Fig. 19-5. Seminiferous tubules by SEM. Testis has been fractured to permit view. Small amounts of connective tissue can be seen around periphery of each tubule. Adjacent tubules exhibit different stages of spermatid development, as reflected by presence of flagellae. (×70.)

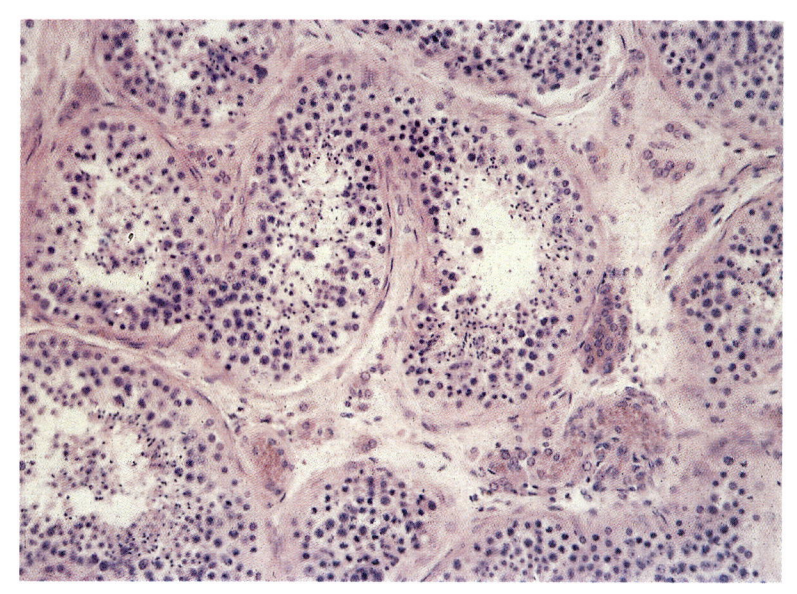

Fig. 19-6. LM of seminiferous tubules demonstrating layer of myoid cells surrounding each tubule. Epithelium consists of Sertoli cells and germinative cells in various stages of development (see Fig 19-9). Look for blood vessels, lymphatics, and clusters of acidophilic interstitial cells of Leydig between tubules. (H&E; ×125.)

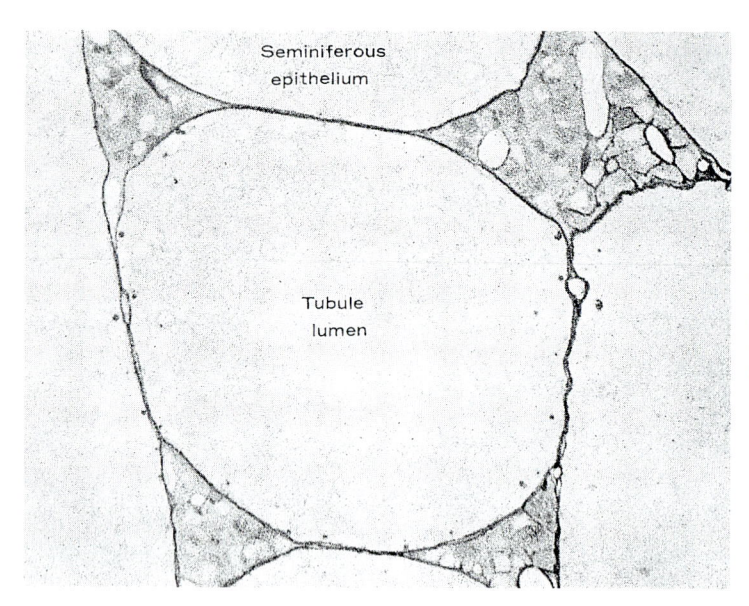

Fig. 19-7. LM of seminiferous tubules after intravascular injection of horseradish peroxidase. Dense reaction product for peroxidase enzyme is present within interstitial issue and surrounds seminiferous tubules. No peroxidase can be found within lumen of seminiferous tubules, suggesting presence of a blood-testis barrier. (×250.)

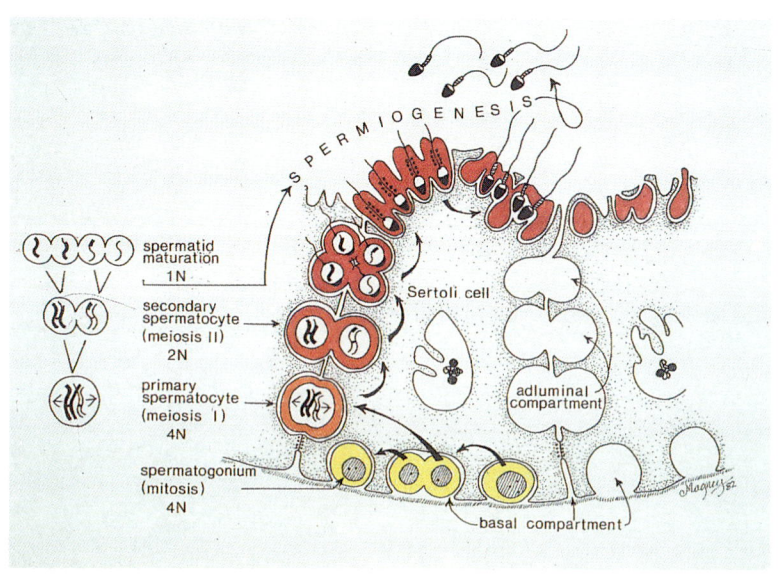

Fig. 19-8. Stages of spermatogenesis and spermiogenesis. Study division of chromosomes and segregation of DNA during meiosis *(left).*

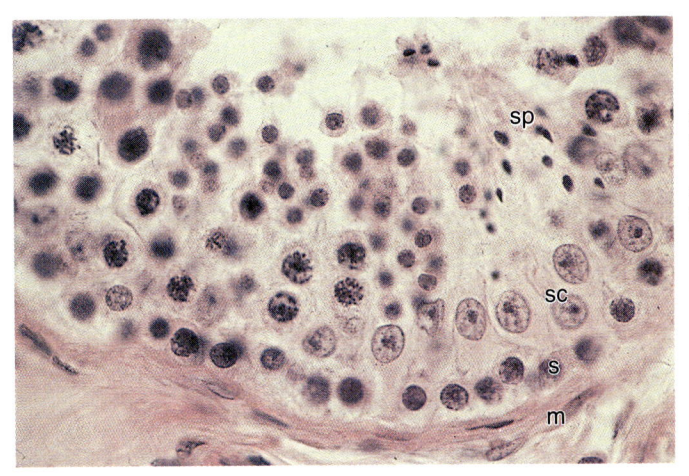

Fig. 19-9. LM of seminiferous tubule. Compare this to Fig. 19-8. Locate myoid cells *(m)*, spermatogonia *(s)*, Sertoli cells containing prominent nucleoli *(sc)*, stages of developing spermatocytes, and spermatids *(sp)*. (H&E; ×800.)

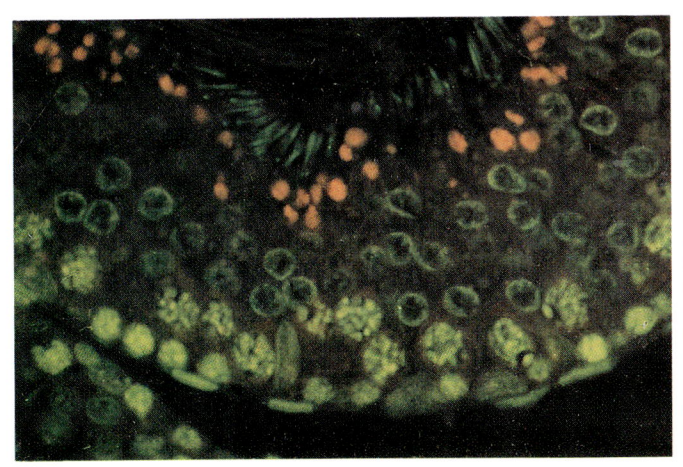

Fig. 19-10. Fluorescent LM of seminiferous tubule stained with acridine orange. Variation in staining of nuclear chromatin defines stages of spermatogenesis. Compare this figure to Figs. 19-8 and 19-9 and locate following cells: myoid cells—elongate nuclei beneath and parallel to base of epithelium; spermatogonia—round, smooth green nuclei in row at base of epithelium; primary spermatocytes—large nuclei with clumped, green chromatin lying directly above basal row of spermatogonia; secondary spermatocytes—smaller, round nuclei with peripherally arranged green heterochromatin, luminal to primary spermatocytes; spermatids—small, elongate, green, rod-shaped nuclei in luminal position. Orange fluorescence represents phagocytic uptake of spermatic cytoplasmic droplets by Sertoli cell. (×800.)

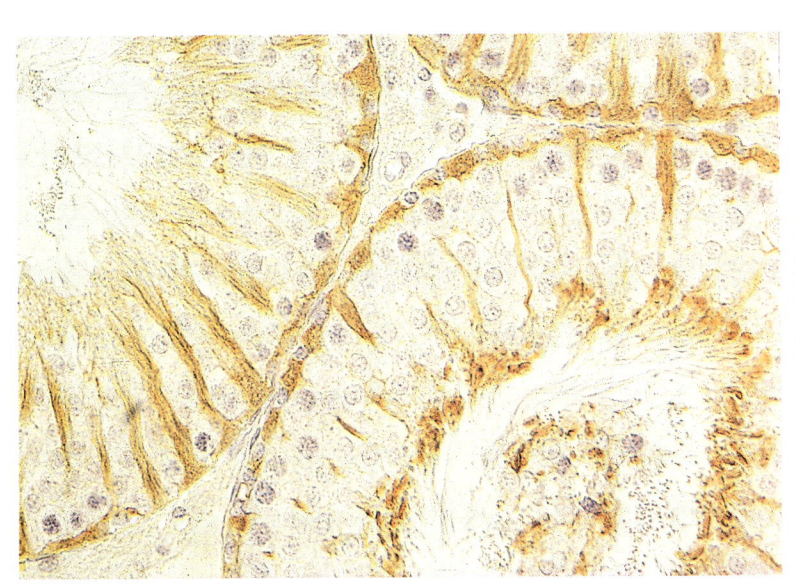

Fig. 19-11. Sertoli cells within seminiferous epithelium demonstrated by immunocytochemical localization of enzyme aldose reductase within cytoplasm. Observe tall columnar nature of Sertoli cell (in left tubule) as it extends from basement membrane to lumen of tubule. Spermatids (in lower right tubule) are embedded within apical invaginations of Sertoli cell. (×400.)

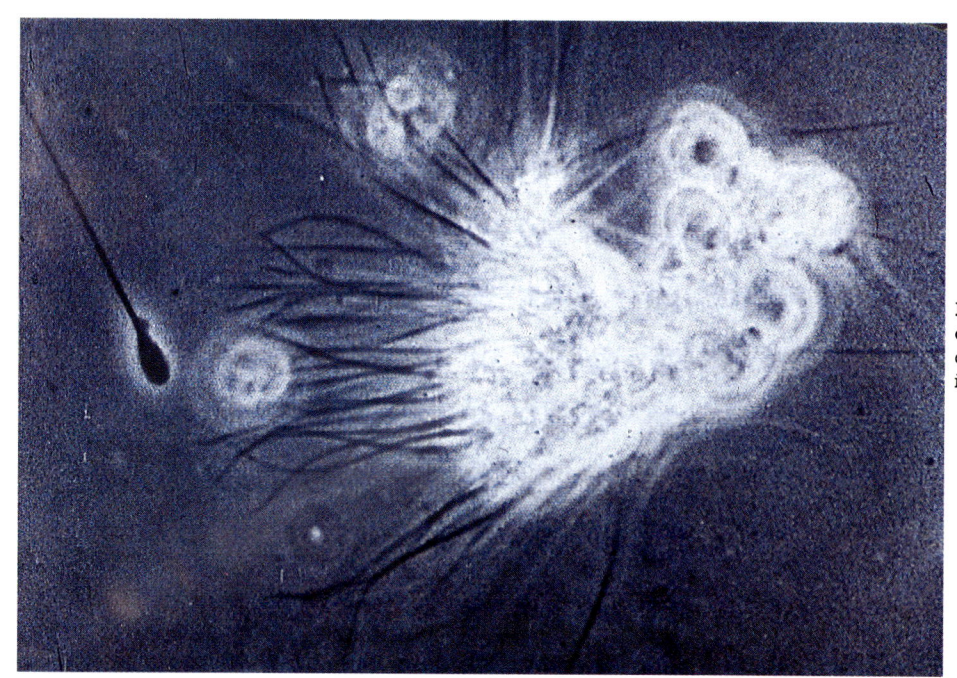

Fig. 19-12. LM of isolated Sertoli cell. Note luminal surface *(left)* and developing spermatids within invaginations of apical cytoplasm. (×800.)

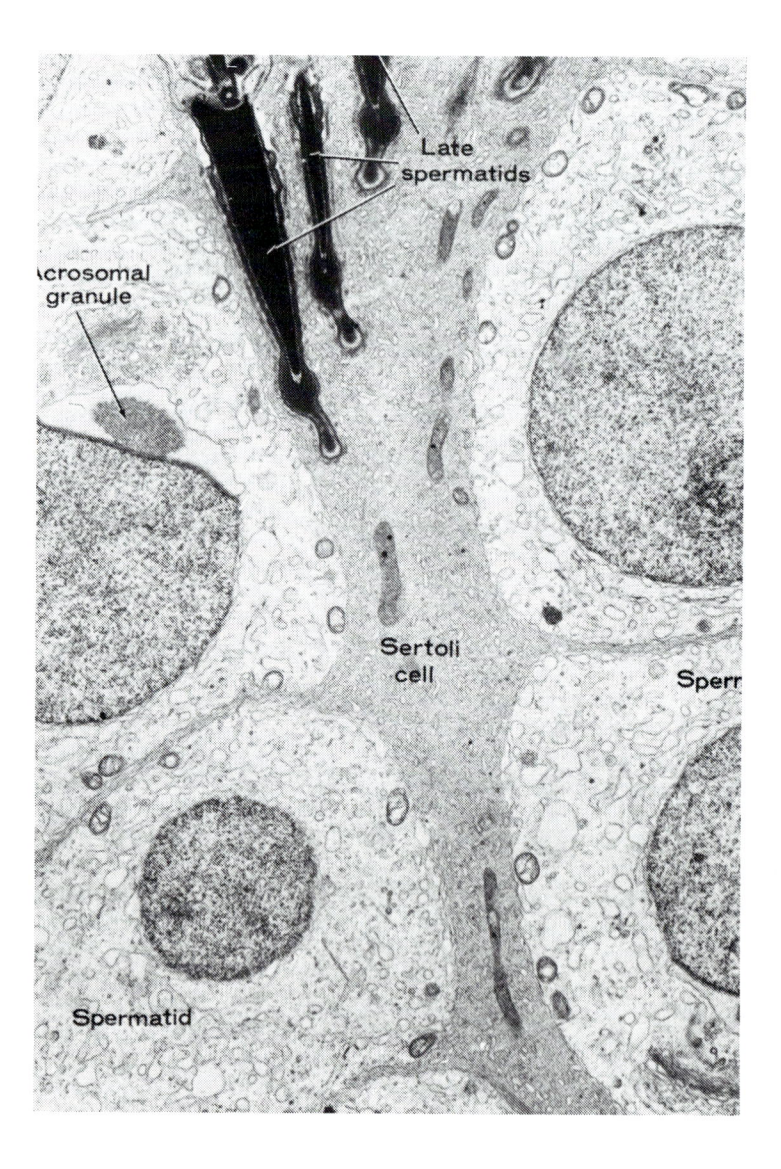

Fig. 19-13. TEM of Sertoli cell showing relationships of developing spermatids to Sertoli cell cytoplasm. More mature spermatids appear embedded in apical surface. (×5,500.)

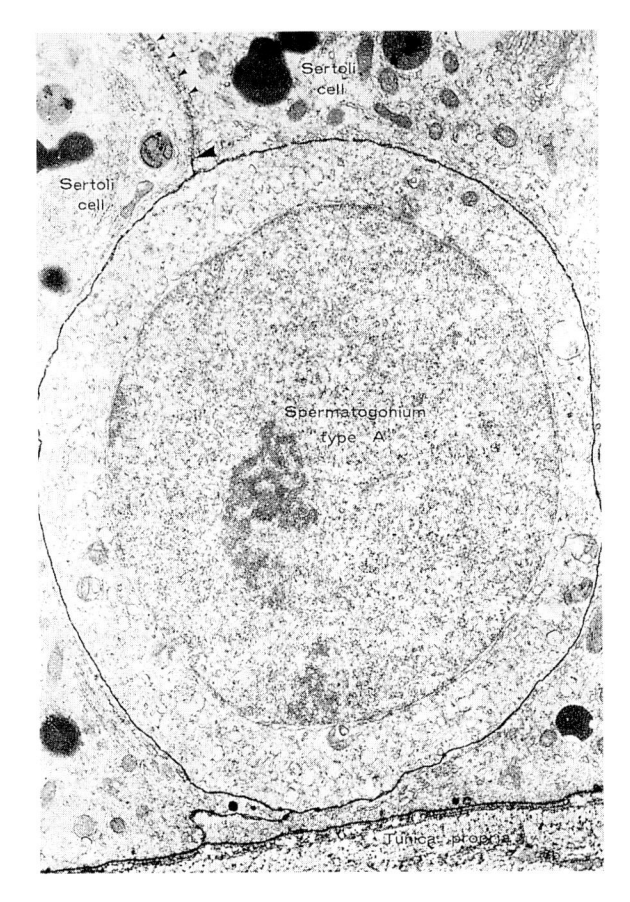

Fig. 19-14. TEM of spermatogonium in seminiferous tubule of primate. Outline of cell is defined by electron-dense tracer lanthanum nitrate. Presence of junctional complexes between adjacent Sertoli cells *(arrowheads)* above spermatogonium prevents electron-opaque tracer from penetrating deeper into seminiferous epithelium. Thus, circulating plasma proteins are excluded from adluminal compartment of seminiferous tubule, and it is likely that the Sertoli-Sertoli junctional complexes are morphologic site of this (blood-testis) barrier. ($\times 8,200$.)

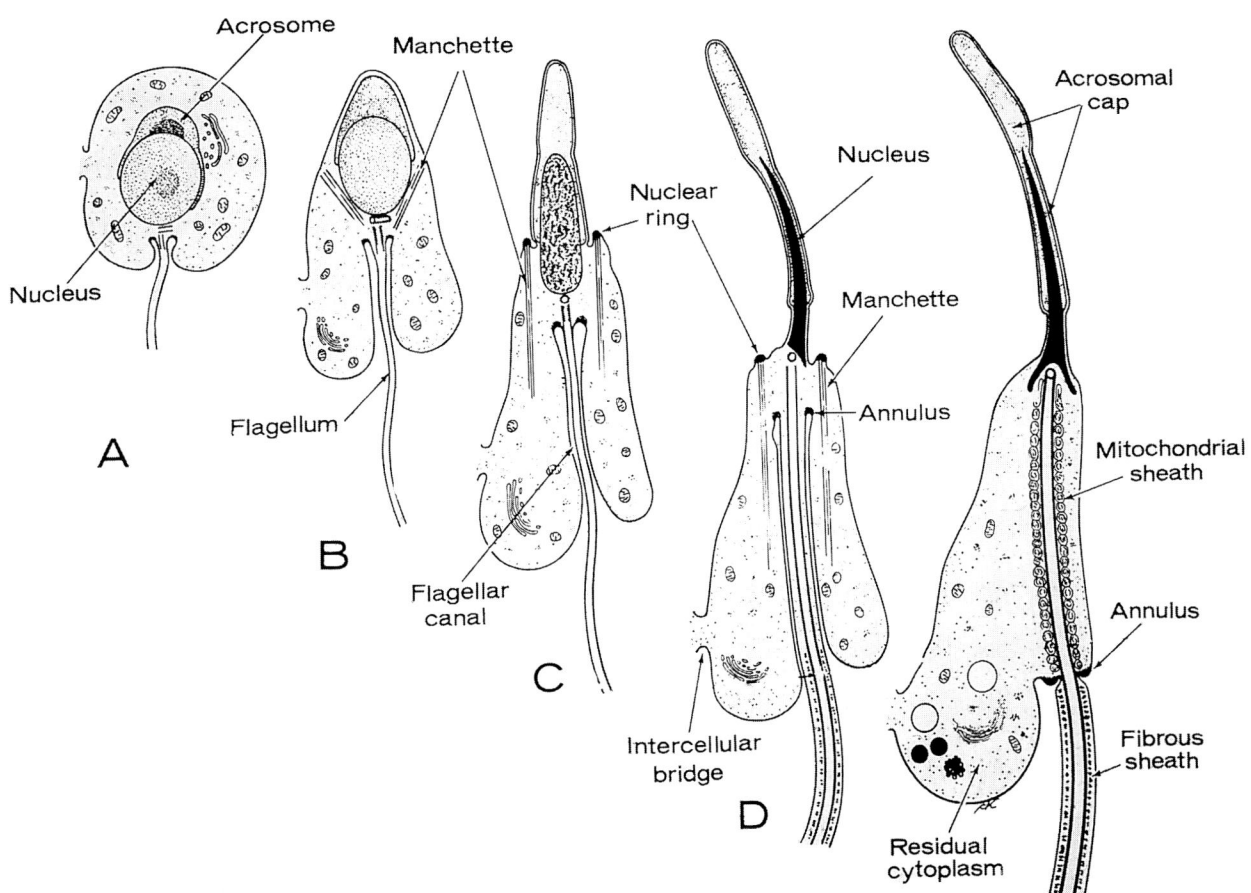

Fig. 19-15. Various stages of spermiogenesis in guinea pig. Spermiogenesis in human is similar, but the acrosomal cap is reduced in size.

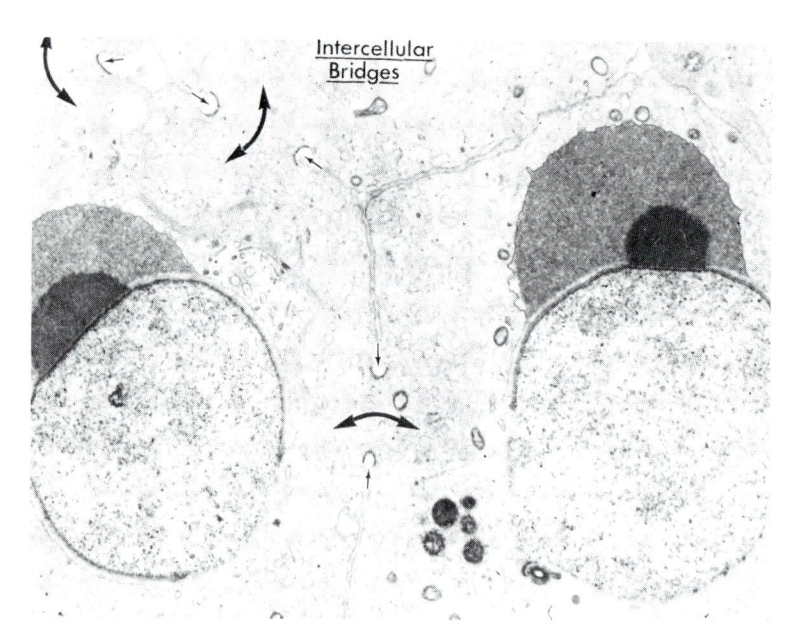

Fig. 19-16. TEM of developing spermatids within seminiferous epithelium. Note accumulation of electron-dense material within acrosomal cap of spermatids and presence of intercellular bridges. ($\times 3{,}800$.)

Fig. 19-17. TEM of spermatids in primate testis showing changes in nuclear condensation and acrosome formation. Cap phase spermatid is illustrated *(left)*, with arrowheads indicating acrosomal cap. Spermatid in acrosomal phase is observed *(center)*; note intimate association of smooth endoplasmic reticulum *(arrowheads)* with spermatid tail. Also shown is spermatid in maturation phase *(right)*. Compare condensation of nuclear chromatin in all three stages, as well as shape of acrosome. All these stages occur while spermatids reside within deep apical invaginations of Sertoli cell. *G*, Acrosomal granule; *SER*, smooth endoplasmic reticulum. ($\times 3{,}500$.)

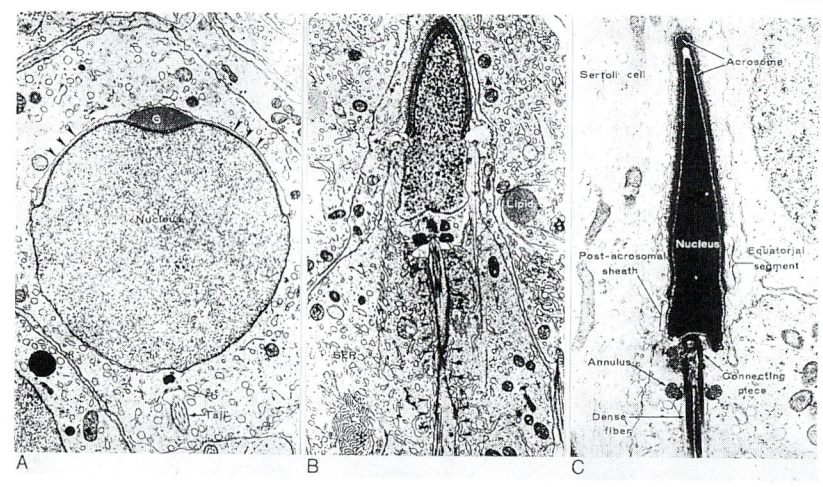

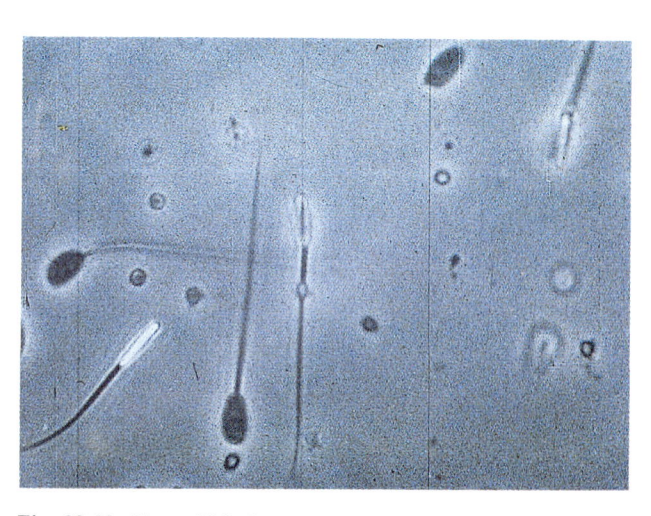

Fig. 19-18. Phase LM of spermatozoa showing flattened heads of spermatozoa in different planes. Observe small amount of residual cytoplasm in middlepiece region of one spermatozoon *(center)*. ($\times 600$.)

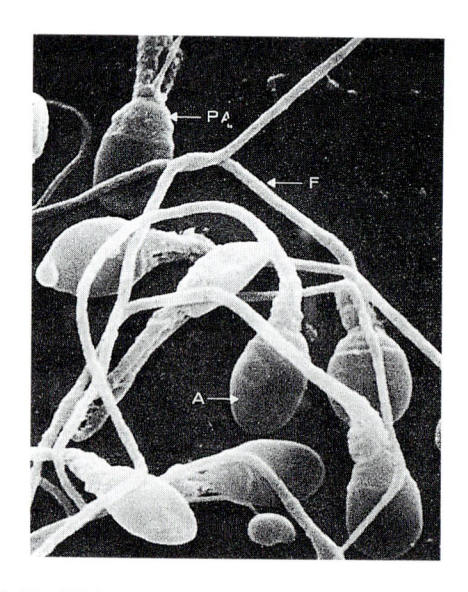

Fig. 19-19. SEM of spermatozoa. Extent of acrosome and postacrosomal segment of sperm head is evident. Note that sperm heads have typical ovoid profile, while little surface detail is seen in flagellum. *A*, acrosomal cap; *PA*, postacrosomal segment; *F*, flagellum. ($\times 1{,}800$.)

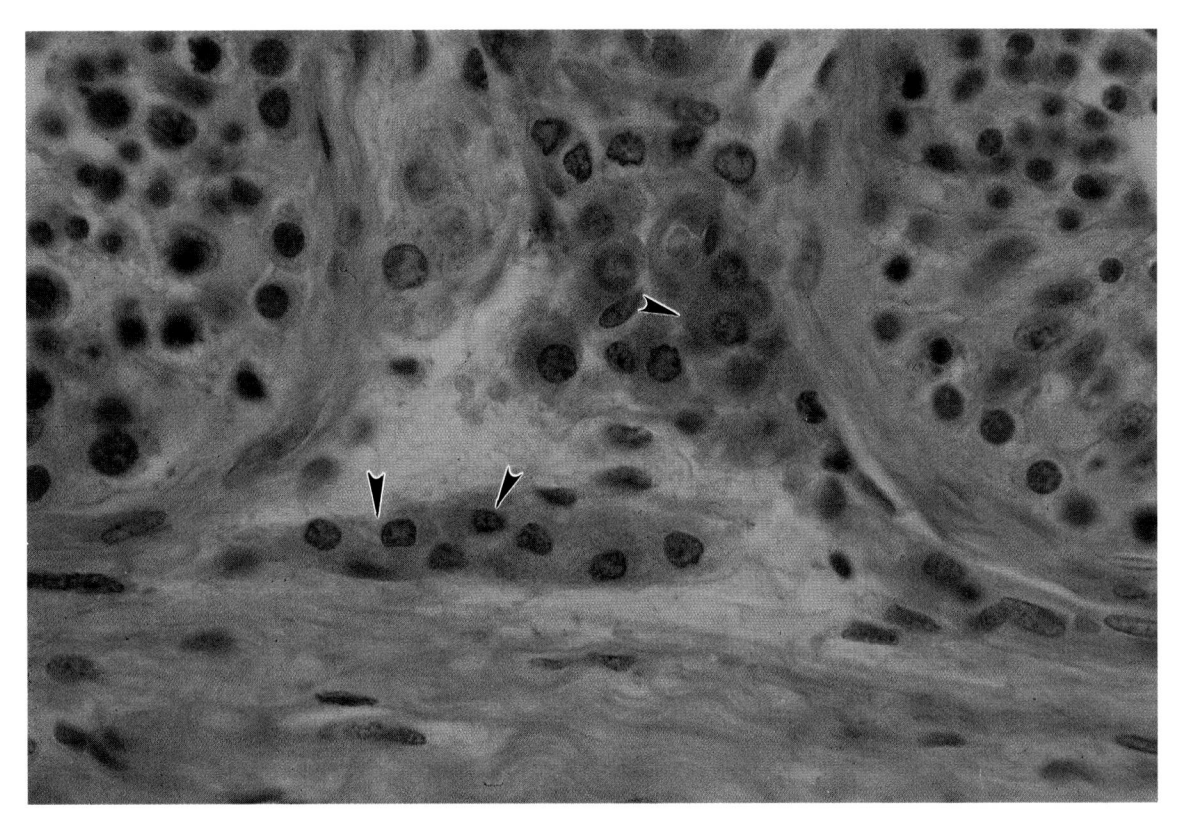

Fig. 19-20. LM of interstitial space between seminiferous tubules in testis. Acidophilic Leydig cells *(arrowheads)* are present in this space, together with vessels and lymphatics. (H&E; ×800.)

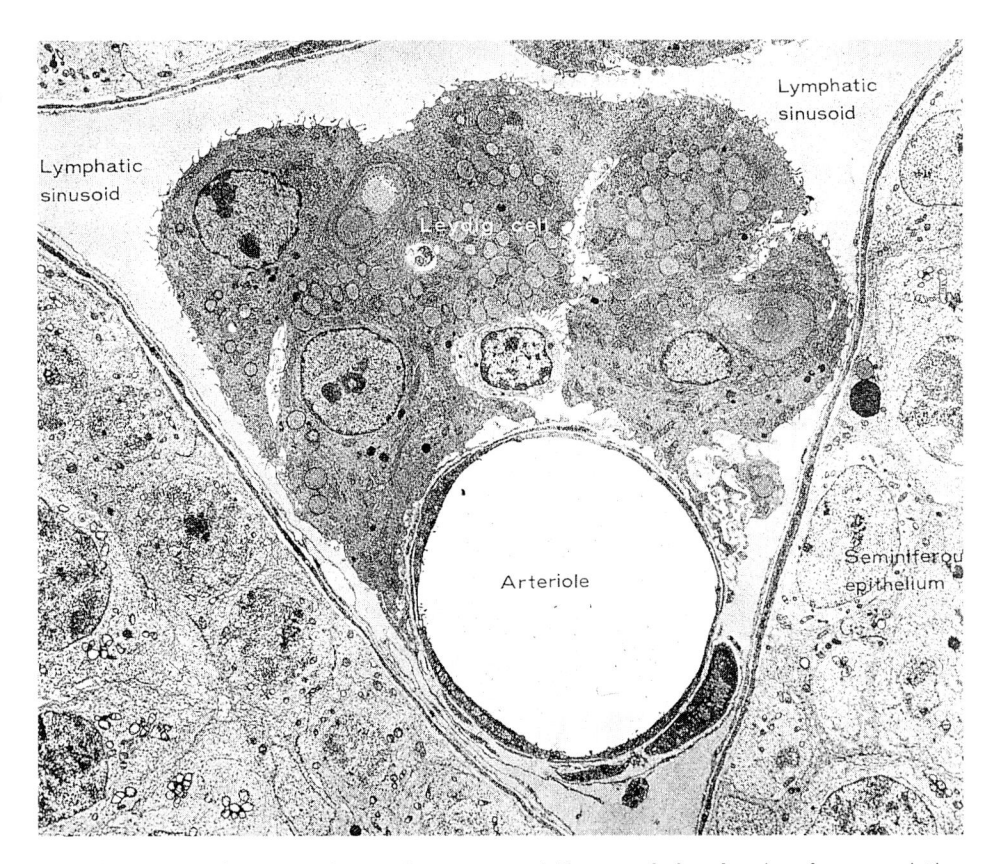

Fig. 19-21. TEM of interstitial space between seminiferous tubules showing close association between Leydig cells and blood vessels. Leydig cells also appear to be directly exposed to lymph in lymphatic sinusoids. (×2,400.)

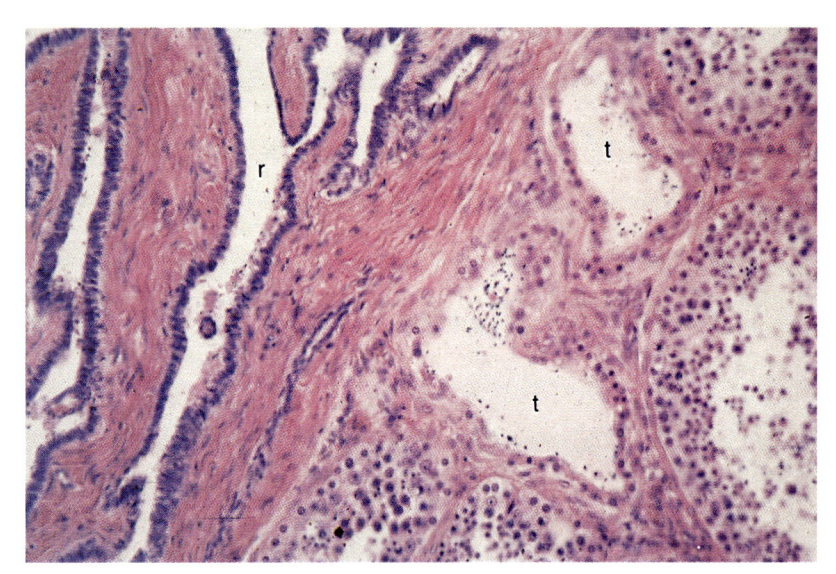

Fig. 19-22. LM of testis showing transition from seminiferous tubules to short tubuli recti (t). Latter open into network of epithelial-lined channels, called rete testis (r), which lies in mediastinum of testis. Compare Fig. 19-1. (H&E; ×125.)

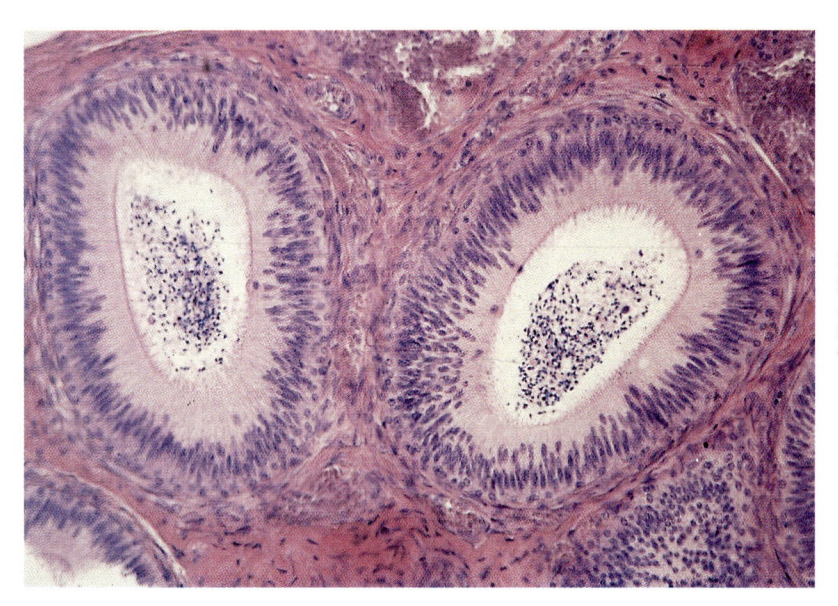

Fig. 19-23. LM of tubules in epididymis. Epithelium is pseudostratified columnar, rests on basal lamina, and is surrounded by smooth muscle fibers arranged in circular fashion. Spermatozoa can be seen within lumina of tubules (H&E; ×125.)

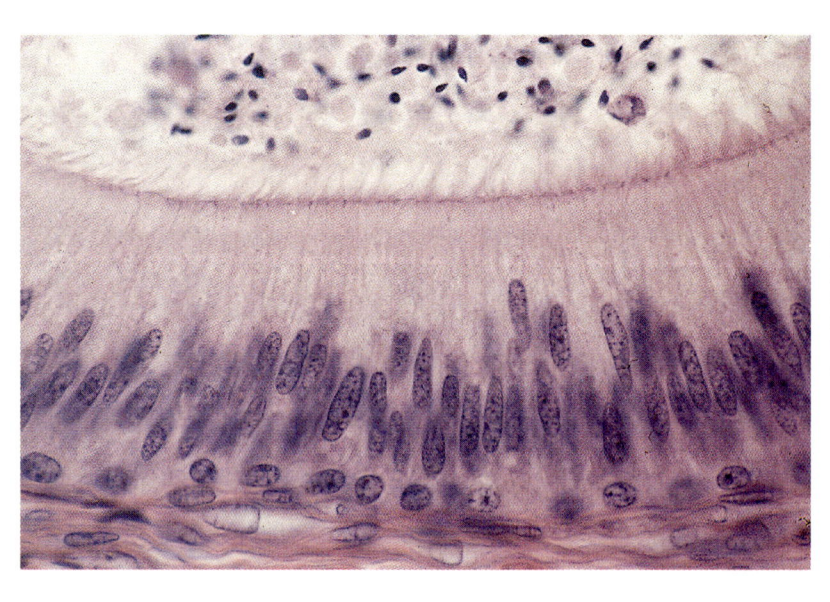

Fig. 19-24. Higher-magnification LM of pseudostratified columnar epithelium of epididymis. Luminal surface of epithelium bears long, nonmotile microvilli called stereocilia. Small round cells containing spherical nuclei are seen at base of epididymal epithelium. (H&E; ×800.)

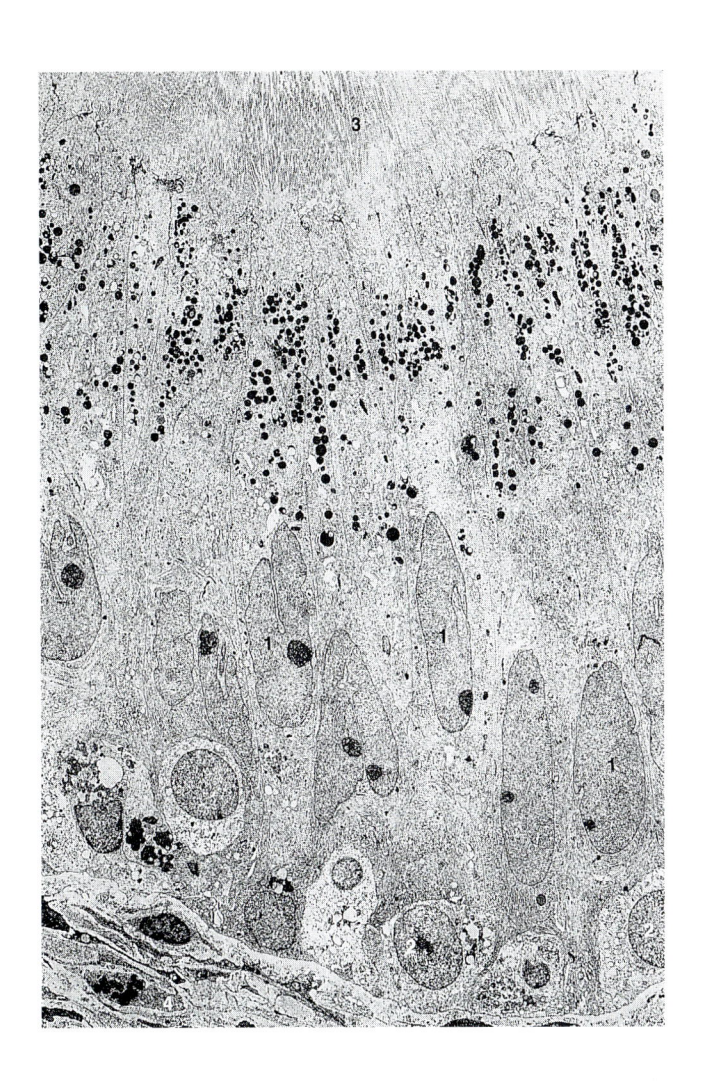

Fig. 19-25. TEM of pseudostratified columnar epithelium of ductus epididymis. Rounded basal cells and columnar principal cells are visible. Supranuclear cytoplasm has many electron-dense vesicles, multivesicular bodies, and lysosomes. Stereocilia emanate from apical surface of cells. ($\times 1,800$.)

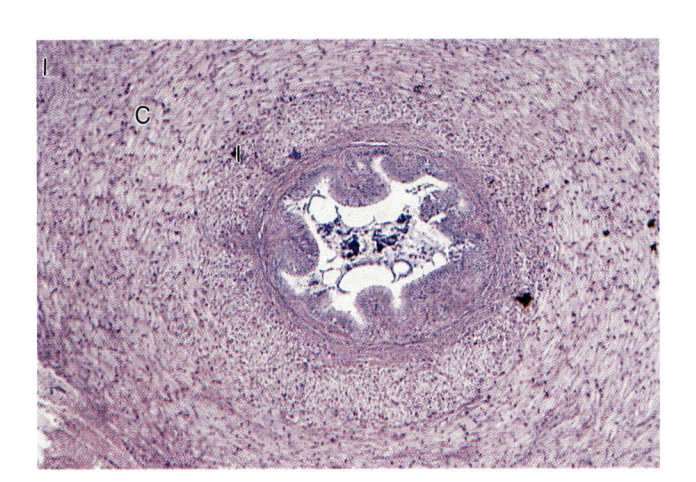

Fig. 19-26. LM of ductus deferens in cross section. Mucosa protrudes into lumen in several low folds. Structure of epithelium is similar to that seen in epididymis, but epithelial cells are not as tall. Surrounding mucosa of ductus deferens are three layers of smooth muscle cells. Fibers of inner and outer layers are arranged longitudinally *(l)*; those of middle layer, circularly *(c)*. (H&E; $\times 150$.)

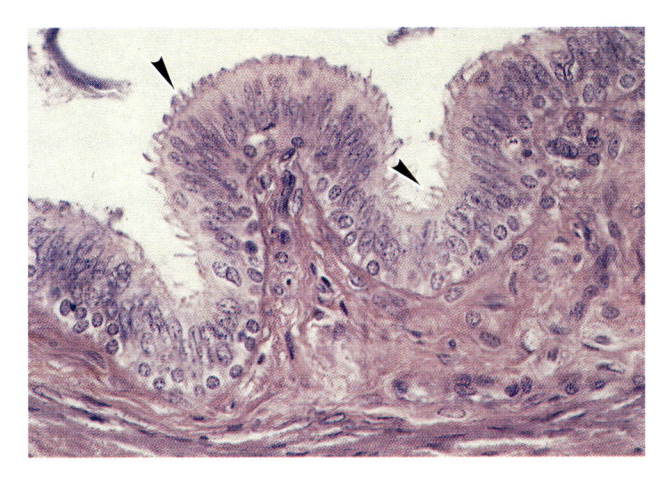

Fig. 19-27. Higher-magnification LM of mucosal surface within ductus deferens. Epithelium is pseudostratified columnar and contains stereocilia projecting from apical cytoplasm. Frequently stereocilia *(arrowheads)* are matted together and form conelike structures. (H&E; $\times 350$.)

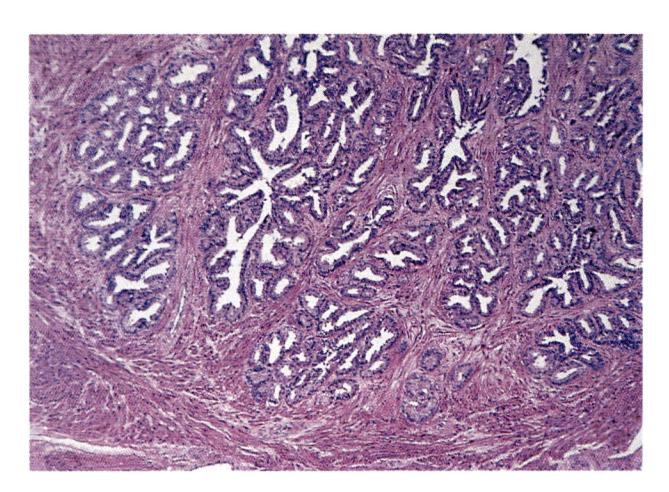

Fig. 19-28. LM of seminal vesicle illustrating branching and anastomosing of secondary and tertiary folds of mucosa, which join to form numerous irregular channels within lumen of gland. Lamina propria contains many elastic fibers, and smooth muscle cells course through connective tissue. (H&E; ×50.)

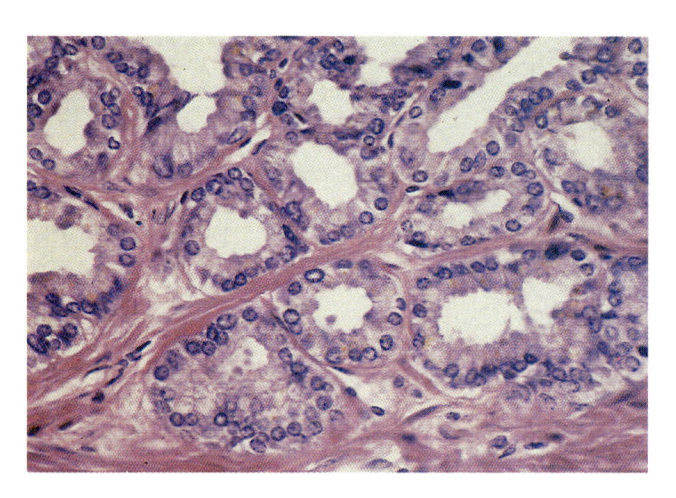

Fig. 19-29. LM of secretory epithelium within seminal vesicle. It is usually pseudostratified columnar epithelium, but occasionally it may appear to be simple columnar epithelium. (H&E; ×350.)

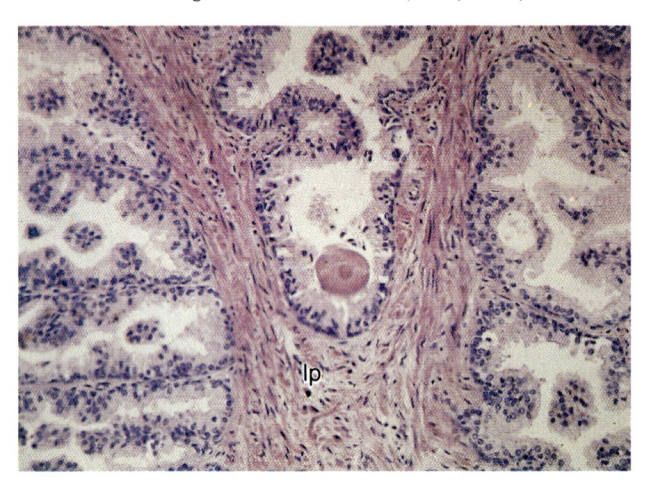

Fig. 19-30. LM of prostate gland. Mucosa of gland forms series of folds, and concretion granules are present within lumen. Lamina propria *(lp)* consists of fibromuscular stroma. (H&E; ×150.)

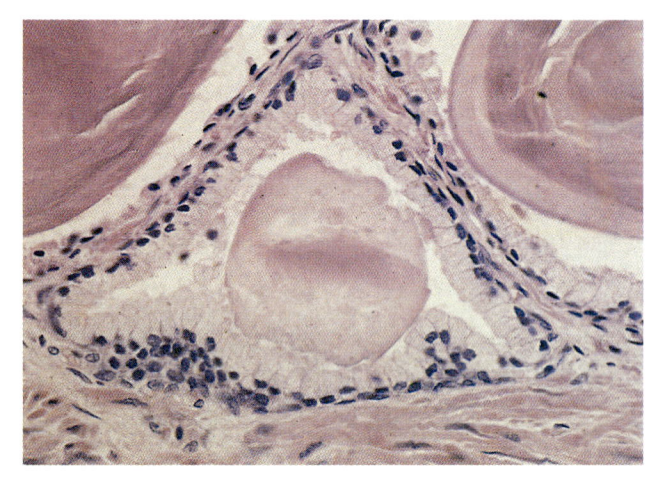

Fig. 19-31. Higher-magnification LM of prostatic alveoli showing large concretion granules within lumina. Epithelium is normally either simple columnar or pseudostratified columnar. (H&E; ×350.)

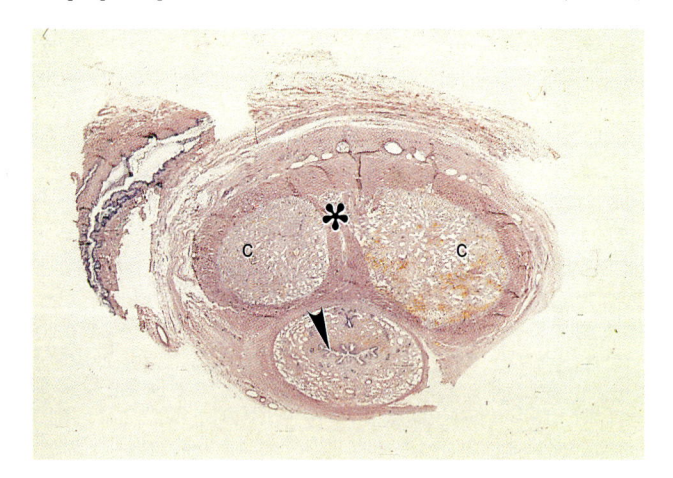

Fig. 19-32. Macrophotograph of penis in cross section. Note incomplete septum (*) dividing corpora cavernosa *(c)*, and observe urethra *(arrowhead)* within corpus spongiosum. Dense fibroelastic connective tissue layer, tunica albuginea, binds three cavernous bodies together and also provides attachment to skin overlying shaft of penis. (H&E; ×4.)

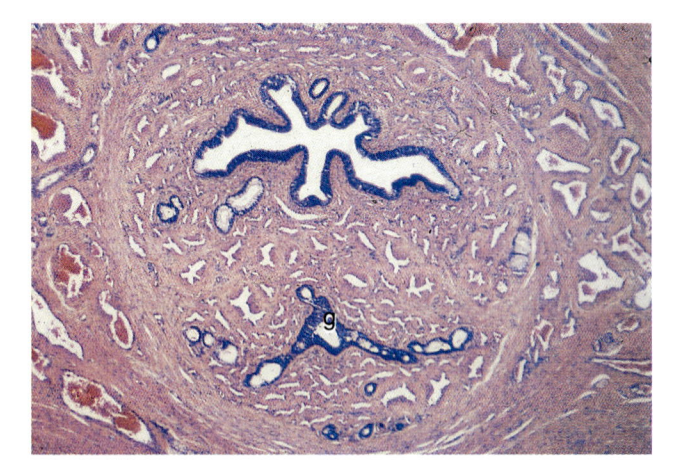

Fig. 19-33. Higher-magnification LM of corpus spongiosum showing location of penile urethra. Portions of seromucous glands *(g)* and small ducts are seen in lower part of field. (H&E; ×25.)

CHAPTER 20

FEMALE REPRODUCTIVE TRACT

ORGANS OF THE female reproductive tract that are directly associated with reproduction are the paired ovaries and uterine tubes, the uterus, and the vagina. The lactating mammary glands are often included in a discussion of the female reproductive tract because of their importance in nourishing the newborn.

1. **Ovaries** function as exocrine glands by producing a female germ cell, the oocyte. Acting as endocrine glands, ovaries secrete estrogens and progesterone, which are involved with development of the germ cells and preparation of the uterus to receive the conceptus.
2. An **oviduct** (**uterine** or **fallopian tube**) receives the ovulated oocyte and transports it to the uterus. En route, the oocyte may be fertilized; if it is, it is called an ovum.
3. The **uterus** undergoes cycling of the epithelial lining to provide a site for implantation and nutritional support for the ovum if fertilization occurs.
4. At term, the fetus passes from the uterus through the fibromuscular **vagina**, or birth canal. The vagina also functions as the female copulatory organ.

OVARIES

Like the testes, ovaries develop in the abdominal cavity. They descend only as far as the lateral walls of the pelvis minor, to which they are attached by a fold of the broad ligament called the **mesovarium** and the **suspensory ligament** of the ovary, which also transmits ovarian blood vessels. As with the testes, ovarian arteries derive from the abdominal aorta and ovarian veins are tributary to the inferior vena cava.

A simple cuboidal mesothelium covering the ovary is called the **germinal epithelium**, but this is a misnomer since the cells are strictly an epithelial lining and not germ (or stem) cells. Beneath this mesothelial layer is the **tunica albuginea**, a dense connective tissue capsule surrounding the **cortex** and **medulla**. Blood vessels enter at a hilum and pass into the medulla. Approximately 400,000 **primordial follicles** are present within the cortex at birth. Each consists of a **primary oocyte** surrounded by a single layer of squamous **follicular cells** joined by desmosomes and separated from the surrounding stroma by a basement membrane. **Follicle-stimulating hormone** causes maturation of one or more primordial follicles during each cycle.

Oocytes grow rapidly and follicular cells multiply, forming a multilaminar **primary follicle.** Follicular cells become cuboidal and secrete estrogens, which promote development of the **primary oocyte** and growth of the uterine mucosa. They are now called **granulosa cells.** Continued development produces a larger **secondary follicle** containing a fluid-filled antrum surrounded outside the basement membrane by stromal cells arranged into concentric layers called the **theca interna** and **theca externa.** At **ovulation,** a mature secondary or graffian follicle releases the **secondary oocyte** into the peritoneal cavity. Thereafter, the ovulated follicle develops into a **corpus luteum** and produces **estrogens** and **progesterone** to prepare the uterus for implantation of the fertilized ovum.

OVIDUCT (UTERINE OR FALLOPIAN TUBE)

The ovulated oocyte, in the peritoneal cavity, must be directed into the **oviduct** and conveyed to the uterus. Finger-like **fimbria,** evaginations of the distal end (**infundibulum**) of the oviduct, sweep across the ovary at ovulation and move the oocyte into the oviduct. The tubular oviduct is subdivided into **infundibulum,** a funnel-shaped end close to the ovary, which narrows to become the **ampulla,** where fertilization usually takes place. The next segment, called the **isthmus,** gives way to the **intramural** portion of the tube as it enters the uterus. The oviduct wall is composed of mucous membrane, muscularis, and serosa.

The **mucous membrane** is thrown into folds that

project into the lumen. These folds form a complex labyrinth and are most prominent in the infundibulum and the ampulla. The epithelium consists of two types of simple columnar cells: **ciliated cells** assist in moving the oocyte along the tube, while **secretory cells** provide a fluid medium in which the oocyte is suspended, nourished, and protected. A highly vascular loose connective tissue **lamina propria** attaches the epithelium to underlying smooth muscle, which is arranged in inner circular and outer longitudinal layers. Peristaltic contraction of the **muscularis** propels the oocyte toward the uterus. A **serosa** covers the uterine tube.

UTERUS

This thick-walled pear-shaped organ consists of **fundus, body,** and **cervix.** The oviducts enter laterally where fundus and body meet. The uterine wall is composed of a mucous membrane (**endometrium**), smooth muscle in three layers (**myometrium**), and an outer serosa or adventitia (**epimetrium**). The endometrium contains simple columnar ciliated and secretory cells arranged in tubular glands with deep and apical regions. The uterine endometrium undergoes a series of changes, referred to as the uterine cycle, in response to hormonal stimulation from the developing follicle and corpus luteum.

After menstruation, the remaining deep portion of the glands, the **pars basalis,** responds to estrogen by regenerating the epithelial lining and the uterine glands (proliferative phase of the uterine cycle). The **pars functionalis** consists of the apical regions of the uterine glands. Following ovulation, the glandular endometrium produces a nutrient-rich secretion (secretory phase of uterine cycle). If implantation does not occur, the pars functionalis portion of the endometrium is shed by hemorrhage at menstruation as a result of ischemia produced by the contraction of coiled arteries deep in the endometrium (menstrual phase of the uterine cycle).

VAGINA

The vagina is a thick-walled fibromuscular tube that forms the last segment of the female reproductive tract. It connects the uterus to the outside of the body. The mucosa of the vagina contains a thick, stratified, squamous, nonkeratinized epithelium and a lamina propria composed of fibroelastic tissue. Variable numbers of white blood cells, including numerous lymphocytes, may be encountered in the mucosa during different parts of the uterine cycle, with increased numbers present during ovulation and menses. No glands are found in the vagina, so any mucus present is derived from glands found within the cervix of the uterus or uterine glands. The **muscularis** consists of indistinct, intertwined smooth muscle bundles and is surrounded by an **adventitia** of dense fibroelastic connective tissue that blends with adjacent pelvic fascia.

MAMMARY GLANDS

The lactating **mammary gland** consists of a branching duct system terminating in secretory tubuloalveolar glands. Contraction of myoepithelial cells surrounding the alveoli expresses milk into large anastomosing collecting ducts (10 to 25), which form lactiferous sinuses and terminate in the nipple. Milk is the watery secretion of the lactating mammary gland; it consists of proteins (casein, lactalbumin), fats (triglycerides, phosphoproteins, cholesterol), carbohydrates (lactose, galactose), immunoglobulins (secretory IgA), minerals, and salts. The first milk produced, called colostrum, is especially rich in immunoglobulin.

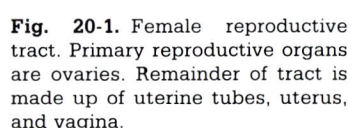

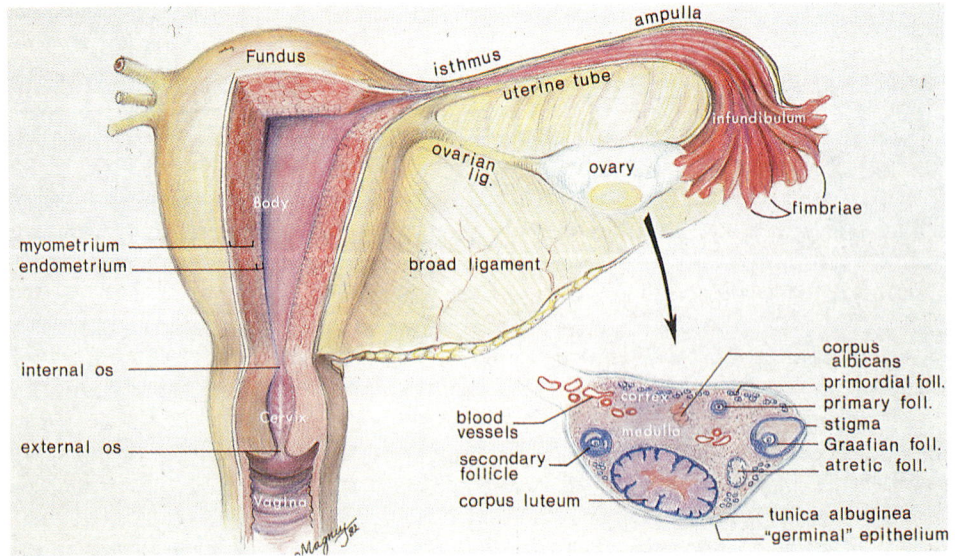

Fig. 20-1. Female reproductive tract. Primary reproductive organs are ovaries. Remainder of tract is made up of uterine tubes, uterus, and vagina.

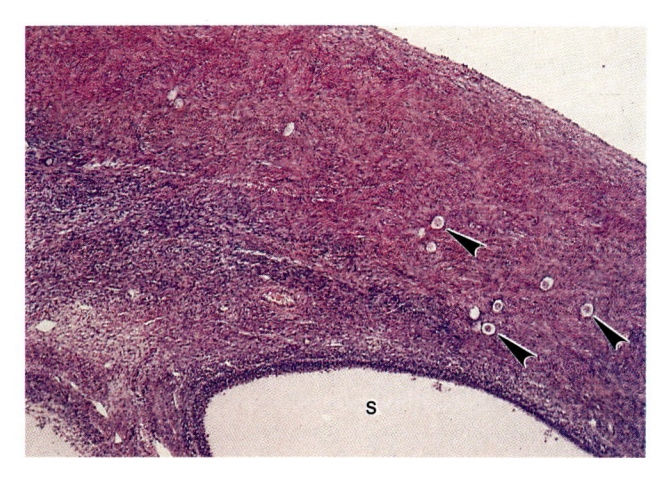

Fig. 20-2. LM of ovarian cortex showing capsule, primordial follicles *(arrowheads)*, and large secondary follicles *(s)*. Stroma is densely populated by spindle-shaped cells, which are characteristic throughout female reproductive tract. (H&E; ×30.)

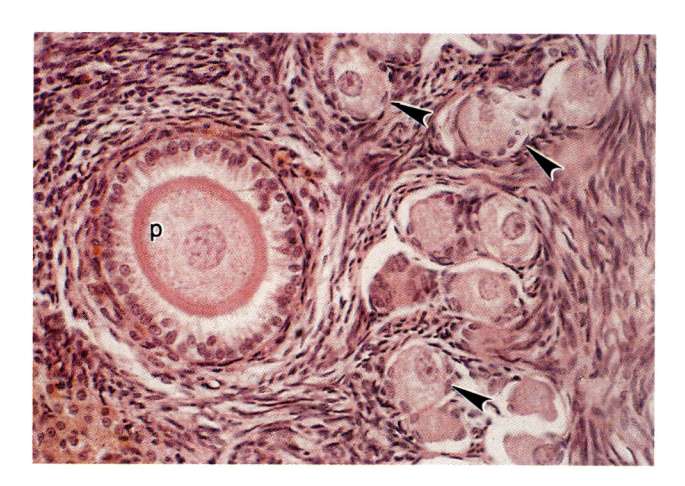

Fig. 20-3. LM of ovary showing many examples of primordial follicles and transitional stages between primordial *(arrowheads)* and primary *(p)* follicles. Follicular cells divide to form multiple layers in primary follicle, and zona pellucida becomes well defined. (H&E; ×300.)

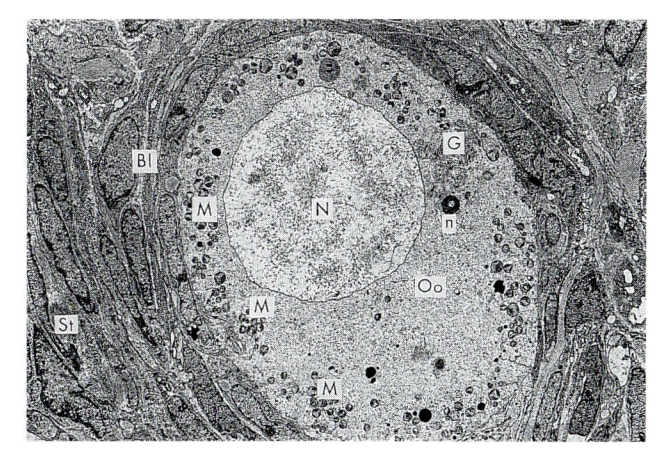

Fig. 20-4. TEM of primordial follicle. Primary oocyte is surrounded by single layer of closely apposed, flattened follicular (pregranulosa) cells. Basal lamina surrounds primordial follicle and separates it from adjacent connective tissue stroma of ovarian cortex. *St*, stroma; *Bl*, basal lamina; *M*, mitochondria; *N*, nucleus; *G*, Golgi; *Oo*, oocyte; *n*, nuclear-like body. (×800.)

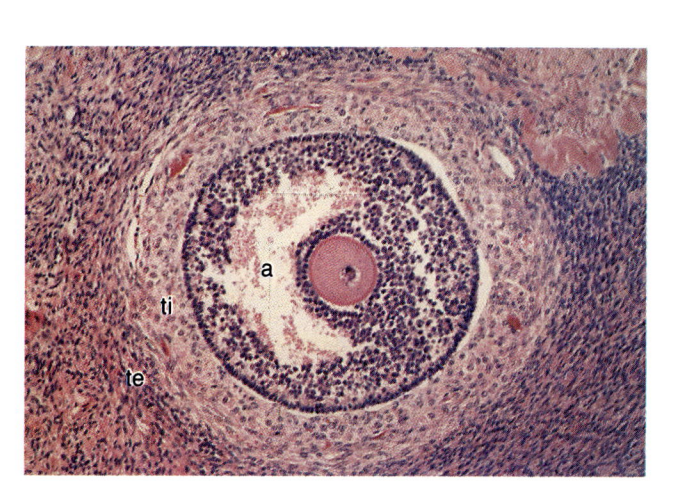

Fig. 20-5. LM of developing secondary follicle. There are now multiple layers of granulosa cells, and an antrum has begun to form *(a)*. At this stage stromal cells are well organized into theca interna *(ti)* and theca externa *(te)*. (H&E; ×150.)

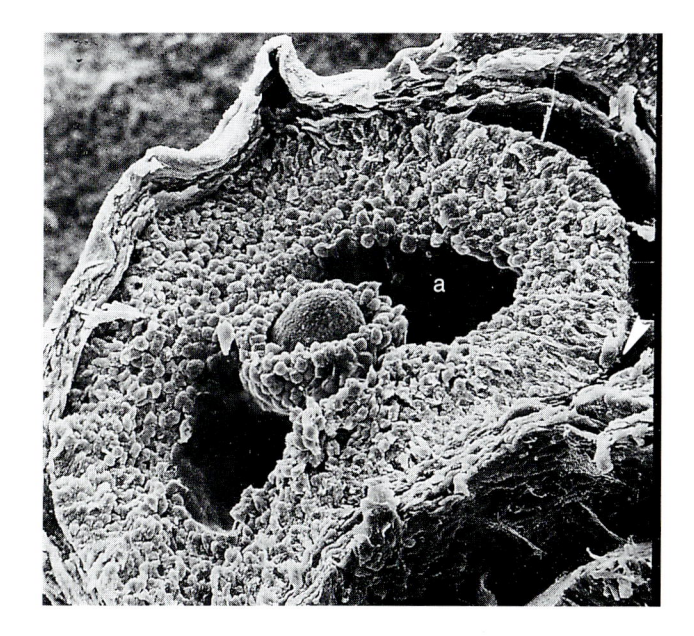

Fig. 20-6. SEM of developing secondary follicle similar to that seen in Fig. 20-5. Observe antrum *(a)* and basal lamina *(arrowhead)*, which separates granulosa cells from theca interna. (×250.)

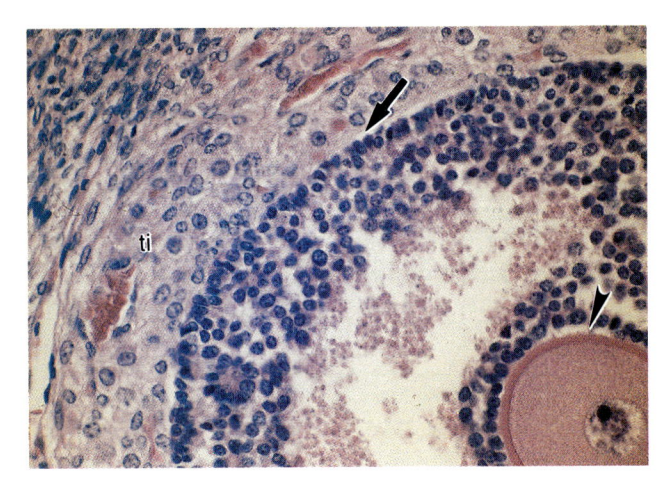

Fig. 20-7. Higher-magnification LM of secondary follicle seen in Fig. 20-5. Note vascularity of theca interna *(ti)*. Primary oocyte *(lower right)* is surrounded by well-developed zona pellucida *(arrowhead)* and adjacent granulosa cells. *Large arrow* indicates region of basement membrane separating avascular granulosa cells from theca interna, (H&E; ×400.)

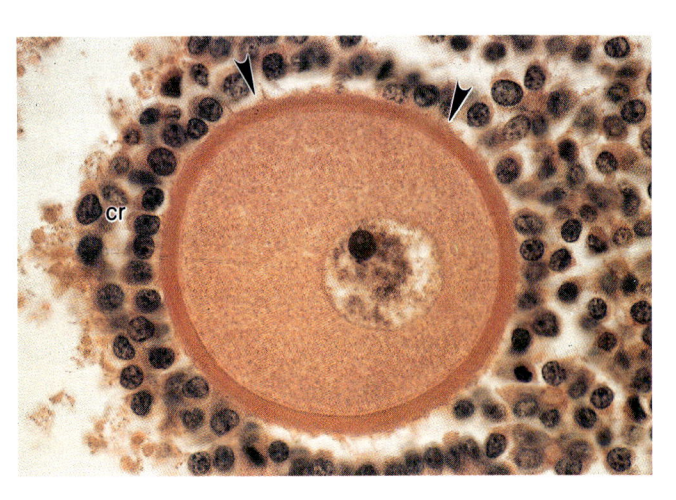

Fig. 20-8. High-magnification LM of a primary oocyte in secondary follicle. Oocyte is surrounded by corona radiata *(cr)* and supported by cumulus oophorus *(right)*; both structures are composed of granulosa cells. Well-developed zona pellucida *(arrowheads)* appears acidophilic. Nucleus and nucleolus are evident within oocyte. (H&E; ×750.)

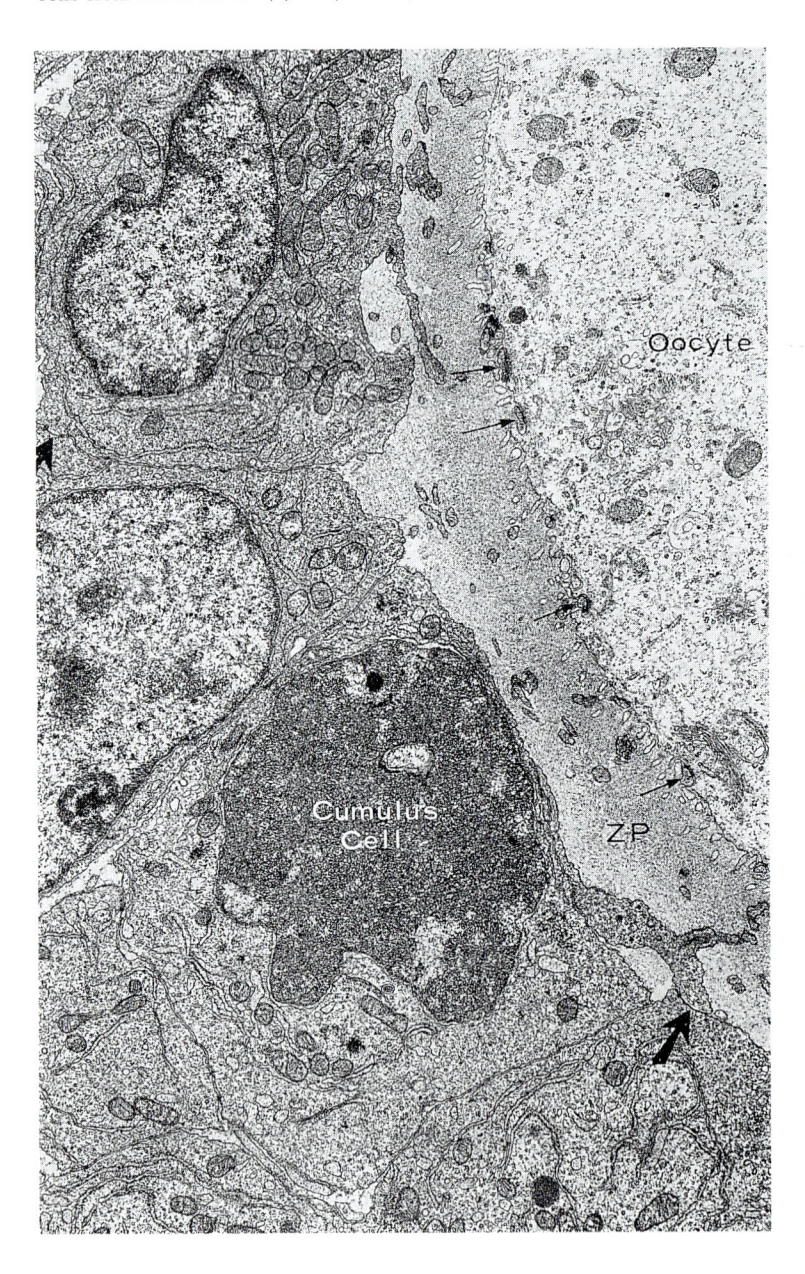

Fig. 20-9. TEM of granulosa cells in cumulus-oocyte complex of large nonpreovulatory follicle from rat. Innermost granulosa cells in cumulus layer (corona radiata) send processes through zona pellucida *(ZP)* to form contacts (gap junctions) with plasma membrane of secondary oocyte *(small arrows)*. Adjacent granulosa cells are also joined by gap junctions *(large arrows)*. (×8,700.)

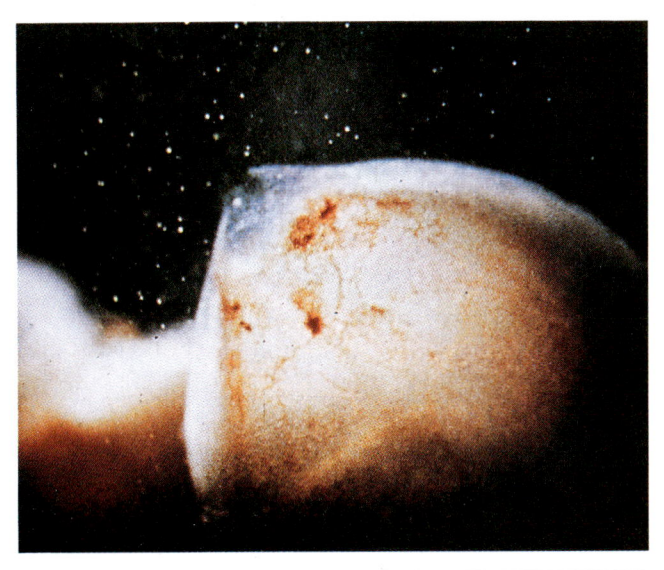

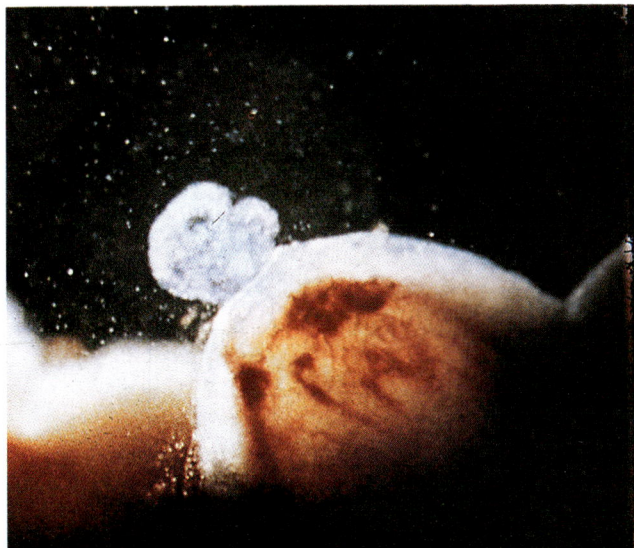

Fig. 20-10 to 20-12. Series of three motion picture frames illustrating stages in ovulation. Shown in Fig. 20-10 is initial rupture of follicle. In Fig. 20-11 cumulus cells are expressed from follicle; secondary oocyte-cumulus complex can be seen as small white ball just beyond opening of ruptured follicle. In Fig. 20-12 entire cumulus mass is about to be picked up by fimbriae of infundibulum as they sweep over surface of ovary.

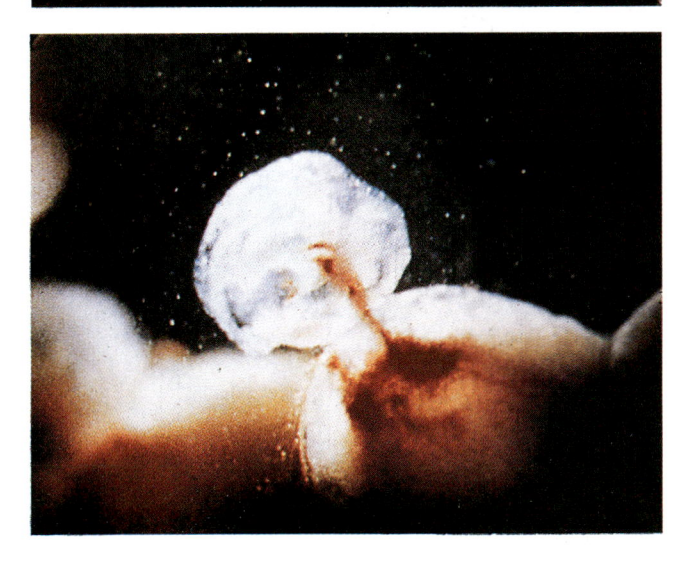

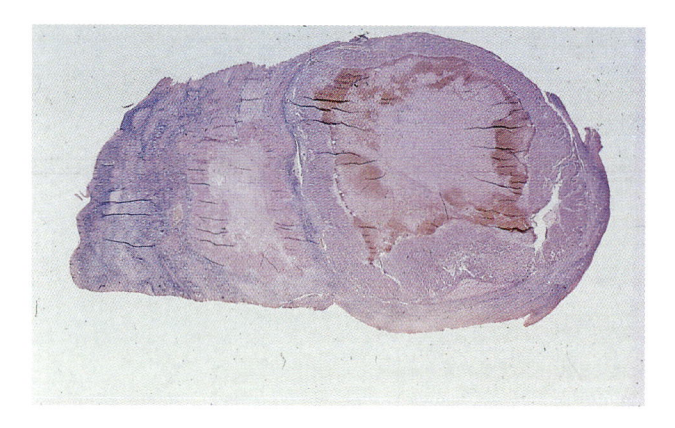

Fig. 20-13. Macrophotograph of section of ovary showing two large corpora lutea. One on right can be considered a corpus hemorrhagicum, since portions of red cell clot can be seen within lumen. Corpus luteum on left is from a previous month's ovulation; it is undergoing regression and does not contain viable luteal cells. (H&E; ×3.)

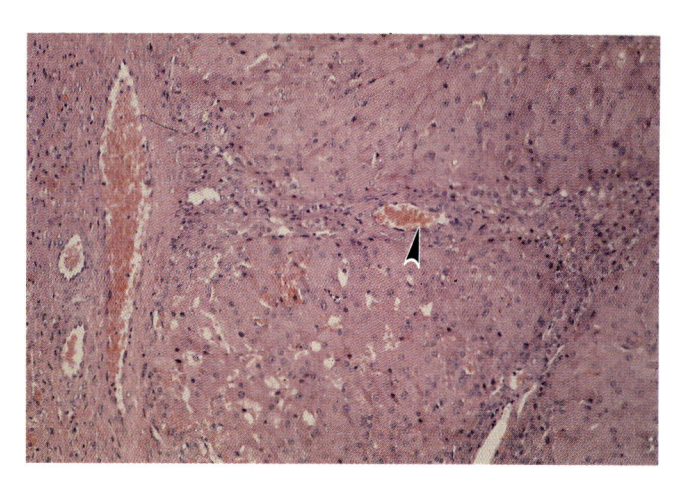

Fig. 20-14. LM of corpus luteum. Large granulosa luteal cells are visible *(middle)*. Vessels in stroma surrounding corpus luteum are sending small branches *(arrowhead)* accompanied by theca luteal cells into previously avascular corpus luteum. (H&E; ×150.)

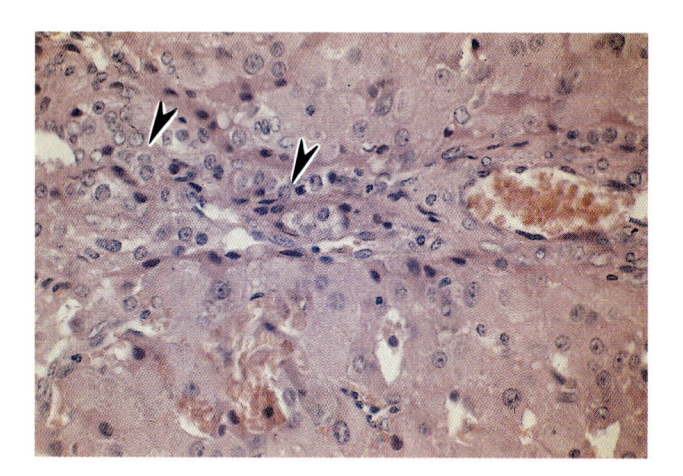

Fig. 20-15. Higher-magnification LM of corpus luteum illustrating smaller theca luteal cells *(arrowheads)* and larger granulosa luteal cells *(g)*. (H&E; ×350.)

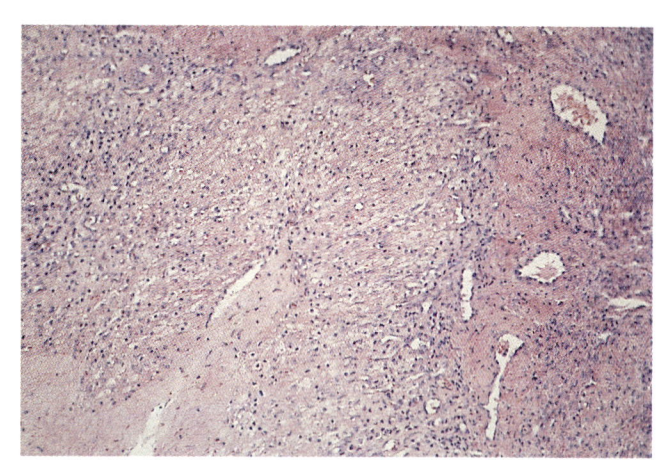

Fig. 20-16. LM of regressing corpus luteum. Ovarian stroma can be seen *(right)*, and luteal wall now contains infiltrating mononuclear cells involved in phagocytosis of degraded luteal cells. (H&E; ×150.)

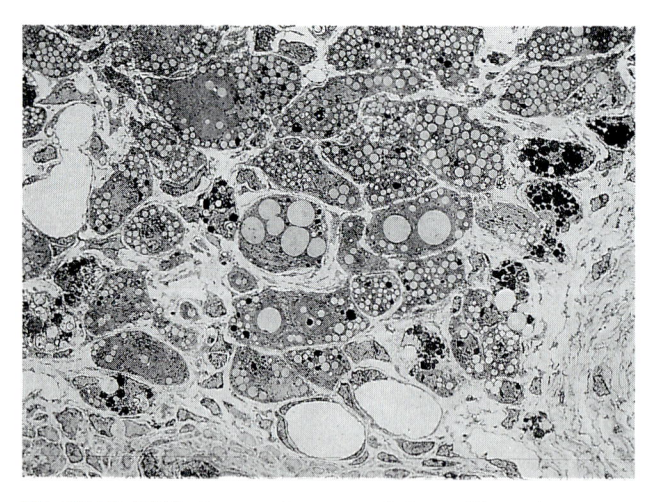

Fig. 20-17. TEM of regressing corpus luteum. Macrophages can be distinguished from luteal cells by presence of numerous dense bodies within their cytoplasm. Note that macrophages appear to be particularly abundant along edge of corpus luteum, a finding consistent with symmetrical centripetal shrinkage that occurs as this structure involutes. Aging luteal cells contain numerous lipid droplets, many of which have been extracted by solvents used during processing of tissue for microscopy. (×550.)

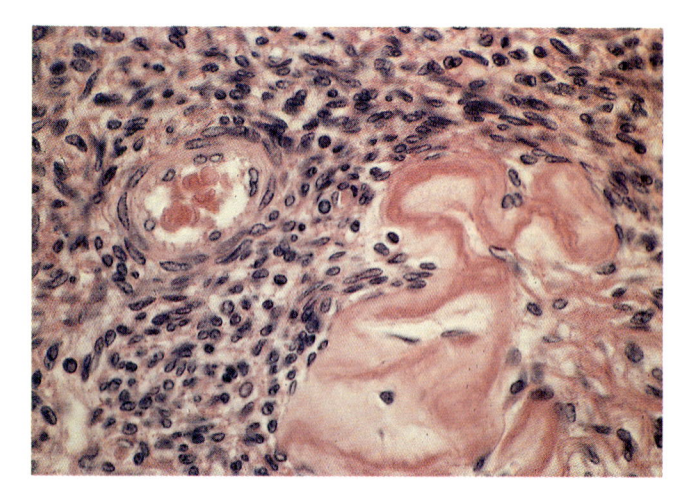

Fig. 20-18. LM of corpus albicans in ovary. After lysis of luteal cells, all that remains of corpus luteum is small scar consisting of collagen fibers, macrophages, a few fibroblasts, and occasionally some cells that bear a superficial resemblance to luteal cells. (H&E; ×400.)

FEMALE REPRODUCTIVE TRACT 167

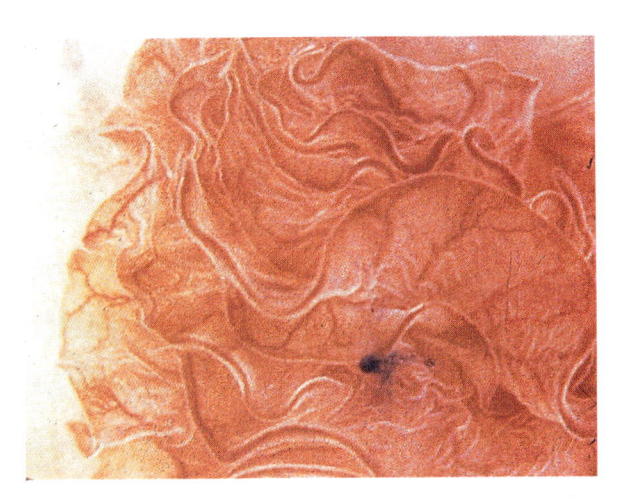

Fig. 20-19. Macrophotograph of infundibular region of uterine tube during ovulation. Oocyte and attached cumulus cells *(stained blue)* are seen in transit toward ostium of tube. If no cumulus cells surround oocyte at this particular time, it will not be transported by ciliary action into uterine tube.

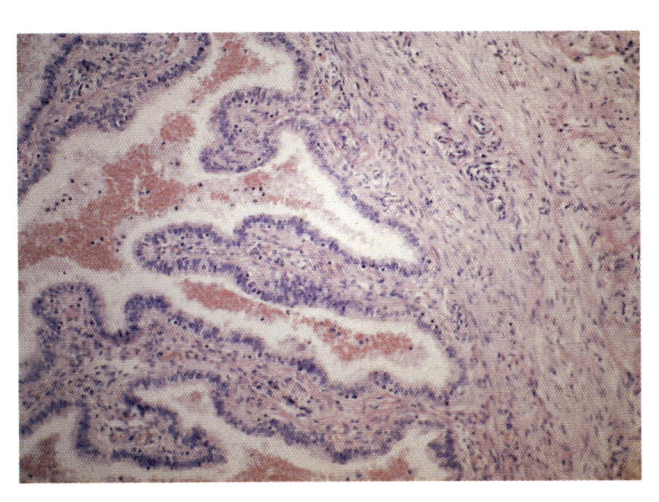

Fig. 20-20. LM of wall of uterine tube. Mucosal folds, projecting into lumen, are common in infundibular region, and lumen (as shown here) often contains red blood cells as a result of hemorrhage at time of surgical removal of specimen. (H&E; ×150.)

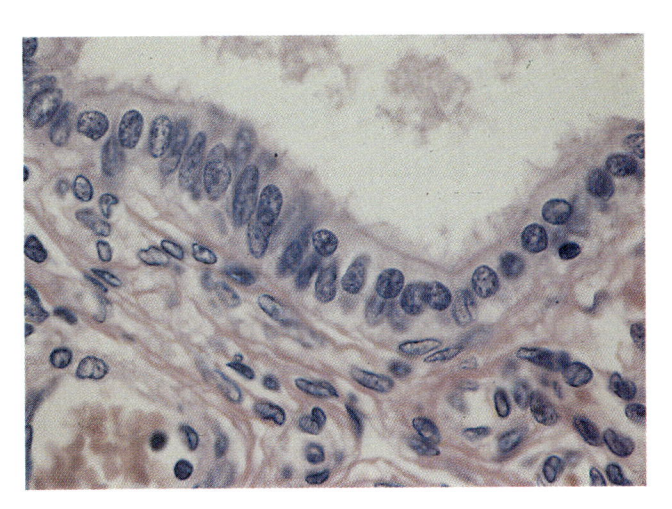

Fig. 20-21. Higher-magnification LM of uterine tube. Epithelial lining consists of simple columnar ciliated cells and other nonciliated cells (bearing microvilli) that are considered to have secretory function. (H&E; ×750.)

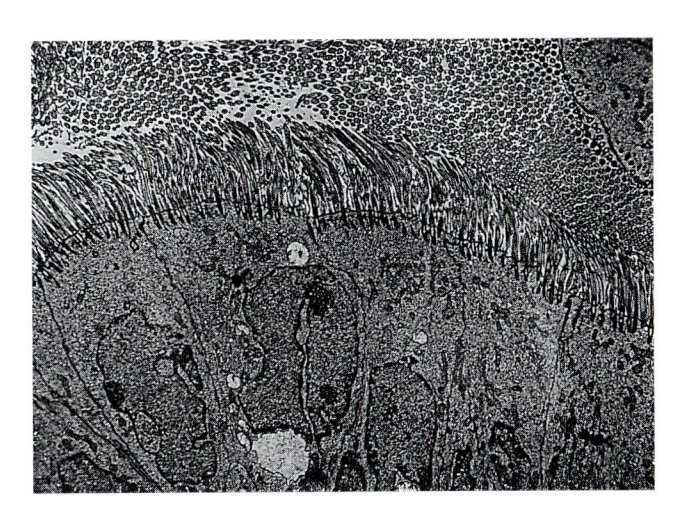

Fig. 20-22. TEM of epithelial cells in uterine tube showing both cilia and microvilli associated with apical surface. (×2,000.)

Fig. 20-23. High-magnification SEM of luminal surface of uterine tube epithelium showing presence of spermatozoa. Fertilization usually takes place in ampullo-isthmic junction of uterine tube. Compare size of microvilli, cilia, and sperm flagella. *fl*, Flagellum; *MP*, midpiece of spermatozoon. (×2,500.)

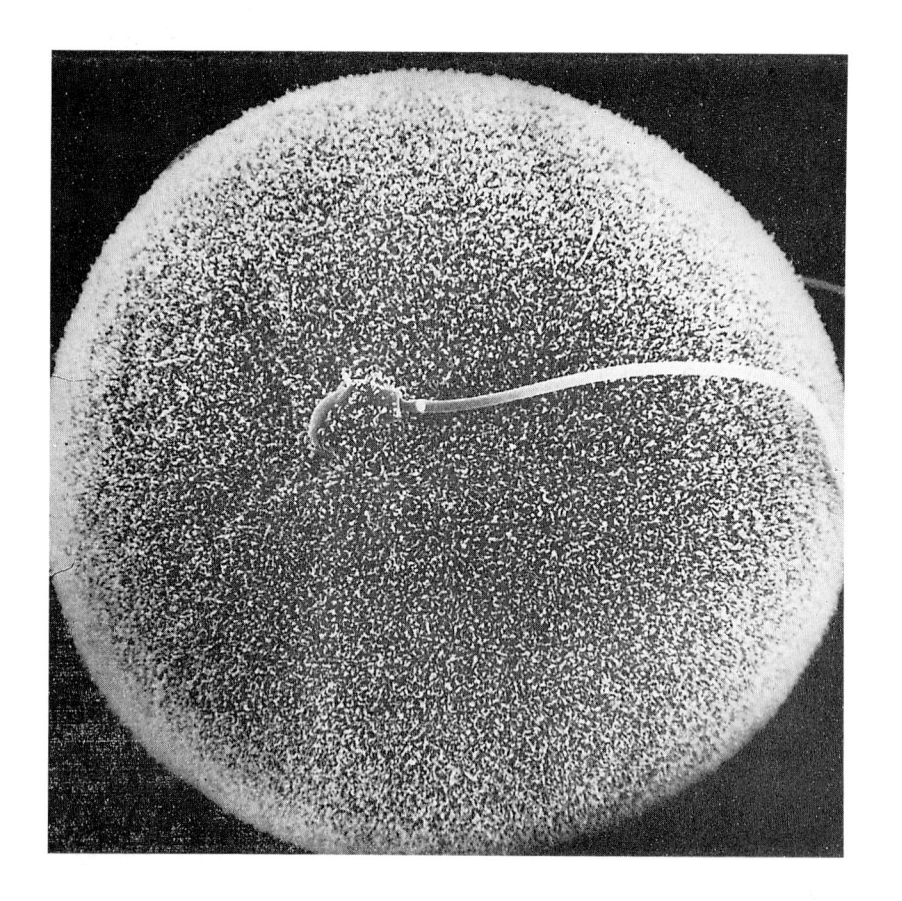

Fig. 20-24. SEM of oocyte and attached spermatozoon. In mammals, fertilization occurs when spermatozoon fuses by its lateral surface with microvilli on surface of oocyte. (×2,000.)

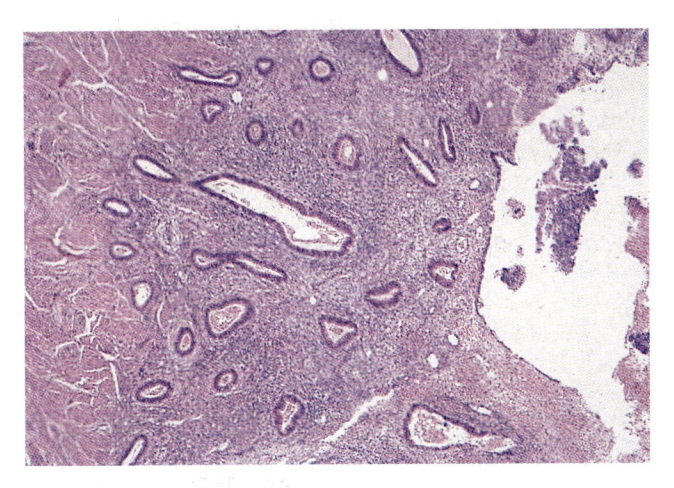

Fig. 20-25. LM of uterine endometrium during menstrual phase of uterine cycle. Uterine surface is still partially denuded of epithelium. Note straight glands extending through endometrium. (H&E; ×50.)

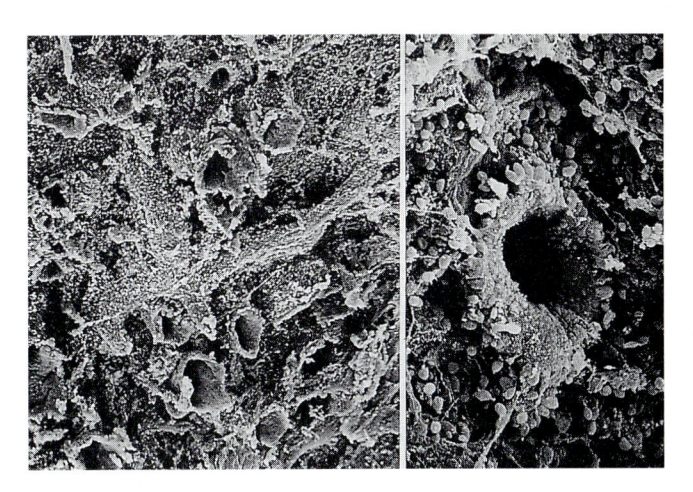

Fig. 20-26. SEM of surface of uterus during menstruation. In low-magnification SEM of uterine surface *(left)*, several openings of tubular uterine glands can be seen. At higher magnification *(right)*, epithelial cells have begun to re-cover surface of uterus through continual cell division and migration of cells over denuded surface. (Left ×75; right ×150.)

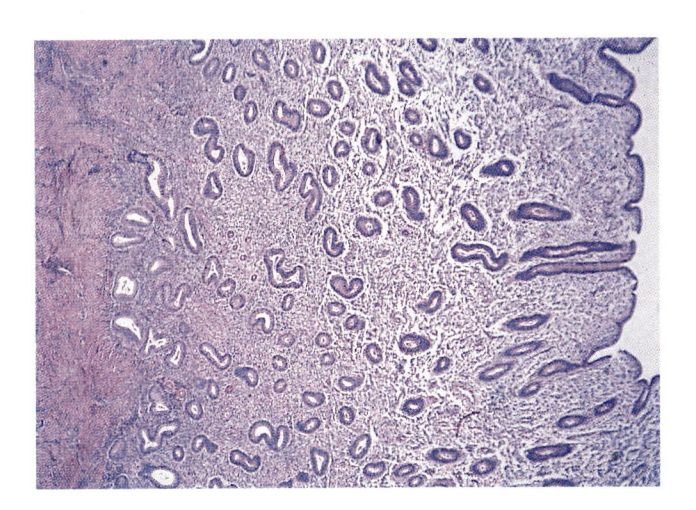

Fig. 20-27. LM of uterine endometrium during proliferative phase of uterine cycle. Observe increased thickness of endometrium and coiled glands. Pars basalis region of endometrium can be distinguished at far left. (H&E; ×50.)

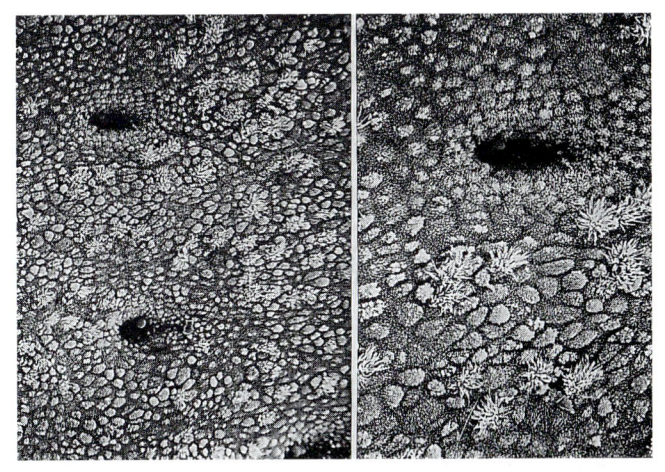

Fig. 20-28. SEM of uterine surface during proliferative phase of uterine cycle. Reepithelialization of surface has been completed, and small numbers of ciliated cells are beginning to appear. Several gland openings are seen in low-magnification SEM at left; single gland is shown at higher magnification on right. (Left ×75; right ×150.)

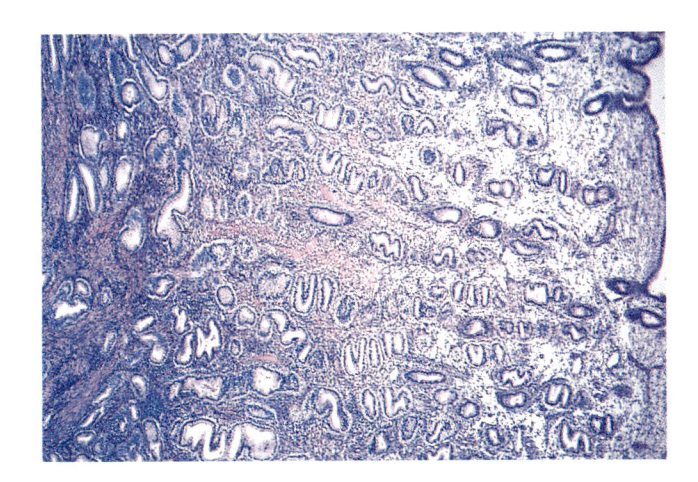

Fig. 20-29. LM of uterine endometrium during secretory phase of uterine cycle. Note edematous accumulation of fluid within endometrium and highly coiled uterine glands. Increased numbers of stromal cells are visible within lamina propria of endometrium. (H&E; ×50.)

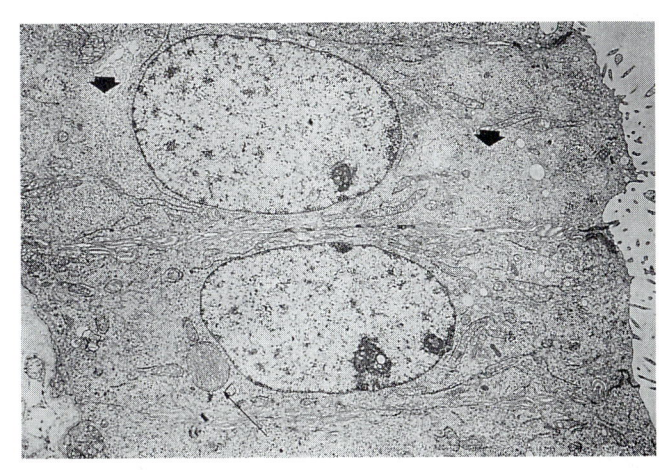

Fig. 20-30. TEM showing several nonciliated uterine epithelial cells. Note simple columnar arrangement of epithelium. Deposits of glycogen can be seen at large arrow and mitochondria at small arrow. (×3,600.)

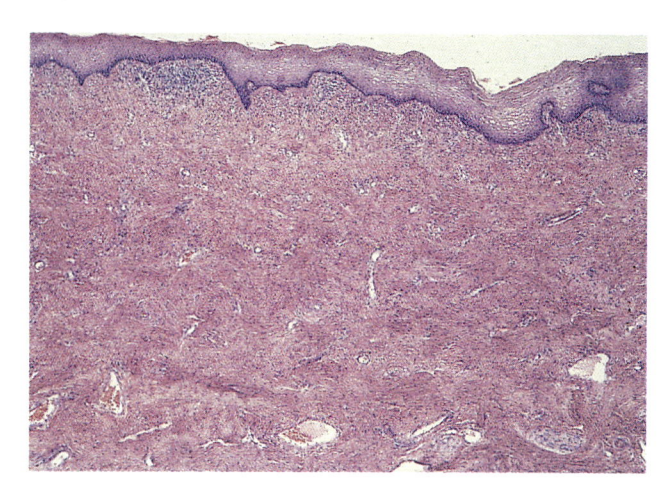

Fig. 20-31. Low-magnification LM of vagina. Epithelium is nonkeratinized stratified squamous. Although vaginal wall resembles esophagus, it does not contain a muscularis mucosa or mucous glands. Likewise, although muscularis consists of smooth muscle cells, there is no apparent organization of bundles into well-defined layers. (H&E; ×50.)

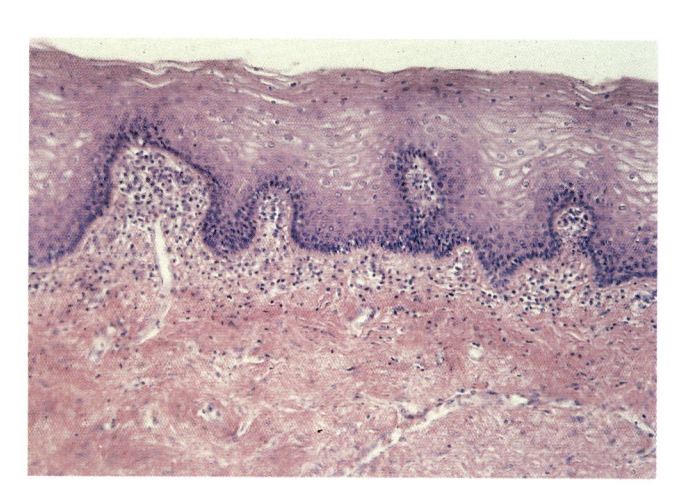

Fig. 20-32. Higher-magnification LM of vagina demonstrating nonkeratinized, stratified squamous epithelium. Lymphocytic infiltration can be seen in lamina propria immediately beneath epithelium. Underlying connective tissue is of loose fibroelastic nature. (H&E; ×150.)

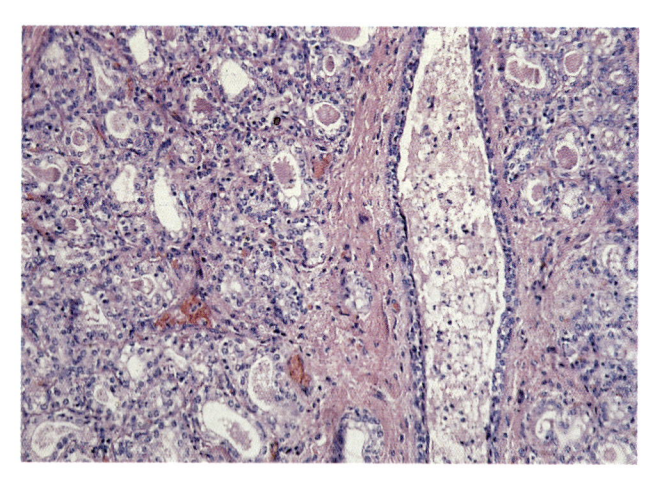

Fig. 20-33. LM of mammary gland. Secretory acini are of variable size and contain a heterogeneous mottled secretory product in lumen. Large ducts surrounded by connective tissue are also present. (H&E; ×150.)

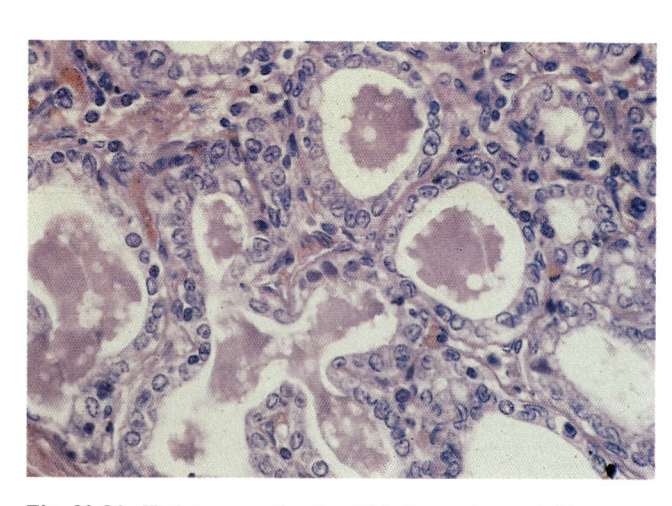

Fig. 20-34. Higher-magnification LM of secretory acini in mammary gland. Observe irregular appearance of secretory product within lumen and branching of acini and ducts. (H&E; ×350.)

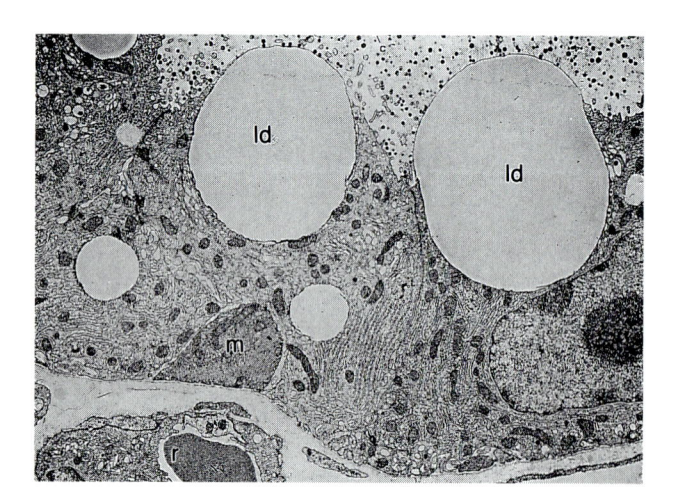

Fig. 20-35. TEM of epithelium lining alveolus in lactating mammary gland. Two large lipid droplets are present within apical cytoplasm of cells. Eventually lipid droplets will be released into lumen, where casein protein droplets are evident. At base of epithelium, myoepithelial cell process can be seen, and in lamina propria continuous capillary containing RBC is present. *C*, casein; *ld*, lipid droplets; *m*, myoepithelial cell process; *r*, red blood cell. (×4,600.)

The following figures have been published previously in the University of Minnesota Press publication: HUMAN HISTOLOGY: A MICROFICHE ATLAS, Volumes I and II, by Stanley L. Erlandsen, PhD and Jean E. Magney.

Figure #

			Figure #		
1-2	4-12	8-20	11-29	15-21	18-22
1-7		8-21	11-31	15-22	18-24
1-8	5-1	8-24	11-32	15-27	18-31
1-10	5-2	8-25	11-33	15-33	18-32
1-11	5-4	8-27		15-37	
1-20	5-12	8-31	12-4	15-41	19-2
1-22	5-15	8-32	12-5		19-4
1-23	5-16	8-33	12-7	16-1	19-5
1-24	5-23		12-9	16-4	19-7
1-25	5-24	9-5	12-17	16-6	19-10
1-26		9-10	12-21	16-7	19-11
1-27	6-2	9-14		16-8	19-12
1-28	6-4	9-15	13-5	16-12	19-13
1-34	6-6	9-16	13-11	16-15	19-14
	6-8	9-18	13-12	16-16	19-15
2-5	6-10	9-21	13-20		19-16
2-7	6-12	9-22	13-28	17-3	19-17
2-8		9-26	13-29	17-9	19-18
2-9	7-3	9-27	13-34	17-13	19-19
2-13	7-4			17-14	19-21
2-15	7-10	10-6	14-4	17-15	19-25
2-19	7-12	10-15	14-5	17-16	
2-27	7-13	10-16	14-6	17-17	20-4
2-29	7-19	10-20	14-8	17-23	20-6
2-30	7-20	10-21	14-10	17-24	20-9
2-32	7-21	10-22	14-15	17-26	20-10
2-33	7-26	10-23	14-16		20-11
		10-24		18-7	20-12
3-1	8-5	10-26	15-9	18-8	20-17
3-5	8-9	10-28	15-10	18-9	20-19
3-11	8-10		15-11	18-10	20-22
3-20	8-12	11-10	15-12	18-13	20-23
3-23	8-13	11-11	15-13	18-15	20-24
3-25	8-15	11-15	15-15	18-16	20-30
3-29	8-17	11-17	15-18	18-18	20-35
	8-18	11-22	15-20	18-19	
	8-19	11-23		18-20	
		11-27			

ILLUSTRATION CREDITS

CHAPTER 1

Fig. 1-2
p. 2
Reproduced with permission from *Gray's Anatomy,* 35th British edition, R. Warwick and P.L. Williams, editors, Longman, Edinburgh, Scotland, 1973.

Fig. 1-7
p. 4
Courtesy of Dr. Ross Johnson, Department of Genetics and Cell Biology, University of Minnesota, Minneapolis, Minnesota.

Fig. 1-8
p. 4
Reproduced with permission from W.T. Daems and P. Brederoo: *Mononuclear Phagocytes,* R. van Furth, editor, Blackwell Scientific Publications, Oxford, England, 1970.

Fig. 1-10
p. 5
Courtesy of Dr. Paul C. Letorneau, Department of Anatomy, Medical School, University of Minnesota, Minneapolis, Minnesota.

Fig. 1-11
p. 5
Courtesy of Dr. Daniel Branton, Biology Laboratory, Harvard University, Cambridge, Massachusetts.

Fig. 1-19
p. 7
Courtesy of Dr. Phyllis M. Novikoff, Department of Pathology, Albert Einstein College of Medicine, Yeshiva University, Bronx, New York.

Fig. 1-20
p. 7
Courtesy of Dr. Keiichi Tanaka, Department of Anatomy, Tottori University School of Medicine, Yonago, Japan.

Fig. 1-21
p. 8
Courtesy of Dr. Phyllis M. Novikoff, Department of Pathology, Albert Einstein College of Medicine, Yeshiva University, Bronx, New York.

Fig. 1-22
p. 8
Courtesy of Dr. Keiichi Tanaka, Department of Anatomy, Tottori University School of Medicine, Yonago, Japan.

Fig. 1-23
p. 8
Courtesy of Dr. Keiichi Tanaka, Department of Anatomy, Tottori University School of Medicine, Yonago, Japan.

Fig. 1-24
p. 9
Courtesy of Gwen Crabbe, Department of Laboratory Medicine and Pathology, University of Minnesota, Minneapolis, Minnesota.

Fig. 1-25
p. 9
Courtesy of Dr. David Chase, Cell Biology Research Laboratory, Veteran's Administration Hospital, Sepulveda, California.

Fig. 1-26
p. 9
Courtesy of Dr. Judith Schollmeyer, Roman Kruska USDA Meat Animal Research Laboratory, Clay Center, Nebraska.

Fig. 1-27
p. 9
Courtesy of Dr. John E. Heuser, Department of Physiology and Biophysics, Washington University School of Medicine, St. Louis, Missouri.

Fig. 1-28
p. 10
Redrawn from Douglas E. Kelly: Bailey's Textbook of Histology, 17th edition, W.M. Copenhaver, D.E. Kelly, and R.L. Wood, editors, Williams and Wilkins, Baltimore, Maryland.

Fig. 1-29
p. 11
Courtesy of Dr. Carol Wells, Department of Laboratory Medicine and Pathology, University of Minnesota School of Medicine, Minneapolis, Minnesota.

Fig. 1-30
p. 11
Courtesy of Dr. Carol Wells, Department of Laboratory Medicine and Pathology, University of Minnesota School of Medicine, Minneapolis, Minnesota.

Fig. 1-32
p. 11
Courtesy of Dr. Phyllis M. Novikoff, Department of Pathology, Albert Einstein College of Medicine, Yeshiva University, Bronx, New York.

Fig. 1-33
p. 11
Courtesy of Dr. Mark C. Willingham, Chief, Ultrastructural Cytochemistry Section, Laboratory of Molecular Biology, National Cancer Institute, Bethesda, Maryland.

Fig. 1-34
p. 11
Courtesy of Dr. Keiichi Tanaka, Department of Anatomy, Tottori University School of Medicine, Yonago, Japan.

CHAPTER 2

Fig. 2-5
p. 13
Courtesy of Dr. Jeanette Lopez-Lewellyn, Wayne State Medical School, Detroit, Michigan.

Fig. 2-7
p. 14
Courtesy of Dr. David Chase, Cell Biology Research Laboratory, Veteran's Administration Hospital, Sepulveda, California.

Fig. 2-8
p. 14
Courtesy of Dr. David Chase, Cell Biology Research Laboratory, Veteran's Administration Hospital, Sepulveda, California.

Fig. 2-9
p. 14
Reproduced with permission from Nobutaka Hirokawa et al: *Journal of Cell Biology* 94:425-43, August 1982.

Fig. 2-11
p. 15
Courtesy of Dr. Judith St. George and Dr. Charles Plopper, Department of Anatomy, School of Veterinary Medicine, University of California—Davis, Davis, California.

Fig. 2-13
p. 15
Courtesy of Dr. Keith Porter, Department of Molecular, Cellular, and Developmental Biology, Biosciences of Colorado, Boulder, Colorado.

Fig. 2-15
p. 15
Courtesy of Dr. Karen Holbrook, Department of Biological Structure, University of Washington School of Medicine, Seattle, Washington.

Fig. 2-19
p. 16
Courtesy of Dr. Ellen Roter Dirksen, Department of Anatomy, University of California School of Medicine, Los Angeles, California.

Fig. 2-25
p. 18
Redrawn from Douglas E. Kelly: Bailey's Textbook of Histology, 17th edition, W.M. Copenhaver, D.E. Kelly, and R.L. Wood, editors, Williams and Wilkins, Baltimore, Maryland.

Fig. 2-27
p. 19
Courtesy of Dr. Judson Sheridan, Department of Anatomy, Medical School, University of Minnesota, Minneapolis, Minnesota.

Fig. 2-29
p. 20
Reproduced with permission from Douglas E. Kelly: *Bailey's Textbook of Histology,* 17th edition, W.M. Copenhaver, D.E. Kelly, and R.L. Wood, editors, Williams and Wilkins, Baltimore, Maryland.

Fig. 2-30
p. 20
Courtesy of Dr. John E. Heuser, Department of Physiology and Biophysics, Washington University School of Medicine, St. Louis, Missouri.

Fig. 2-32
p. 20
Courtesy of Dr. David Chase, Cell Biology Research Laboratory, Veteran's Administration Hospital, Sepulveda, California.

Fig. 2-33
p. 20
Reproduced with permission from Adolfo Martinez-Palomo: *Electron Microscopy,* 9th International Congress on Electron Microscopy, vol. 3, Microscopical Society of Canada, Toronto, Canada, 1978.

CHAPTER 3

Fig. 3-1
p. 23
Reproduced with permission from Gretchen Hascall and Vincent Hascall: *Cell Biology of Extracellular Matrix,* Elizabeth D. Day, editor, Plenum Press, New York, New York. The model for fibronectin is redrawn and appears courtesy of Dr. Kenneth Yamada, Chief, Membrane Biochemistry Section, Department of Health, Education, and Welfare, National Institutes of Health, Bethesda, Maryland.

ILLUSTRATION CREDITS 175

Fig. 3-5 Courtesy of Dr. Jerry A. Maynard, Department of Orthopedic Surgery,
p. 24 Carver Pavillion, College of Medicine, University of Iowa, Iowa City, Iowa.

Fig. 3-11 Courtesy of Dr. Daniel H. Bodley, Department of Anatomy, Chicago College
p. 25 of Osteopathic Medicine, Chicago, Illinois.

Fig. 3-20 Reproduced with permission from Tatsuo Ebe and S. Kobayashi: *Fine*
p. 27 *Structure of Human Cells and Tissues,* T. Ebe and S. Kobayashi, editors, Igaku-Shoin, Tokyo, Japan.

Fig. 3-23 Reproduced with permission from J.-P. Revel, M. Rabinovitch, and M.J.
p. 27 DeStefano: *Histology,* 4th edition, L. Weiss and R.O. Greep, editors, McGraw-Hill, New York, New York.

Fig. 3-25/ Courtesy of Dr. David Chase, Cell Biology Research Laboratory, Veteran's
Fig. 3-29 Administration Hospital, Sepulveda, California.
p. 28

CHAPTER 4

Fig. 4-6 Reproduced with permission from Dr. E.B. Hunziker: Improved cartilage
p. 30 fixation by ruthenium hexamine trichloride (RHT), *Journal of Ultrastructural Research* 81:1-12, 1982.

Fig. 4-11 Reproduced with permission from Dr. Giuliano Quintarelli: Fibrogenesis
p. 31 and biosynthesis of elastin in cartilage, *Connective Tissue Research* 7:1-19, 1979.

Fig. 4-12 Reproduced with permission from Marie Yamada: *Archivum Histologicum*
p. 31 39:347, 1976.

CHAPTER 5

Fig. 5-1 Reproduced with permission from *Gray's Anatomy,* 35th British edition, R.
p. 33 Warwick and P.L. Williams, editors, Longman, Edinburgh, Scotland, 1973.

Fig. 5-2 Reproduced with permission from Donald W. Fawcett: *A Textbook of*
p. 34 *Histology,* 10th edition, W. Bloom and D.W. Fawcett, Saunders, Philadelphia, Pennsylvania.

Fig. 5-4 Reproduced with permission from C.P. Leblond: *Histology,* 8th edition,
p. 34 A.W. Ham and D.H. Cormack, editors, Lippincott, Philadelphia, Pennsylvania, 1979.

Fig. 5-12 Courtesy of Dr. Jerry A. Maynard, Department of Orthopedica Surgery,
p. 35 Carver Pavillion, College of Medicine, University of Iowa, Iowa City, Iowa.
and
Fig. 5-15/
Fig. 5-16
p.36

Fig. 5-23 Courtesy of Dr. Robert Schenk, Institute of Anatomy, University of Bern,
p. 37 Bern, Switzerland.

Fig. 5-24 Reproduced with permission from Robert Schenk: *Journal of Cell Biology*
p. 37 34:279, 1967.

CHAPTER 6

Fig. 6-2 Courtesy of Dr. David Chase, Cell Biology Research Laboratory, Veteran's
p. 40 Administration Hospital, Sepulveda, California.

Fig. 6-4 Courtesy of Dr. Janet Parkin, Department of Laboratory Medicine and
p. 40 Pathology, University of Minnesota, Minneapolis, Minnesota.

Fig. 6-6 Reproduced with permission from J.C. Cawley and F.G.J. Hayhoe:
p. 40 *Ultrastructure of Haemic Cells,* Saunders, London, England, 1973.

Fig. 6-8 Courtesy of Dr. Janet Parkin, Department of Laboratory Medicine and
p. 41 Pathology, University of Minnesota, Minneapolis, Minnesota.

Fig. 6-10 *p. 41*	Courtesy of Dr. David Chase, Cell Biology Research Laboratory, Veteran's Administration Hospital, Sepulveda, California.
Fig. 6-12 *p. 41*	Courtesy of Dr. Janet Parkin, Department of Laboratory Medicine and Pathology, University of Minnesota, Minneapolis, Minnesota.

CHAPTER 7

Fig. 7-3 *p. 44*	Courtesy of Dr. L. Weiss, Department of Animal Biology, University of Pennsylvania, Philadelphia, Pennsylvania, and Dr. L.T. Chen, Department of Anatomy, University of South Florida, Tampa, Florida.
Fig. 7-4 *p. 44*	Courtesy of Dr. L.T. Chen, Department of Anatomy, University of South Florida, Tampa, Florida, and Dr. L. Weiss, Department of Animal Biology, University of Pennsylvania, Philadelphia, Pennsylvania.
Fig. 7-10 *p. 46*	Courtesy of Dr. G. Adolph Ackerman, Department of Anatomy, Ohio State University, Columbus, Ohio.
Fig. 7-12/ **Fig. 7-13** *p. 46*	Courtesy of Dr. Kenneth Campbell, Department of Pathology, Reproductive Biology Program, University of Michigan, Ann Arbor, Michigan.
Fig. 7-19 *p. 48*	Reproduced with permission from J.C. Cawley and F.G.J. Hayhoe: *Ultrastructure of Haemic Cells,* Saunders, London, England, 1973.
Fig. 7-20 *p. 48*	Reproduced with permission from Dorothy Bainton: *Developmental Biology* 44:223-227, 1975.
Fig. 7-21 *p. 48*	Reproduced with permission from J.C. Cawley and F.G.J. Hayhoe: *Ultrastructure of Haemic Cells,* Saunders, London, England, 1973.
Fig. 7-26 *p. 49*	Courtesy of Dr. G. Adolph Ackerman, Department of Anatomy, Ohio State University, Columbus, Ohio.

CHAPTER 8

Fig. 8-5 *p. 52*	Courtesy of Dr. Frederic S. Fay, Department of Physiology, University of Massachusetts, Worchester, Massachusetts.
Fig. 8-9 *p. 53*	Courtesy of Dr. J.H. Venable, Department of Anatomy, Colorado State University, Fort Collins, Colorado.
Fig. 8-10 *p. 53*	Reproduced with permission from Lawrence P. McCallister and Robert Hadek: *Journal of Ultrastructural Research* 33:360, 1977. (Special thanks expressed to Evjes Equipment Co., Chicago, Illinois, for technical assistance.)
Fig. 8-12 *p. 54*	Courtesy of Ms. Barbara Zweber, St. Paul, Minnesota.
Fig. 8-13 *p. 54*	Reproduced with permission from M.S. Forbes: *Journal of Ultrastructural Research* 60:306, 1977.
Fig. 8-15 *p. 54*	Reproduced with permission from David Smith: *Muscle,* Academic Press, New York, New York.
Fig. 8-17 *p. 55*	Courtesy of Dr. Paul C. Letourneau, Department of Anatomy, Medical School, University of Minnesota, Minneapolis, Minnesota.
Fig. 8-18 *p. 55*	Reproduced with permission from Tsuneo Fujita: *SEM Atlas of Cells and Tissues,* T. Fujita, K. Tanaka, and J. Tokunaga, editors, Igaku-Shoin, Tokyo, Japan.
Fig. 8-19 *p. 56*	Courtesy of Drs. Rosemary Mazanet and Clara Franzini-Armstrong, Department of Biology, University of Pennsylvania, Philadelphia, Pennsylvania.
Fig. 8-20 *p. 56*	Courtesy of Dr. J.E. Heuser, Department of Physiology and Biophysics, Washington University School of Medicine, St. Louis, Missouri.

ILLUSTRATION CREDITS 177

Fig. 8-21 Reproduced with permission from Steven J. Burden: *Journal of Cell Biology*
p. 56 82:412-425, August 1979.

Fig. 8-24 Courtesy of Dr. David Chase, Cell Biology Research Laboratory, Veteran's
p. 57 Administration Hospital, Sepulveda, California.

Fig. 8-25 Reproduced with permission from *Gray's Anatomy,* 35th British edition, R.
p. 57 Warwick and P.L. Williams, Longman, Edinburgh, Scotland, 1973.

Fig. 8-27 Courtesy of Dr. David Chase, Cell Biology Research Laboratory, Veteran's
p. 57 Administration Hospital, Sepulveda, California.

Fig. 8-31 Reproduced with permission from S. Viragh: *Ultrastructure of the*
p. 58 *Mammalian Heart,* C.E. Challice and S. Viragh, editors, Academic Press, Orlando, Florida.

Fig. 8-32 Courtesy of Dr. S. Viragh, Department of Pathology, Postgraduate Medical
p. 58 School, Budapest, Hungary.

Fig. 8-33 Courtesy of Dr. David Chase, Cell Biology Research Laboratory, Veteran's
p. 58 Administration Hospital, Sepulveda, California.

CHAPTER 9

Fig. 9-5 Reproduced with permission from Michael J. Cullen: *Tissue and Cell* (1):1-
p. 61 10, 1977.

Fig. 9-10 Courtesy of Dr. Glenn Giesler, Department of Anatomy, Medical School,
p. 62 University of Minnesota, Minneapolis, Minnesota.

Fig. 9-14 Reproduced with permission from Jean Babel, A. Bischoff, and H. Spoendlin:
p. 63 *Ultrastructure of the Peripheral Nervous System and Sense Organs,* A. Bischoff, editor, Georg Thieme Verlag, Stuttgart, Germany, 1970.

Fig. 9-15 Reproduced with permission from Pietro M. Motta, *Atlante di microscopia*
p. 63 *elettronica a scansione,* Piccin Nuova Libraria S.p.A., Padova, Italy.

Fig. 9-16 Reproduced with permission from Jean Babel, A. Bischoff, and H. Spoendlin:
p. 63 *Ultrastructure of the Peripheral Nervous System and Sense Organs,* A. Bischoff, editor, Georg Thieme Verlag, Stuttgart, Germany, 1970.

Fig. 9-18 Reproduced with permission from Giorgio Gabella: *Structure of the*
p. 64 *Autonomic Nervous System,* Chapman and Hall, London, England, 1976.

Fig. 9-21 Reproduced with permission from M. Costa, J.B. Furness, A.C. Cuello, A.A.J.
p. 65 Verhofstad, H.W.J. Steinbusch, and R.P. Elde: *Neuroscience,* Vol. 7, No. 2, February 1982.

Fig. 9-22 Reproduced with permission from Giorgio Gabella: *Structure of the*
p. 65 *Autonomic Nervous System,* Chapman and Hall, London, England, 1976.

Fig. 9-26 Reproduced with permission from Koji Uchizono: Excitation and Inhibition,
p. 66 *Synaptic Morphology,* Igaku-Shoin, Tokyo, Japan, 1975.

Fig. 9-27 Reproduced with permission from Sanford Palay and Victoria Chan-Palay:
p. 66 *Handbook of Physiology,* Section 1, vol. 1, The American Physiological Society, Bethesda, Maryland, 1977.

CHAPTER 10

Fig. 10-6 Reproduced with permission from Jona C. Thaemert: *American Journal of*
p. 71 *Anatomy* 136:62, 1973.

Fig. 10-15 Reproduced with permission from Melvyn Weinstock: *Histology,* 8th edition,
p. 72 A.W. Ham and D.W. Cormack, editors, Lippincott, Philadelphia, Pennsylvania, 1979.

Fig. 10-16 Courtesy of Dr. Richard Wood, Department of Anatomy, University of
p. 72 Southern California School of Medicine, Los Angeles, California.

Fig. 10-20 Courtesy of Dr. David Chase, Cell Biology Research Laboratory, Veteran's
p. 74 Administration Hospital, Sepulveda, California.

Fig. 10-21 Reproduced with permission from Dr. Albert L. Jones and E. Spring Mills:
p. 74   *Histology,* 5th edition, Leon Weiss, editor, New York, Elsevier, 1983.

Fig. 10-22 Reproduced with permission from P.M. Motta: *The Liver. An Atlas of SEM,*
p. 74   P.M. Motta, M. Muto, and T. Fujita, editors, Igaku-Shoin, Tokyo, Japan,
            1978.

Fig. 10-23/ Courtesy of Drs. Rosemary Mazanet and Clara Franzini-Armstrong,
Fig. 10-24   Department of Biology, Faculty of Arts and Sciences, University of
p. 75   Pennsylvania, Philadelphia, Pennsylvania.

Fig. 10-26 Reproduced with permission from G.D. Levine: *Histology,* 4th edition, L.
p. 75   Weiss and R.O. Greep, editors, McGraw-Hill, New York, New York, 1977.

Fig. 10-28 Reproduced with permission from Nicolae Simonescu and Maia Simonescu:
p. 75   *Histology,* 4th edition, L. Weiss and R.O. Greep, editors, McGraw-Hill, New
            York, New York, 1977.

CHAPTER 11

Fig. 11-10/ Courtesy of Dr. Lee Leek, Department of Anatomy, Howard University
Fig. 11-11   College of Medicine, Washington, DC.
p. 81

Fig. 11-15 Reproduced with permission from Tsuneo Fujita: *SEM Atlas of Cells and*
p. 83   *Tissues,* T. Fujita, K. Tanaka, and J. Tokunaga, editors, Igaku-Shoin, Tokyo,
            Japan, 1981.

Fig. 11-17 Reproduced with permission from Wei S. Hwang: *Laboratory Investigation*
p. 83   31:481, 1974.

Fig. 11-22 Reproduced with permission from Tsuneo Fujita: *Archivum Histologicum*
p. 85   *Japonicum* 37(3):187-216, 1974.

Fig. 11-23 Reproduced with permission from Tsuneo Fujita: *SEM Atlas of Cells and*
p. 85   *Tissues,* T. Fujita, K. Tanaka, and J. Tokunaga, editors, Igaku-Shoin, Tokyo,
            Japan, 1981.

Fig. 11-27 Reproduced with permission from Tatsuo Ebe and S. Kobayashi: *Fine*
p. 87   *Structures of Human Cells and Tissues,* T. Ebe and S. Kobayashi, editors,
            Igaku-Shoin, Tokyo, Japan, 1972.

Fig. 11-29 Reproduced with permission from R.M. Bearman: *Anatomical Record*
p. 87   190:769, 1978.
  and
Fig. 11-31
p. 88

Fig. 11-32/ Reproduced with permission from Elio Raviola: *Journal of Experimental*
Fig. 11-33   *Medicine* 136:466, 1972.
p. 88

CHAPTER 12

Fig. 12-4/ Courtesy of Dr. J.R. Garrett, Department of Oral Pathology and Oral
Fig. 12-5   Medicine, Dental School, Kings College Hospital Medical School, London,
p. 91   England.

Fig. 12-7 Courtesy of Dr. I. Joel Leeb, Department of Endodontics, School of
p. 92   Dentistry, University of North Carolina, Chapel Hill, North Carolina.

Fig. 12-9 Reproduced with permission from Bernard Tandler: *Anatomical Record*
p. 92   184:115, 1976.

Fig. 12-17 Courtesy of Dr. Robert S. Redman, Dental Service, Veteran's
p. 93   Administration Hospital, Washington, DC.

Fig. 12-21 Reproduced with permission from Arthur R. Hand: *Anatomical Record*
p. 94   173:135, 1972.

ILLUSTRATION CREDITS

CHAPTER 13

Fig. 13-5
p. 97
Courtesy of Dr. Damon C. Herbert, Department of Anatomy, The University of Texas Health Science Center at San Antonio, San Antonio, Texas.

Fig. 13-11
p. 98
Courtesy of Dr. Peter Gould, Whitstable, Kent, England.

Fig. 13-12
p. 98
Courtesy of Dr. Hisao Fujita, Department of Anatomy, Hiroshima University School of Medicine, Hiroshima, Japan.

Fig. 13-19
p. 100
Courtesy of Dr. Sandford Roth, Department of Pathology, School of Medicine, Northwestern University, Chicago, Illinois.

Fig. 13-20
p. 100
Courtesy of Dr. Peter Gould, Whitstable, Kent, England.

Fig. 13-28
p. 101
Courtesy of Dr. John A. Long, Department of Anatomy, School of Medicine, University of California, San Francisco, California.

Fig. 13-29
p. 101
Reproduced with permission from Odile Grynszpan-Winograd: *Handbook of Physiology,* Section 7, vol. 6, American Physiological Society, Bethesda, Maryland, 1975.

Fig. 13-32/
Fig. 13-33
p. 102
Courtesy of Drs. Orion Hegre and Robert Sorenson, Department of Cell Biology and Neuroanatomy, University of Minnesota Medical School, Minneapolis, Minnesota.

Fig. 13-34
p. 103
Reproduced with permission from Lars-Inge Larsson: *Diabetologia* 12:233, 1976.

CHAPTER 14

Fig. 14-4
p. 106
Courtesy of Drs. Gary Gorbsky, Hisato Shida, and Malcolm Steinberg, Department of Biology, Princeton University, Princeton, New Jersey.

Fig. 14-5
p. 106
Courtesy of Dr. Karen Holbrook, Department of Biological Structure, University of Washington School of Medicine, Seattle, Washington.

Fig. 14-6
p. 106
Courtesy of Drs. Christine Skerrow and David Skerrow, Department of Dermatology, University of Glasgow, Glasgow, Scotland.

Fig. 14-8/
Fig. 14-10
p. 107
Courtesy of Dr. Karen Holbrook, Department of Biological Structure, University of Washington School of Medicine, Seattle, Washington.

Fig. 14-15
p. 108
Courtesy of Dr. Karen Holbrook, Department of Biological Structure, University of Washington School of Medicine, Seattle, Washington.

Fig. 14-16
p. 108
Reproduced with permission from Richard A. Ellis: *Ultrastructure of Normal and Abnormal Skin,* A.S. Zelickson, editor, Lea and Febiger, Philadelphia, Pennsylvania, 1967.

CHAPTER 15

Fig. 15-9/
Fig. 15-10
p. 113
Reproduced with permission from J.E. Magney, S.L. Erlandsen, M.L. Bjerknes, and H. Cheng: *American Journal of Anatomy* 177:43-53, 1986.

Fig. 15-11
p. 114
Reproduced with permission from L.C. Junqueira, J. Carneiro, and R.O. Kelly: Basic Histology, 6th edition, Appleton and Lange, 1989, Norwalk, Connecticut.

Fig. 15-12
p. 114
Reproduced with permission from Tatsuo Ebe and S. Kobayashi: *Fine Structure of Human Cells and Tissues,* T. Ebe and S. Kobayashi, editors, Igaku-Shoin, Tokyo, Japan, 1972.

Fig. 15-13
p. 115
Reproduced with permission from Walter Rubin: *Laboratory Investigation* 19:598, 1968.

Fig. 15-15 Reproduced with permission from Tatsuo Ebe and S. Kobayashi: *Fine Structure of Human Cells and Tissues,* T. Ebe and S. Kobayashi, editors, Igaku-Shoin, Tokyo, Japan, 1972.
p. 115

Fig. 15-18 Reproduced with permission from J.E. Magney, S.L. Erlandsen, M.L. Bjerknes, and H. Cheng: *American Journal of Anatomy* 177:43-53, 1986.
p. 117

Fig. 15-20 Courtesy of Dr. David Chase, Cell Biology Research Laboratory, Veteran's Administration Hospital, Sepulveda, California.
p. 117

Fig. 15-21 Reproduced with permission from Susumu Ito: *The Cell,* 2nd edition, D.W. Fawcett, editor, Saunders, Philadelphia, Pennsylvania, 1981.
p. 117

Fig. 15-22 Reproduced with permission from Adolfo Martinez-Palomo: *Electron Microscopy,* 1978, Ninth International Congress on Electron Microscopy, vol. 3, Microscopical Society of Canada, Toronto, Canada.
p. 117

Fig. 15-27 Reproduced with permission from Tomas Hokfelt and Marianne Schultzberg: *Nature,* Vol. 284, Macmillan Journals, London, England, April 1980.
p. 118

Fig. 15-31 Courtesy of Dr. David Chase, Cell Biology Research Laboratory, Veteran's Administration Hospital, Sepulveda, California.
p. 120

Fig. 15-33 Reproduced with permission from Shigeru Kobayashi: *Archivum Histologicum Japonicum* 31:477, 1970.
p. 121

Fig. 15-37 Courtesy of Dr. Robert L. Owen, Department of Medicine, Veteran's Administration Hospital, San Francisco, California.
p. 122

Fig. 15-41 Courtesy of Dr. Marian Neutra, Department of Anatomy, Harvard Medical School, Boston, Massachusetts.
p. 123

CHAPTER 16

Fig. 16-1 Reproduced with permission from A.D. Hally and Sybil M. Lloyd: *Clinical Science,* Biochemical Society, London, England, 1968.
p. 125

Fig. 16-4 Reproduced with permission from Tsuneo Fujita: *SEM Atlas of Cells and Tissues,* T. Fujita, K. Tanaka, and J. Tokunaga, editors, Igaku-Shoin, Tokyo, Japan, 1981.
p. 126

Fig. 16-6 Reproduced with permission from H.D. Fahimi: *Laboratory Investigation* 16:736, 1967.
p. 126

Fig. 16-7 Reproduced with permission from Tsuneo Fujita: *SEM Atlas of Cells and Tissues,* T. Fujita, K. Tanaka, and J. Tokunaga, editors, Igaku-Shoin, Tokyo, Japan, 1981.
p. 127

Fig. 16-8 Courtesy of Dr. Richard Wood, Department of Anatomy, University of Southern California School of Medicine, Los Angeles, California.
p. 127

Fig. 16-12 Courtesy of Dr. Ann L. Hubbard, Department of Cell Biology and Anatomy, Johns Hopkins School of Medicine, Baltimore, Maryland.
p. 128
and
Fig. 16-15
p. 129

Fig. 16-16 Reproduced with permission from P.M. Motta: *The Liver. An Atlas of SEM,* P.M. Motta, M. Muto, and T. Fujita, editors, Igaku-Shoin, Tokyo, Japan, 1978.
p. 129

CHAPTER 17

Fig. 17-3 Reproduced with permission from Lennart Nilsson: *Behold Man,* Little, Brown, Boston, Massachusetts, 1973.
p. 132

Fig. 17-9 Reproduced with permission from Ernest Cutz: *Cell and Tissue Research* 158:425, 1975.
p. 134

Fig. 17-13 *p. 135*	Courtesy of Dr. Charles Kuhn III, Department of Pathology, Washington University School of Medicine, St. Louis, Missouri.
Fig. 17-14 *p. 135*	Reproduced with permission from Sergei P. Sorokin: *Anatomical Record* 181:607, 1975.
Fig. 17-15/ **Fig. 17-16** *p. 135*	Reproduced with permission from D. Zucker-Franklin et al: *Atlas of Blood Cells,* vol. 1, Edi Ermes S.R.L., Milano, Italy, 1981.
Fig. 17-17 *p. 136*	Reproduced with permission from Sergei P. Sorokin: *Histology,* 4th edition, L. Weiss and R.O. Greep, editors, McGraw-Hill, New York, New York, 1977.
Fig. 17-23 *p. 137*	Reproduced with permission from Marianne Bachofen: *American Review of Respiratory Diseases,* vol. 3, American Lung Association, New York, New York, 1975.
Fig. 17-24 *p. 137*	Reproduced with permission from Lelio Orci: *Freeze Etch Histology,* L. Orci and A. Perrelet, editors, Springer-Verlag, New York, New York, 1975.
Fig. 17-26 *p. 137*	Reproduced with permission from James O. Shaw: *American Journal of Pathology* 101:283, 1980.

CHAPTER 18

Fig. 18-7 *p. 142*	Courtesy of Dr. Masayuki Miyoshi, Department of Anatomy, Fukuoka University, School of Medicine, Fukuoka, Japan.
Fig. 18-8 *p. 142*	Reproduced with permission from Marilyn Farquhar, Kidney International 8:197, 1975.
Fig. 18-9 *p. 142*	Reproduced with permission from Tsuneo Fujita, *SEM Atlas of Cells and Tissues,* T. Fujita, K. Tanaka, and J. Tokunaga, editors, Igaku-Shoin, Tokyo, Japan, 1981.
Fig. 18-10 *p. 142*	Courtesy of Dr. Franco Spinelli, Medical Research Department, Hoffman-LaRoche, Ltd., Basel, Switzerland.
Fig. 18-13 *p. 144*	Reproduced with permission from Arvid B. Maunsbach, *Electron Microscopy in Human Medicine,* vol. 9, J.V. Johannessen, editor, McGraw-Hill, New York, New York, 1979.
Fig. 18-15 *p. 144*	Courtesy of Dr. Ruth Bulger, Department of Pathology and Laboratory Medicine, University of Texas Health Science Center, Houston, Texas.
Fig. 18-16 *p. 144*	Courtesy of Dr. Lydia Osvaldo, Karokinska Institutet, Stockholm, Sweden.
Fig. 18-18 *p. 145*	Reproduced with permission from Melvin Schwartz, Kidney International 6:193, 1974.
Fig. 18-19 *p. 145*	Courtesy of Dr. Ruth Bulger, Department of Pathology and Laboratory Medicine, University of Texas Health Science Center, Houston, Texas.
Fig. 18-20 *p. 145*	Courtesy of Dr. Marco Celio, Department of Anatomy, University of Zurich, Zurich, Switzerland.
Fig. 18-22 *p. 145*	Courtesy of Dr. Luciano Barajas, Department of Pathology, UCLA School of Medicine, Torrance, California.
Fig. 18-24 *p. 146*	Courtesy of Dr. Ruth Bulger, Department of Pathology and Laboratory Medicine, University of Texas Health Science Center, Houston, Texas.
Fig. 18-26 *p. 146*	Reproduced with permission from Arvid B. Maunsbach, *Electron Microscopy in Human Medicine,* vol. 9, J.V. Johannessen, editor, McGraw-Hill, New York, New York, 1979.
Fig. 18-31 *p. 147*	Reproduced with permission from Myron Tannenbaum, *Electron Microscopy in Human Medicine,* vol. 9, J.V. Johannessen, editor, McGraw-Hill, New York, New York, 1979.

Fig. 18-32 Reproduced with permission from Keith Porter, *Protoplasma* 63:262, 1967.
p. 147

Fig. 18-33/ Courtesy of Drs. Y. Ikeuchi and T. Kanaseki, Department of Genetics,
Fig. 18-34 Tokyo Metropolitan Institute for Neurosciences, Tokyo, Japan.
p. 147

CHAPTER 19

Figs. 19-2/ Courtesy of Dr. Richard Blandau, Department of Biological Structure,
Fig. 19-4 University of Washington School of Medicine, Seattle, Washington; from
p. 151 his film *Sperm Maturation in the Male Reproductive Tract: Development of Motility,* 1968.

Fig. 19-5 Courtesy of Dr. A. Kent Christensen, Department of Anatomy, University of
p. 151 Michigan School of Medicine, Ann Arbor, Michigan.

Fig. 19-7 Reproduced with permission from Martin Dym, *Anatomical Record* 175:639,
p. 151 1973.

Fig. 19-10 Courtesy of Dr. D. Szabo, Institute of Experimental Medicine, Hungarian
p. 153 Academy of Sciences, Budapest, Hungary.

Fig. 19-11 Courtesy of Dr. Mark Ludvigson, U.S. Army Medical Corps, St. Paul,
p. 153 Minnesota.

Fig. 19-12 Courtesy of Dr. Richard Blandau, Department of Biological Structure,
p. 154 University of Washington School of Medicine, Seattle, Washington; from his film *Sperm Maturation in the Male Reproductive Tract: Development of Motility,* 1968.

Fig. 19-13 Reproduced with permission from D.W. Fawcett, *Handbook of Physiology,*
p. 154 Section 7, vol. 5, *Male Reproductive Tract,* D.W. Hamilton and R.O. Greep, editors, American Physiological Society, Bethesda, Maryland, 1975.

Fig. 19-14 Reproduced with permission from Martin Dym: *Basic Reproductive*
p. 155 *Medicine,* vol. 2, D.W. Hamilton and F. Naftolin, editors, MIT Press, Cambridge, Massachusetts, 1982.

Fig. 19-15 Reproduced with permission from D.W. Fawcett, W.A. Anderson, and D.M.
p. 155 Phillips, *Developmental Biology* 26:220, 1971.

Fig. 19-16 Reproduced with permission from Donald W. Fawcett, *A Textbook of*
p. 156 *Histology,* 10th edition, W. Bloom and D.W. Fawcett, editors, Saunders, Philadelphia, Pennsylvania, 1975.

Fig. 19-17 Reproduced with permission from Martin Dym: *Basic Reproductive*
p. 156 *Medicine,* vol. 2, D.W. Hamilton and F. Naftolin, editors, MIT Press, Cambridge, Massachusetts, 1982.

Fig. 19-18 Courtesy of Dr. Richard Blandau, Department of Biological Structure,
p. 156 University of Washington School of Medicine, Seattle, Washington; from his film *Sperm Maturation in the Male Reproductive Tract: Development of Motility,* 1968.

Fig. 19-19 Reproduced with permission from Gary Olson: *Basic Reproductive*
p. 156 *Medicine,* vol. 2, D.W. Hamilton and F. Naftolin, editors, MIT Press, Cambridge, Massachusetts, 1982.

Fig. 19-21 From the collection of Dr. R. Vitale, whom we have been unable to locate
p. 157 to obtain his permission.

Fig. 19-25 Courtesy of Dr. A.F. Holstein, Department of Microscopical Anatomy,
p. 159 University of Hamburg, Hamburg, West Germany.

CHAPTER 20

Fig. 20-4 Courtesy of Dr. Jonathan Van Blerkom, Department of Molecular, Cellular
p. 163 and Developmental Biology, University of Colorado, Boulder, Colorado.

Fig. 20-6 Courtesy of Dr. P. Bagavandoss, Department of Anatomy, University of
p. 163 Michigan, Ann Arbor, Michigan.

Fig. 20-9 Reproduced with permission from Norton B. Gilula, Journal of Cell Biology
p. 164 78:58, 1978.

Fig. 20-10/ Courtesy of Dr. Richard Blandau, Department of Biological Structure,
Fig. 20-11/ University of Washington School of Medicine, Seattle, Washington; from
Fig. 20-12 his film *Ovulation and Egg Transport in Mammals,* 1973.
p. 165

Fig. 20-17 Courtesy of Dr. Laurie G. Paavola, Department of Anatomy, Temple
p. 166 University School of Medicine, Philadelphia, Pennsylvania.

Fig. 20-19 Courtesy of Dr. Richard Blandau, Department of Biological Structure,
p. 167 University of Washington School of Medicine, Seattle, Washington; from
his film *Ovulation and Egg Transport in Mammals,* 1973.

Fig. 20-22 Courtesy of Dr. Ellen R. Dirksen, Department of Anatomy, University of
p. 167 California School of Medicine, Los Angeles, California.

Fig. 20-23 Reproduced with permission from Pietro M. Motta, *Atlanta di microscopia*
p. 168 *elettronica a scansione,* Piccin Nuova Libraria S.p.A., Padova, Italy.

Fig. 20-24 Reproduced with permission from David Phillips, *The Cell,* ed. 2, D.W.
p. 168 Fawcett, editor, Saunders, Philadelphia, Pennsylvania, 1981.

Fig. 20-30 Courtesy of Dr. Alex Ferenczy, McGill University, Montreal, Canada.
p. 169

Fig. 20-35 Courtesy of Dr. Judy Strum, Department of Anatomy, University of
p. 170 Maryland School of Medicine, Baltimore, Maryland.

INDEX

A
A band of skeletal muscle, 50
A cells, 97
Absorptive cells of small intestine, 110
Accessory glands of male reproductive system, 150
Accessory organs of digestion, 111
Acetylcholine and muscle contraction, 50
Acidophilia, 1
Acinar exocrine glands, 89
Acinus
  liver, 124
  of mammary gland, 170
  pancreatic, 7, 94
ACTH; see Adrenocorticotrophic hormone
Actin
  in cell, 1
  filaments of, 9, 14, 50
  localization of, 9
  in muscle, 50
Adenohypophysis, 95
Adipocytes, 21, 26, 27
Adipose connective tissue, 22, 26
Adluminal compartment of testis, 149
Adrenal cortex, 100
Adrenal gland, 100, 101
Adrenocorticotrophic hormone, 96
Adventitia, 109
  of vagina, 162
Adventitial cells, 42
Afferent arteriole, 138, 140
Agranular leukocytes, 38
Aldosterone, 96, 139
Alimentary canal, 109
Alpha cells, 97, 102, 103
Alveolar ducts, 131
Alveolar epithelial cell, 137
Alveolar exocrine glands, 89
Alveolar macrophages, 131, 135
Alveolar pores, 131, 137
Alveolar sacs, 131
Alveoli
  of lungs, 131, 137
  of mammary glands, 162, 170
Amino acids as hormones, 95
Ampulla
  of oviduct, 161
  of vas deferens, 149
Androgens, production of, 96
Annuli fibrosi, 69
Antibodies, formation of, 77
Antidiuretic hormone, 139
Antigen presenting cells, 77
Aorta, 71
Apocrine glands, 104
Apocrine secretion of exocrine glands, 89
Appendix, 110, 122
Appositional growth of cartilage, 29
Arcuate arteries of kidney, 138
Area cribrosa, 139
Areolar connective tissue, 22
Arterial portal system, 73

Arteries, 67-68
  bronchial, 130
  central, of white pulp, 78
  hepatic, 124
  muscular, 25, 72, 76
  ovarian, 161
  pulmonary, 130
  renal, 138, 141
  smooth muscle of, 52
  splenic, 78
  testicular, 149
Arterioles, 67, 68, 72
  afferent, 138, 140
  efferent, 138
  penicillar, of spleen, 78
Arteriovenous anastomosis, 68
Ascending colon, 110
Ascending thin limb of loop of Henle, 139
Astrocytes, 60
Atria, 67, 70
Atrial cardiac muscle cell, 58
Atrial natriuretic peptide, 67
Atrioventricular bundle, 58
Atrioventricular node, 58, 67, 71
Auerbach, myenteric plexus of, 65
Auerbach's ganglia of small intestine, 110
Autonomic nervous system, 59, 64
Autophagy, 10
Axoaxonic region, 59
Axodendritic region, 59
Axo-IS region, 59
Axon, 55, 60
  of neuron, 59
  in peripheral nervous system, 62
  surrounded by myelin, 63
Axon hillock, 59
Axon terminal, presynaptic, 59
Axoplasm, 59
Axosomatic region, 59
Azure granules, 38, 40, 47

B
B cells, 97
  and humoral immunity, 77
Bacteria, endocytosis of, 11
Band form of granulocyte, 43
Bands of skeletal muscle, 50
Basal bodies in cell, 1
Basal compartment of testis, 149
Basal lamina
  of basal membrane, 12
  of basement membrane, 17
  of muscle, 50
Basal region of stratified squamous epithelium, 17
Basement membrane, 2, 12, 17
  of epithelium, drawing of, 17
  glomerular, 139
Basophilic myelocytes, 43
Basophilic normoblasts, 42, 46
Basophilic staining of cell, 1
Basophils, 38, 39, 41, 43

185

Bertin, renal columns of, 138
Beta cells, 97, 102, 103
Bile, 124
Bile canaliculi, 124, 127
Bile ductules, 124
Billroth, cords of, 78
Bladder, urinary, 138, 139, 148
  transitional epithelium of, 148
Blood
  peripheral, 38-41
    cells of, types of, 39
  proteins in, 38
  serum of, 38
Blood-air barrier, 131
Blood cells, 38
  developing, 21
  maturation of, comparison of, 49
Blood-testis barrier, 149
Blood-thymus barrier, 78, 88
B-lymphocytes, 38, 77
Bone, 32-37
  cancellous, 32, 34
  cells of, 32
  compact, 32, 34, 36
  ground, 34, 35
  immature, 32
  lacunae of, 32
  long, 34
    growth of, 33
    lamellae of, 32
    macrophotograph of, 36
  mature, microstructure of, 33
  primary, 32
  remodeling of, 32-33
  secondary, 32
  spongy, 32, 34
  woven, 32
Bone marrow, 44
  cells of, 48
  functions of, 42
  and hemopoiesis, 42-49
  megakaryocyte in, 49
  plasma cell in, 48
  vasculature and circulation in, 43
Bowman's capsule, 138, 141
Branched exocrine glands, 89
Bronchial arteries, 130
Bronchiole, 135
  respiratory, 130-131, 136
  terminal, 136
Bronchus, 130, 135
Brunner's glands of small intestine, 110
"Brush border," 2, 12, 139, 144
Bundle of His, 58, 67
Bundle branches, 58

C

C cells of thyroid gland, 95
Calcification, zone of, of epiphyseal plate, 37
Calcium phosphate, amorphous, in bone, 32
Calyces of kidney, 138, 140
Canaliculi, 32
  bile, 124, 127
Cancellous bone, 32, 34
Capillaries, 68, 73, 74
  fenestrated, 74
  glomerular, 142
  lymphatic, 76, 78, 81
  sinusoidal, 74
Capillary loops, glomerular, 142
Capillary plexus, peritubular, 138
Capsular matrix in cartilage, 29
Capsule cells of neuron, 60
Capsule
  Bowman's, 138, 141
  connective tissue, around spleen, 78
  of thymus, 78
Cardiac glands of esophagus, 109
Cardiac muscle, 50, 51, 57, 58, 73
Cardiac skeleton, 51
Cardiovascular system, 67-76
Cartilage, 29-31
  growth by, 29

Cartilage—cont'd
  of respiratory system, 130
  resting, 36
  types of, 29
Cavity
  nasal, 130
  oral, 109
Cecum, 110
Cell, 1-11
  A, 97
  absorptive, of small intestine, 110
  adjacent, freeze fracture of, 4
  adventitial, 42
  alpha, 97, 102, 103
  antigen presenting, 77
  B, 97
  beta, 97, 102, 103
  blood, 38
    developing, 21
  bone, 32
  bone marrow, 48
  C, of thyroid gland, 95
  capsule, of neuron, 60
  cardiac muscle, 51, 57, 58
  cartilage, 29
  chief, 110, 115
  chondrogenic, 30
  chromaffin, 96, 100
  ciliated, of oviduct, 162
  columnar, simple, 2, 3
  components of, 1
  composite, drawing of, 2
  connective tissue, 21
  D, 97
  delta, 97, 102, 103
  dorsal root ganglion, 62
  dust, 131
  effector, 77
  endothelial, of kidney, 138
  enteroendocrine, of small intestine, 110
  epithelial; see Epithelial cells
  examination of, 1
  follicular, of ovary, 161
  goblet, 2, 3, 110
  granulosa, of ovary, 161, 164
  hematogenous, 21
  hemopoietic, of bone marrow, 44
  interstitial, of Leydig, 149
  juxtaglomerular, 139, 145, 146
  of kidney, 138-139
  Kupffer, 124, 129
  Langerhans, 104
  Leydig, 157
  liver, cytoplasm of, 8
    lysosomes in, 11
  M, of small intestine, 110
  mast, in connective tissue, 23, 28
  memory, 77
  Merkle, 104
  mesangial, of kidney, 138
  mesenchymal, 21
  microglial, 60
  of mucosa of gallbladder, 125
  mucous, of stomach, 109
  mucous neck, 110
  muscle, ultrastructure of, 54
  myoepithelial, 89
  natural killer (NK), 77
  nerve, 59
  osteogenic, 37
  osteoprogenitor, 32
  oxyphil, in parathyroid gland, 100
  pancreatic islet, innervation of, 103
  Paneth, 110, 119
  parafollicular, of thyroid gland, 95
  parietal, of stomach, 110, 114
  peripheral blood, types of, 39
  plasma, 21, 28, 77
    in bone marrow, 48
    in lamina propria, 120
    of small intestine, 110
  polymorphonuclear, 38
  PP, 97
    of respiratory system, 130-131

Cell—cont'd
  PP—cont'd
    reticular, 21
      epithelial, of thymus, 78
    satellite, of neuron, 60
    Schwann, 55, 60, 62, 63
    secretory, of oviduct, 162
    Sertoli, 149, 154, 155
      of skeletal muscle, 51, 53
      of smooth muscle, 51
    stem; see Stem cells
    T, 38
    TEM and freeze fracture of, comparison of, 4
    T-helper, 77
    thyrocalcitonin (parafollicular), 99
    T-suppressor, 77
    umbrella, of transitional epithelium, 15, 148
Cell body, 60
  neuronal, parasympathetic, 65
Cell membrane, drawing of, 4
Cell nests, isogenous, in cartilage, 29, 30
Cell-mediated immunity and T-lymphocytes, 77
Cellular immunity, cells involved in, 38
Cementing substance, 32
Central arteries of white pulp, 78
Central nervous system, 59
Central vein of liver, 124, 126, 129
Centriole, 1, 9
  triplet arrangement of microtubules in, 9
Cerebral cortex, neuron in, 61
Cervix of uterus, 162
Chemical synapses, 59
Chief cells, 110, 115
Cholecystokinin, 125
Cholesterol, 124
Chondroblasts, 29, 30
Chondrocytes, 29, 30
  in elastic cartilage, 31
  in epiphyseal plate, 37
Chondrogenic cells, 30
Chondronectin, 22, 23
  in cartilage, 29
Chromaffin cells, 96, 100
Chyme, 109
Cilia, 16
  in cell, 1
  in epithelium, 12
Ciliated cells of oviduct, 162
Ciliated epithelium, simple columnar, 16
Circulation
  portal, 110
  systemic, 69
Circumferential lamellae of long bone, 32
Cisternae
  of Golgi apparatus, 7
  parallel, of rough endoplasmic reticulum, 8
  of rough endoplasmic reticulum, 8
Classic hepatic lobule, 124
Clathrin-coated pits, 11
Clefts
  of Schmidt-Lantermann, 63
  subneural, 55
  synaptic, 55, 59
Closed circulation model of splenic blood flow, 78
Cold-insoluble globulin; see Fibronectin
Collagen, 21
  in extracellular matrix of connective tissue, 21
  fibers of, 24
    in fibrocartilage, 31
  formation of, steps in, 24
  type I, 21
    in bone, 32
    in cartilage, 29
  type II, 21
    in cartilage, 29
  type III, 12, 21; see also Reticular fibers
    of basement membrane, 17
  type IV, 12, 21
    of basement membrane, 17
  type V, 21
  type VII, 21
  type X, 21
Collecting duct of kidney, 138, 139, 147
Colloid, 95

Colon, 110, 123
  epithelium of, 123
  mucosa of, 123
Colony stimulating factors, 44
Colostrum, 162
Columnar cells, simple, 2, 3
  three-dimensional representation of, 2
Columnar epithelium, 12
  pseudostratified, 15, 17
  simple, 14
  simple ciliated, 16
Committed stem cells, 42, 44
Compact bone, 32, 34, 36
Composite cell, drawing of, 2
Compound exocrine glands, 89
Conducting portion of respiratory system, 130, 131
Conducting system of heart, 58
Conducting tubules and ducts of male reproductive system, 149-150
Conductivity of neurons, 59
Connective tissue, 1, 21-28
  adipose, 22, 26
  areolar, 22
  cells of, categories of, 21
  classification of, 22
  components of, 21
  dense, 22, 26
  functions of, 21
  loose, 22, 26
  mast cell in, 23
  mucous, 22
  reticular, 22
  specialized, 22
  subcutaneous, 104
  unmyelinated nerve in, 64
Connective tissue capsule around spleen, 78
Continuous capillaries, 68
Contractile proteins in cell, 1
Contraction
  of skeletal muscle, 50
  of smooth muscle, 50, 52
Convoluted tubules
  distal, 139, 147
  proximal, 139, 144, 147
Cord
  of Billroth, 78
  spermatic, 149
  vocal, 130, 132
Corpora cavernosa, 150
Corpus albicans, 166
Corpus hemorrhagicum, 166
Corpus luteum, 161, 166
Corpus spongiosum, 150, 160
Corpuscle
  Hassall's, 78
    in thymus, 87
  Meissner's, 60, 65, 108
  pacinian, 60, 65, 108
  renal, 138, 141, 142, 145
Cortical ascending thick limb of loop of Henle, 139
Cortical labyrinth of kidney, 139
Cortical lobule of kidney, 139
Corticosterone, 96
Cortisol, 96
Crypts
  intestinal, 116, 119
  of Leiberkühn, 110, 121
Crystals, hydroxyapatite, in bone, 32
Cuboidal epithelium, 12
  simple, 13
  stratified, 16
Cystic duct, 125
Cytodifferentiation
  of erythrocytes, 45
  of granulocytes, 47
Cytoplasm, 1
  intestinal epithelial cell, 6
  liver cell, 8
    lysosomes in, 11
  neuron, 61
  staining of, 1
Cytoskeletal organelles in cell, 1
Cytotoxic T cells, 38

D

D cells, 97
Delta cells, 97, 102, 103
Dendrites of neuron, 59
Dendritic spines, 59
Dense bodies of muscle, 50
Dense connective tissue, 22, 26
Dermis, 26, 104, 105
Descending colon, 110
Descending thin limb of loop of Henle, 139
Desmosomal complexes in epidermis, 106
Desmosomes, 20
    tonofilaments of, 14, 20
Detumescence, 150
Diaphragm-covered pores in nuclear envelope, 5
Diastole, 67
Diffuse lymphatic tissue, 77
Digestion
    accessory organs of, 111
    intracellular, lysosomal system in, diagram of, 10
Digestive enzymes, 117
Digestive system, 109-110
Disks, intercalated, 51
    of cardiac muscle, 57
Disse, space of, 124
Distal convoluted tubule, 139, 147
Dorsal root ganglion, cells of, 62
Duct
    alveolar, 131
    collecting, of kidney, 138, 139, 147
    cystic, 125
    ejaculatory, 149-150
    of exocrine glands, 89, 90
    interlobular, 90, 92
    intralobular, 90
    of male reproductive system, 149-150
    of multicellular exocrine glands, 89
    pancreatic, simple cuboidal epithelium of, 13
    parotid, 92
    stratified cuboidal epithelium of, 16
    thoracic, 81
Duct systems
    of exocrine glands, 90
    of mammary glands, 162
Ductules
    bile, 124
    efferent, of male reproductive system, 149
Ductus deferens, 159
Ductus epididymis, 159
Duodenal mucosa, 116
Duodenum, 110
Dust cells, 131

E

Eccrine sweat gland, 108
Effector cells, 77
Efferent arteriole, 138
Efferent ductules of male reproductive system, 149
Ejaculatory duct, 149-150
Elastic arteries, 67
Elastic cartilage, 29, 31
Elastic fibers
    of connective tissue, 21, 25
        formation of, steps in, 24
    of respiratory system, 130
Elastic lamina of muscular artery, 25
Elastin, 21, 71
Electron microscopy, 1; *see also* Transmission electron microscopy
Embryonic mesoderm, 96
End bulb of Krause, 60
End plate, motor, 50, 55, 56, 59
Endocardium, 67, 70
Endochondral ossification, 32-33
Endocrine glands, 12, 95-103
Endocytic uptake, 10
Endocytosis
    of bacteria, 11
    receptor-mediated, 10, 11
Endometrium of uterus, 162, 169
Endomysium, 50-51
Endoneurium, 60, 62, 63
Endoplasmic reticulum
    of liver, 124
    rough, 1, 8

Endoplasmic reticulum—cont'd
    smooth, 1
Endosomes, 10
    formation of, 11
Endosteum, 32
Endothelial cells of kidney, 138
Endothelial venules, high, 68
Enkephalins, 96
Enteroendocrine cells of small intestine, 110
Enzymes
    digestive, 117
    of stomach, 110
Eosinophilia, 1
Eosinophilic myelocytes, 43
Eosinophils, 38-39, 41, 43
Epicardium, 67, 70
Epidermis, 104, 105, 106, 107
Epididymis, 149, 158
Epiglottis, 130
Epimetrium of uterus, 162
Epimysium, 51
Epinephrine, 96
Epineurium, 60, 62, 63
Epiphyseal plate, 36, 37, 44
Epithelial cells
    alveolar, 137
    drawing of, 2
    intestinal, cytoplasm of, 6
    of kidney, 142
    reticular, thymus, 78
    simple columnar, of gallbladder, 3
    surface specializations of, diagram of, 18
    of uterus, 169
Epithelium, 1, 2, 12-20
    of alimentary canal, 109
    basement membrane of, drawing of, 17
    bronchiolar, 135
    characteristics of, 12
    classification of, 12, 13
    colonic, 123
    columnar, 12
        pseudostratified, 15, 17
        simple, 14
        simple ciliated, 16
    cuboidal, 12
        simple, 13
        stratified, 16
    of epididymis, 158
    functions of, 12
    germinal, of ovary, 161
    intestinal
        with goblet cell, 3
        of simple columnar cells, 2
    of intestinal villus, 116
    of kidney, 138-139
    laryngeal, 132
    parietal, of kidney, 138
    prostatic, 160
    pseudostratified, 13
    respiratory, 130
    seminiferous, of testes, 149
    simple, 12
    squamous, 12
        simple, 13
        stratified, 17, 20, 80, 106
        stratified keratinized, 15
        stratified nonkeratinized, 16, 109
    stratified, 12
        squamous, 17, 20, 80, 106
    tonsillar, 80
    tracheal, 133, 134
    transitional, 13
        of urinary bladder, 15, 148
        of urinary tract, 139
    of vagina, 170
    of villi, 117
    visceral, of kidney, 138
Erythroblast, 42; *see also* Normoblast
Erythrocytes, 38, 39, 40
    cytodifferentiation of, 45
    lifespan of, 49
    polychromatophilic, 42-43
Erythropoiesis, 42
Esophageal glands, 111

Esophagus, 109
  layers of, 111
  mucosa of, 40
  stratified squamous nonkeratinized epithelium of, 16
Estrogens, 161
Excitation-contraction coupling, 50
Excitatory neurotransmittors, 59
Exocrine glands, 12, 89-94
  classification of, 89
  structure and activities of, 90
Exocrine secretion, neural regulation of, 94
Exocytosis, 89
External respiration, 130
Extracellular matrix
  of bone, 32
  of cartilage, 29
  of connective tissue, 21, 25
  of peripheral blood, 38

F

Facial nerve, 63
Fallopian tube; *see* Oviduct
False vocal cords, 132
Fascicles of skeletal muscle cells, 50-51, 53
Fatty acids, 117
Female reproductive tract, 161-170
  diagram of, 162
Fenestrated capillaries, 68, 74
Fibers
  collagen, in fibrocartilage, 31
  of connective tissue, 21
  elastic; *see* Elastic fibers
  myelinated, of sciatic nerve, 63
  nerve, 60
  Purkinje, 51, 67, 71
  reticular, 21; *see also* Collagen, type III
    of connective tissue, 25
    of lymph node, 25
    of skeletal muscle, 50-51
  Sharpey's, 32
  skeletal muscle, 53
  stress, 9
Fibroblasts, 21, 24, 28
  of bone, 32
  drawing of, 24
Fibrocartilage, 29
  collagen fibers in, 31
Fibronectin, 22, 23
Fibrous astrocytes, 60
Filaments
  actin, 9, 14
  intermediate, 1
  of skeletal muscle, 50
Filtration barrier, 139
  glomerular, 143
Filtration slits, 139
Fimbriae of oviduct, 161
Flagella in cell, 1
Follicle
  hair, 104, 105
  ovarian, 161, 163
  primordial, 163
  secondary, 163, 164
  of thyroid gland, 95, 99
Follicle-stimulating hormone, 161
Follicular cells of ovary, 161
Fractured tracheal wall, 133
Free ribosomes of cell, 1
Freeze fracture of cell, 4
Freeze-fracture technique, 1

G

GAGs; *see* Glycosaminoglycans
Gallbladder, 125
  and liver, 124-129
  mucosa of, 129
  simple columnar epithelial cells of, 3
Ganglia, Auerbach's, of small intestine, 110
Ganglion cells, dorsal root, 62
Gap junctions, 18, 19, 50
Gastric glands, 109-110, 112, 113, 114
Gastric pits, 109-110, 112, 113, 115
Gastrointestinal tract, 111
Germinal center of lymphatic nodule, 77

Germinal epithelium of ovary, 161
Gland
  accessory, of male reproductive system, 150
  adrenal, 100, 101
  of alimentary canal, 109
  apocrine, 104
  Brunner's, of small intestine, 110
  cardiac, of esophagus, 109
  endocrine, 12, 95-103; *see also* Endocrine glands
  esophageal, 111
  exocrine, 12, 89-94; *see also* Exocrine glands
  gastric, 109-110, 112, 113, 114
  intestinal, 110
  mammary, 162, 170
  parathyroid, 96, 99, 100
  parotid, 89, 90, 91, 92
    innervation of, 94
  pituitary, 95, 97
    hypothalamus and, relationships between, 96
  prostate, 150, 160
  pyloric, 115
  salivary, 89-90
  sebaceous, 104, 107, 108
  seromucous
    mixed, 93
    of respiratory system, 130
  of skin, 104
  sublingual, 89, 90, 93
  submandibular, 89, 90, 93
  submucosal
    of esophagus, 109
    of small intestine, 110
  suprarenal, 96
  sweat, 104, 108
  thyroid, 95-96, 98, 99
Glans penis, 150
Glisson's capsule, 124
Globulin, cold-insoluble; *see* Fibronectin
Glomerular basement membrane, 139
Glomerular capillaries, 142
Glomerular capillary loops, 142
Glomerular filtration barrier, 143
Glomerulus, 138
Glucagon, 97
Glucocorticoids, production of, 96
Glycocalyx, 110, 117
Glycogen in cell, 1
Glycoproteins, structural, 21-22, 32
Glycosaminoglycans, 21-22
Goblet cells, 2
  intestinal epithelium with, 3
  of small intestine, 110
Golgi apparatus, 7
  of cell, 1
  of liver, 124
Granular leukocytes, 38
Granules, azure, 38, 47
Granulocytes, 21, 45
  cytodifferentiation of, 47
  formation of, 43
  wandering, 3
Granulopoiesis, 42-43
Granulosa cells, 164
  of ovary, 161
Gray matter, 60
Great alveolar cell of respiratory system, 131
Ground bone, 34, 35
Ground substance of connective tissue, 21
  components of, 21-22
  diagram of, 23
Growth
  of cartilage, 29
  of long bone, 33

H

H band of skeletal muscle, 50
Hair follicles, 104, 105
Hair shaft, 107
Hassall's corpuscles, 78, 87
Haustra of colon, 110
Haversian canal, 35
Haversian system, 32
  drawing of, 34
H&E; *see* Hematoxylin and eosin stain

Heart, 67
  conducting system of, 58
  skeleton of, 67, 69
Hematogenous cells, 21
Hematoxylin and eosin stain, 1
Hemopoiesis, 42
  bone marrow and, 42-49
Hemopoietic cells of bone marrow, 44
Hemopoietic compartment of bone marrow, 42
Henle, loop of, 139, 144, 145
Hepatic arteries, 124
Hepatic lobule, classic, 124
Hepatocytes, 124, 126, 127, 128, 129
Herring bodies, 95
Heterophagy, 10
High endothelial venules, 68
His, bundle of, 67
Histologic stains, routine, 1
Holocrine secretion of exocrine glands, 89
Hormones, 95
  adrenocorticotrophic, 96
  antidiuretic, 139
  follicle-stimulating, 161
  functions of, 95
  steroid, 100
  stomach's production of, 110
  thyroid, 95
Howship's lacunae, 32, 36
Humerus, head of, 34
Humoral immunity
  B-cells and, 77
  cells involved in, 38
Hyaline cartilage, 29, 30
Hyaluronic acid in cartilage, 29
Hydrochloric acid
  formation of, 114
  stomach's production of, 110
Hydroxyapatite crystals in bone, 32
Hypertrophy, zone of, of epiphyseal plate, 37
Hypodermis, 104, 105, 108
Hypophyseal portal system, 95
Hypophysis, 95; *see also* Thyroid gland
Hypothalamic-hypophyseal portal system, 96
Hypothalamohypophyseal tract, 95
Hypothalamus and pituitary gland, relationships between, 96

I

I band of skeletal muscle, 50
IgA, secretory, 110, 120
Ileocecal valve, 110
Ileum, 110
Ileus, mucosa of, 118
Immature bone, 32
Immunity
  cell-mediated, and T-lymphocytes, 77
  cellular, cells involved in, 38
  humoral
    B-cells and, 77
    cells involved in, 38
Inclusions, lipid, in cell, 1
Infundibulum of oviduct, 161
Inhibitory neurotransmittors, 59
Inner circumferential lamellae of long bone, 32
Insulin, 97
Interalveolar wall, 137
Intercalated disks, 51, 57
Intercalated ducts of exocrine system, 90
Interlobar arteries of kidney, 138
Interlobular arteries of kidney, 138, 141
Interlobular ducts of exocrine system, 90, 92
Intermediate filaments, 1
Internal respiration, 130
Interspinous ligament, 26
Interstitial cells of Leydig, 149
Interstitial growth of cartilage, 29
Interstitial lamellae of bone, 32
Interterritorial matrix in cartilage, 29
Interventricular septum, membranous, 69
Intestinal crypts, 80, 116, 119
Intestinal epithelium
  with goblet cell, 3
  of simple columnar cells, 2
Intestinal epithelial cell cytoplasm, 6
Intestinal glands, 110

Intestinal mucosa, secretory IgA in, 120
Intestinal villus, epithelium of, 116
Intestine
  large; *see* Colon
  simple columnar epithelium of, 14
  simple squamous epithelium of, 13
  small, 110
    crypts in, 80
Intracellular degradation of particles, 10
Intracellular digestion, lysosomal system in, diagram of, 10
Intralobular ducts of exocrine system, 90
Intramembraneous ossification, 32
Intramural portion of oviduct, 161
Intrinsic factor, stomach's production of, 110
Irritability of neurons, 59
Islets of Langerhans, 96-97, 102, 103
Isogenous cell nests or groups in cartilage, 29, 30
Isthmus of oviduct, 161

J

Jejunum, 110
Junctional complex, 9, 20; *see also* Terminal bar
Junctional folds, 55
Juxtaglomerular apparatus, 139, 145
Juxtaglomerular cells, 139, 145, 146

K

Keratinized epithelium, 12
  stratified squamous, 15
Keratinocytes, 104
Kidney, 138-139
  collecting duct of, 147
  cortex of, 140, 141, 144
  epithelial cells of, 142
  hemisection of, 140
  interlobular artery of, 141
  medulla of, 140, 145
  medullary ray of, 144
  simple squamous epithelium of, 13
Krause, end bulb of, 60
Kupffer cells, 124, 129

L

Lactiferous sinuses, 162
Lacunae
  of bone, 32
  of cartilage, 29, 30
  of compact bone, osteocytes in, 36
  Howship's, 32, 36
Lamellae
  of bone, 34
    interstitial, 32
  of compact bone, 32
Lamina
  basal
    of basal membrane, 12
    of basement membrane, 17
    of muscle, 50
  elastic, of muscular artery, 25
  reticular
    of basal membrane, 12
    of basement membrane, 17
Lamina densa of basement membrane, 17
Lamina propria
  of alimentary canal, 109
  of oviduct, 162
  plasma cells in, 120
Lamina rara of basement membrane, 17
Laminin, 23
Langerhans, islets of, 96-97, 102, 103
Langerhans cell, 104
Large intestine; *see* Colon
Larynx, 130
  epithelium of, 132
Leukocytes, 38
  lifespan of, 49
  polymorphonuclear, 41
Leydig, interstitial cells of, 149, 157
Lieberkühn, crypts of, 110, 121
Ligament
  interspinous, 26
  suspensory, of ovary, 161
Ligamentum nuchae, 26

Light microscopy, 1
    ultrastructural components as viewed by, 2
Lines of skeletal muscle, 50
Lingual tonsils, 78
Lipid inclusions in cell, 1
Lipofuscin pigment in liver cell, 11
Liver, 6, 124
    central vein of, 126
    and gallbladder, 124-129
    lobules of, 125, 127, 129
    major vessels entering and leaving, 125
    parenchyma of, 126, 128
    sinusoids of, 127, 128, 129
Liver acinus, 124
Liver cell, 7, 11
    cytoplasm of, 8
        lysosomes in, 11
LM; see Light microscopy
Lobes of kidney, 138
Lobules
    of kidney, 138, 139
    of liver, 124, 125, 127, 129
    of thymus, 78
Long bone, 34
    growth of, 33
    lamellae of, 32
    macrophotograph of, 36
Loop of Henle, 139, 144, 145
Loose connective tissue, 22, 26
Lower motor neurons, 61
Lung, 136
    alveoli, of, 137
Lymph, 78
Lymph nodes, 25, 78
    diagram of, 82
    postcapillary venule in, 75
Lymphatic capillary, 76, 78, 81
Lymphatic drainage system of body, 81
Lymphatic nodule, 77, 83
    secondary, 82
    of small intestine, 110
Lymphatic organs, 79
Lymphatic sheaths, periarteriolar, 78
Lymphatic tissue, 79
    arrangements of, 79
    dense, 80
    diffuse, 77
Lymphatic vessels, 78
Lymphocytes, 2, 21, 38, 39, 40, 77
    B, 38
    T, 38
    T-cytotoxic, 77
Lymphoid nodules, 77
Lymphoid system, 77-87
Lymphokines, 77
Lymphopoiesis, 43
Lysosomal system, 1
    in intracellular digestion, diagram of, 10
Lysosomes
    of hepatocytes, 124
    in liver cell cytoplasm, 11

M

M cells of small intestine, 110
M line of skeletal muscle, 50
Macrocyte, 43
Macrophage activating factor, 77
Macrophage inhibitory factor, 77
Macrophages, 21, 27, 42, 46, 77
    alveolar, 131, 135
Macula adherens, 20
Macula densa, 139, 145, 146
Major calyx, 138
Male reproductive tract, 149-160
    diagram of, 150
Mammary glands, 162, 170
Marginal zone of spleen, 78
Marrow, bone; see Bone marrow
Mast cells in connective tissue, 23, 28
Matrix
    capsular, in cartilage, 29
    extracellular
        of bone, 32
        of cartilage, 29

Matrix—cont'd
    extracellular—cont'd
        of connective tissue, 21, 25
        of peripheral blood, 38
    interterritorial, in cartilage, 29
    of kidney, 138
    territorial, in cartilage, 29
Maturation
    of blood cells, comparison of, 49
    neutrophilic, 47
Mature bone, microstructure of, 33
Medullary ascending thick limb of loop of Henle, 139
Medullary pyramids, 138
Medullary rays of kidney, 139, 144
Megakaryocyte, 49
Meissner's corpuscle, 60, 65, 108
Meissner's plexus of small intestine, 110
Melanocyte, 104
Membrane
    basement, 2, 12, 17
        of epithelium, drawing of, 17
        glomerular, 139
    cell, drawing of, 4
    mucous, of oviduct, 161-162
    respiratory, 131
Membrane linkers, 20
Membranous interventricular septum, 69
Memory cell, 77
Memory T cells, 38
Menstrual phase of uterine cycle, 169
Menstruation, uterus during, 169
Merkle cell, 104
Merocrine secretion of exocrine glands, 89
Mesangial cells of kidney, 138
Mesenchymal cells, 21
Mesentery, 110
Mesocolon, 110
Mesoderm, embryonic, 96
Mesovarium, 161
Messenger RNA, 8
Metamyelocyte, neutrophilic, 47
Metamyelocyte stage of granulopoiesis, 43
Microcirculatory unit, diagram of, 73
Microfibrils of elastic fibers of connective tissue, 21
Microglial cells, 60
Microscopy, 1-2; see also Transmission electron microscopy
Microtubules in cell, 1
    triplet arrangement of, in centriole, 9
Microvilli, 16, 117
    of epithelial cells, 12
Microvillous border, 2
    of intestinal epithelial cells, absorption across, 117
    of simple columnar epithelium, 14
    of terminal web region, 14
Mineralocorticoids, production of, 96
Minor calyx, 138
Mitochondria, 1, 6
    diagram of, 6
    of hepatocytes, 124
    staining of, 1
Mitosis, polychromatic normoblast in, 46
Mixed seromucous gland, 93
Monocytes, 21, 38, 39, 40
Mononuclear leukocytes, 38
Mononuclear phagocytic system, 38
Motor end plate, 50, 55, 56, 59
    diagram of, 55
Motor neurons
    lower, 61
    in spinal cord, 60
Mucopolysaccharides; see Glycosaminoglycans
Mucosa
    of alimentary canal, 109
    of colon, 110, 123
    of esophagus, 40, 111
    of gallbladder, 125, 129
    ileal, 118
    intestinal, secretory IgA in, 120
    pyloric, 115
    of vagina, 162
Mucous cells of stomach, 109
Mucous connective tissue, 22
Mucous exocrine glands, 89
Mucous membrane of oviduct, 161-162

Mucous neck cell, 110
Mucus, stomach's production of, 110
Multicellular exocrine glands, 89
Multinucleated osteoclast, 49
Muscle, 1, 50-58
  cardiac, 50, 51, 57, 58, 73
  cell of, ultrastructure of, 54
  nuclei of, 50
  skeletal; see Skeletal muscle
  smooth; see Smooth muscle
  tissue of, 50
  types of, 50
Muscular arteries, 25, 67, 68, 72, 76
Muscularis
  of oviduct, 162
  of vagina, 162
Muscularis externa
  of alimentary canal, 109
  of colon, 110
  of esophagus, 109
  of gallbladder, 125
Muscularis mucosa of alimentary canal, 109
Myelin, axons surrounded by, 63
Myelinated nerve fibers, 60
  of sciatic nerve, 63
Myeloblasts, 43, 47
Myelocytes
  basophilic, 43
  eosinophilic, 43
  neutrophilic, 43, 47, 48
Myenteric plexus of Auerbach, 65
Myocardium, 58, 67, 70
Myoepithelial cells, 51, 89
Myofibers, 50
Myofibrils, 50, 51
Myofilaments, 50
Myometrium of uterus, 162
Myosin
  in cell, 1
  in muscle, 50
  of skeletal muscle, 50
Myotendinous junction, 54

N

Naked nerve endings, 60
Nasal cavity, 130
Nasopharynx, 130
Natriuretic peptide, atrial, 67
Natural killer cells, 77
Nephron, 138
Nerve, 1, 59-66
  cells of, 59
  facial, 63
  fibers of, 60
  longitudinal section through, 63
  peripheral, 63
  sciatic, myelinated fibers of, 63
  unmyelinated, in connective tissue, 64
Nerve endings, naked, 60
Nerve tissue, 59
Nervous system, 59
  autonomic, 64
  parasympathetic, 64
  peripheral, 62
  sympathetic, 64
Neural crest, 96
Neural regulation of exocrine secretion, 94
Neurofibrils, 59
Neurohypophysis, 95
Neuronal cell bodies, parasympathetic, 65
Neurons, 59
  in cerebral cortex, 61
  classification of, 59
  cytoplasm of, 61
  motor
    lower, 61
    of spinal cord, 60
  parasympathetic postganglionic, 64
Neurotransmitters, 59
Neurovascular unit, 75
Neutrophilic metamyelocyte, 47
Neutrophilic myelocytes, 43, 47, 48
Neutrophils, 38, 39, 41, 43, 48
  maturation of, 47

Nissl bodies, 59
Nissl substance, 61
Node
  atrioventricular, 58, 67, 71
  lymph; see Lymph nodes
  of Ranvier, 59, 63
  sinoatrial, 58, 67
Nodule
  lymphatic, 77, 83
    secondary, 82
    of small intestine, 110
  lymphoid, 77
Nonkeratinized epithelium, stratified squamous, 16, 80
  of esophagus, 109
Norepinephrine, 96
Normoblast, 42, 45, 46
  basophilic, 42, 46
  orthochromatic, 42
  polychromatic, 42, 45, 46
Nuclear envelope, 5
Nucleus
  of cell, 1
  diagram of, 5
  paraventricular, neurosecretions of, 95
  of Schwann cell, 63
  supraoptic, neurosecretions of, 95
Nutrients, absorption of, 117

O

Oligodendrocytes, 60
Oocyte, 161, 163, 164
  and spermatozoon, 168
Open circulation model of splenic blood flow, 78
Oral cavity, 109
Organelles, 2
  cytoskeletal, in cell, 1
Organs
  of digestion, accessory, 111
  of female reproductive tract, 161
  lymphatic, 79
  of respiratory system, 130
  target, for hormones, 95
Orthochromatic normoblast, 42
Ossification
  endochondral, 32-33
  intramembranous, 32
Ossification centers, 33
Osteoblasts, 32, 35
Osteocalcin in bone, 32
Osteoclasts, 32, 36, 37
  multinucleated, 49
Osteocytes, 32, 35
  in lacunae of compact bone, 36
Osteogenic cells, 37
Osteoid, 35
Osteon, 32, 34
Osteonectin, 22
Osteoprogenitor cells, 32
Outer circumferential lamellae of long bone, 32
Ovarian arteries, 161
Ovarian veins, 161
Ovary, 161, 163-166
  cortex of, 163
  follicles in, 163
Oviduct, 161-162, 167, 168
  simple columnar epithelium from, 16
Ovulation, 161, 162
  stages in, 165
Oxyphil cells in parathyroid gland, 100

P

Pacinian corpuscle, 60, 65, 108
Palatine tonsils, 78
  epithelium of, 80
Pampiniform plexus, 149
Pancreas, 89, 90, 94, 102
Pancreatic acinus, 7, 94
Pancreatic duct, simple cuboidal epithelium of, 13
Pancreatic islet cells, innervation of, 103
Pancreatic polypeptide, 97
Paneth cells, 110, 119
Papilla of kidney, 138
Papillary layer of dermis, 104

Parafollicular cell, 99
  of thyroid gland, 95
Parasympathetic nervous system, 64
Parasympathetic neuronal cell bodies, 65
Parasympathetic postganglionic neuron, 64
Parathormone, 100
Parathyroid gland, 96, 99, 100
Paraventricular nuclei, neurosecretions of, 95
Parenchyma, liver, 126, 128
Parietal cell
  in gastric gland, 114
  of stomach, 110
Parietal epithelial cells of kidney, 142
Parietal epithelium of kidney, 138
Parotid ducts, 92
Parotid gland, 89, 90, 91, 92
  innervation of, 94
Pars basalis of uterus, 162
Pars distalis, 95, 97, 98
Pars functionalis of uterus, 162
Pars intermedia of pituitary gland, 95
Pars nervosa, 95, 98
Pars tuberalis of pituitary gland, 95
Pelvis, renal, 139, 140
Penicillar arterioles of spleen, 78
Penile urethra, 160
Penis, 149, 150, 160
Peptides
  as hormones, 95
  natriuretic, atrial, 67
Periarteriolar lymphatic sheaths, 78
Perichondrium, 29
Pericyte, 75
Perikaryon, 60
Perimysium, 51
Perineurium, 60, 62, 63
Periosteal collar, 33
Periosteum, 32
Peripheral blood, 38-41
  cells of, types of, 39
Peripheral nerve, 63
Peripheral nervous system, 59, 62
Peristalsis, 109
Peritubular capillary plexus, 138
Peroxisomes of cell, 1
Peyer's patches, 77, 110, 122
Phagocytic system, mononuclear, 38
Phagocytosis, 10
  of bacteria by macrophage, 11
Pharyngeal tonsils, 78, 130
Pharynx, 109
Phospholipids, 124
Pigment in cell, 1
  lipofuscin, 11
Pigmentation in skin cells, 107
Pinocytosis, 10
Pituitary gland, 95, 97
  hypothalamus and, relationships between, 96
Plasma, 38
Plasma cells, 21, 28, 77
  in bone marrow, 48
  in lamina propria, 120
  of small intestine, 110
Plasmalemma, 61
  drawing of, 4
Platelets, 38, 39, 40, 49
Plexus
  capillary, peritubular, 138
  Meissner's, of small intestine, 110
  myenteric, of Auerbach, 65
  pampiniform, 149
Plicae circulares, 110, 122
Pluripotent stem cell of bone marrow, 44
PMNs; see Neutrophils
Podocytes, 139, 142
Polychromatic normoblast, 42, 45, 46
  in mitosis, 46
Polychromatophilic erythrocyte, 42-43
Polymorphonuclear cells, 38
Polymorphonuclear leukocytes, 41
Polypeptide, pancreatic, 97
Polyribosomes
  of cell, 1
  in rough endoplasmic reticulum, 8

Pores
  alveolar, 131, 137
  diaphragm-covered, in nuclear envelope, 5
  in nuclear envelope, freeze fracture of, 5
Portal canals, 125, 126
  of liver, 124
Portal circulation, 110
Portal lobule of liver, 124
Portal systems, 68
  arterial, 73
  hypothalamic-hypophyseal, 96
Portal triad, 124, 127, 128
Portal vein, 127, 128
Portal venules of liver, 124
Postcapillary venules, 68, 83
  in lymph node, 75
Postganglionic neuron, parasympathetic, 64
Postsynaptic region of synapse, 59
PP cell, 97
Presynaptic axon terminal, 59
Presynaptic terminals, 66
Primary bone, 32
Primary bronchi, 130
Primary follicles of ovary, 161
Primary oocyte, 161, 163, 164
Primary ossification center, 33
Primordial follicles in ovary, 161, 163
Procollagen, 21
Proelastin, 21
Proerythroblasts, 42
Progesterone, 161
Proliferation, zone of, of epiphyseal plate, 37
Promyelocyte, 43, 47
Pronormoblasts, 42, 45
Prostate gland, 150, 160
Proteins
  blood, 38
  in cell, 1
  as hormones, 95
  synthesis of, 7
Proteoglycan aggregates in cartilage, 29
Proteoglycan molecule, 22
Proteoglycans, 21
  in bone, 32
  of connective tissue, formation of, steps in, 24
  sulfated, in cartilage, 29
Protoplasmic astrocytes, 60
Proximal convoluted tubules, 139, 144, 147
Proximal straight tubules, 144
Pseudostratified columnar epithelium, 15, 17
Pseudostratified epithelium, 13
Pulmonary arteries, 130
Pulmonary circuit of heart, 67
Pulmonary veins, 130
Pulp veins of spleen, 78
Purkinje fibers, 51, 58, 67, 71
Purkinje system, 58, 69
Pyloric gland, 115
Pyloric mucosa, 115
Pyloric sphincter, 109

R

Ranvier, nodes of, 59, 63
Rappaport's lobule of liver, 124
Reaction center of lymphatic nodule, 77
Receptor-mediated endocytosis, 10, 11
Receptors, sensory, of skin, 104
Receptosomes, 10
  formation of, 11
Red blood cells; see Erythrocytes
Red pulp of spleen, 78, 84, 85
Renal artery, 138
Renal calyces, 140
Renal columns of Bertin, 138
Renal corpuscle, 138, 141, 142, 145
Renal pelvis, 138, 139, 140
Renal sinus, 138
Renal tubule, 138
Renal vein, 138
Renin, immunocytochemical localization of, 145
Renin-angiotensin system, 96
Reproductive tract
  female, 161-170
    diagram of, 162

Reproductive tract—cont'd
  male, 149-160
    diagram of, 150
RER; see Rough endoplasmic reticulum
Respiration, 130
Respiratory bronchioles, 130-131, 136
Respiratory epithelium, 130
Respiratory membrane, 131
Respiratory portion of respiratory system, 130-131, 136
Respiratory system, 130-137
Respiratory tract, 131
Resting cartilage, 36
Rete testis, 149, 158
Reticular cells, 21
  epithelial, of thymus, 78
Reticular connective tissue, 22
Reticular fibers, 21; see also Collagen, type III
  of connective tissue, 25
  of lymph node, 25
  of skeletal muscle, 50-51
Reticular lamina
  of basal membrane, 12
  of basement membrane, 17
Reticular layer of dermis, 104
Reticulocytes, 43
Reticulum, endoplasmic; see Endoplasmic reticulum
Ribonucleic acid, messenger, 8
Ribosomes
  free, of cell, 1
  in rough endoplasmic reticulum, 8
Rough endoplasmic reticulum, 1
  cisternae of, 8
  of liver, 124
"Ruffled border," 36
Rugae
  of gallbladder, 125
  of stomach, 109

S

Salivary glands, 89-90
Sarcolemma, 50
Sarcomeres, 50
  of skeletal muscle, 54
Sarcoplasm of skeletal muscle, 50
Sarcoplasmic reticulum
  of sarcomeres, 54
  of skeletal muscle, 50
Satellite cells of neuron, 60
Scanning electron microscopy, 1
Schmidt-Lantermann, clefts of, 63
Schwann cells, 55, 60, 62, 63
  nuclei of, 63
Sciatic nerve, myelinated fibers of, 63
Scrotum, 149
Sebaceous glands, 104, 107, 108
Secondary bone, 32
Secondary follicles of ovary, 161, 163, 164
Secondary oocytes, 161, 164
Secondary ossification center, 33
Secretion
  of exocrine glands, 89
    neural regulation of, 94
  of glucagon, 97
  of insulin, 97
  of mammary glands, 162
  salivary gland, 90
Secretory cells of oviduct, 162
Secretory IgA, 110
  in intestinal mucosa, 120
Secretory unit of exocrine glands, 89
Segmental arteries of kidney, 138
SEM; see Scanning electron microscopy
Semen, 150
Seminal vesicle, 149, 150, 160
Seminiferous epithelium of testes, 149
Seminiferous tubules, 149, 151, 152, 153, 157, 158
Sensory receptors of skin, 104
Septulae testes, 149
SER; see Smooth endoplasmic reticulum
Seromucous gland
  exocrine, 89
  mixed, 93
  of respiratory system, 130

Serosa
  of alimentary canal, 109
  of oviduct, 162
Serous exocrine glands, 89
Sertoli cells, 149, 154, 155
Serum, blood, 38
Sharpey's fibers, 32
Sialomucins of exocrine glands, 89
Sialoprotein in bone, 32
Sigmoid colon, 110
Simple columnar cells
  of epithelium of gallbladder, 3
  intestinal epithelium of, 2
  three-dimensional representation of, 2
Simple columnar ciliated epithelium, 16
Simple columnar epithelium, 14
Simple cuboidal epithelium, 13
Simple epithelium, 12
Simple exocrine glands, 89
Simple squamous epithelium, 13
Sinoatrial node, 58, 67
Sinuses
  lactiferous, 162
  renal, 138
Sinusoidal capillaries, 68, 74
Sinusoids
  of liver, 124, 127, 128, 129
  splenic, 78, 85
Skeletal muscle, 50
  cells of, 51, 53
  of esophagus, 109
  fascicle of, 53
  fibers of, 53
  sarcomeres of, 54
Skeleton, cardiac, 51
Skin, 104-108
  dermis of, 26
  diagram of, 105
  functions of, 104
  pigment in, 107
  stratified squamous epithelium of, 20
    keratinized, 15
  thick, 105, 108
  thin, 105, 107
Small intestine, 110
  crypts in, 80
Smooth endoplasmic reticulum, 1
  of liver, 124
Smooth muscle, 50, 52
  cells of, 51
  contraction of, 52
  of esophagus, 109
  of respiratory system, 130
Soma of neuron, 59
Somatic components of nervous system, 59
Somatomedin, 124
Somatostatin, production of, 97
Space
  of Disse, 124
  urinary, 138
Specialized connective tissue, 22
Specificity of lymphocytes, 77
Spermatic cord, 149
Spermatids, 156
Spermatocytes, 149
Spermatogenesis, 149, 152
Spermatogonia, 149, 155
Spermatozoa, 149, 156, 157
  oocyte and, 168
Spermiogenesis, 152, 155
Sphincter, pyloric, 109
Spinal cord, 60, 62
  motor neuron in, 60
Spines, dendritic, 59
Spleen, 78, 84, 85
Splenic artery, 78
Splenic sinusoids, 78
Splenic vein, 78
Spongy bone, 32, 34
Squamous epithelium, 12
  simple, 13
  stratified, 20, 106
    basal region of, 17
  stratified keratinized, 15

Squamous epithelium—cont'd
  stratified nonkeratinized, 16, 80
    of esophagus, 109
Stain
  hematoxylin and eosin, 1
  histologic, routine, 1
Staining, basophilic, of cell, 1
Stem cells
  committed, 42, 44
  pluripotent, of bone marrow, 44
  totipotent, 42
Stereocilia, 12, 149
Steroid hormones, 100
Steroid molecules as hormones, 95
Stomach, 109-110
  body of, 112
  cardiac regions of, 112
  fundus of, 112, 113
  mucosa of, 115, 116
  pyloric region of, 112
  wall of, divisions of, 112
Straight tubules, proximal, 144
Stratified cuboidal epithelium, 16
Stratified epithelium, 12
Stratified squamous epithelium, 20, 106
  basal region of, 17
  keratinized, 15
  nonkeratinized, 16, 80
    of esophagus, 109
Stratum basalis, 104, 105
Stratum corneum, 104, 105, 106, 107
Stratum germinativum, 104
Stratum granulosum, 104, 105, 106, 107
Stratum spinosum, 20, 104, 105, 106, 107
Stress fibers, 9
Striate border, 2, 12
  of small intestine, 110
Striated ducts of exocrine system, 90
Structural glycoproteins, 21-22
Structural proteins in cell, 1
Subclavian vein, 81
Subcutaneous connective tissue, 104
Sublingual gland, 89, 90, 93
Submandibular gland, 89, 90, 93
Submucosa
  of alimentary canal, 109
  of esophagus, 111
Submucosal glands
  of esophagus, 109
  of small intestine, 110
Subneural clefts, 55
Sulfated proteoglycans in cartilage, 29
Sulfomucins of exocrine glands, 89
Supraoptic nuclei, neurosecretions of, 95
Suprarenal gland, 96
Surface mucous cells of stomach, 109
Surface specializations of epithelial cells, diagram of, 18
Surfactant, 131
Suspensory ligament of ovary, 161
Sweat glands, 104, 108
Sympathetic nervous system, 64
Synapses, 66
  chemical, 59
  structure of, 59-60
Synaptic clefts, 55, 59
Synaptic endings, 66
Synaptic terminals, 59, 66
Synthesis of proteins, 7
Systemic circuit of heart, 67
Systemic circulation, 69
Systole, 67

T

T cells, 38
T tubules, 50, 54, 57
Taenia coli of colon, 110
Target organs for hormones, 95
T-cytotoxic lymphocytes, 77
Telodendria, 59
TEM; *see* Transmission electron microscopy
Tendon, 26
Terminal bars, 20; *see also* Junctional complex
Terminal bronchioles, 130, 136
Terminal web region of cell, 14

Territorial matrix in cartilage, 29
Testes, 149, 151
Testosterone, 149
Tetraiodithyronine, 95
Theca externa, 161
Theca interna, 161
T-helper cells, 77, 38
Thick skin, 104, 105
Thin skin, 104, 105
Thoracic duct, 81
Thymic factors, 78
Thymus, 78, 86, 87, 88
  Hassall's corpuscle, 87
  postcapillary venule in, 83
Thyrocalcitonin, 96
Thyrocalcitonin cell, 99
Thyroglobulin, 95
Thyroid follicle, 99
Thyroid gland, 95-96, 98, 99
Thyroid hormone, 95
Thyroid stimulating hormone, 95
Thyroxine, 95
Tissue
  connective, 1, 21-28; *see also* Connective tissue
  lymphatic, 79
    arrangements of, 79
    dense, 80
    diffuse, 77
  muscle, 50
  nerve, 59
T-lymphocytes, 38, 77, 78
Tonofilaments of desmosomes, 14, 20
Tonsillar epithelium, 80
Tonsils, 77-78
  palatine, epithelium of, 80
  pharyngeal, 130
Totipotent stem cell, 42
Trabeculae
  of spleen, 78
  of thymus, 78
Trabecular arteries of spleen, 78
Trabecular veins of spleen, 78
Trachea, 130
  cartilage of, 30
  cilia and microvilli of, 16
  ciliated pseudostratified columnar epithelium of, 15
  epithelium of, 133, 134
  wall of, 133
    fracture of, 133
Transitional epithelium, 13
  of urinary bladder, 15, 148
  of urinary tract, 139
Transmission electron microscopy, 1
  of cell, comparison of freeze fracture with, 4
  ultrastructural components as viewed by, 2
Transverse colon, 110
Triglycerides, 124
Trigones of heart, 69
Triiodothyronine, 95
Triplet arrangement of microtubules in centriole, 9
True vocal cords, 132
TSH; *see* Thyroid stimulating hormone
T-suppressor cells, 38, 77
Tubal tonsils, 78
Tube, uterine or fallopian; *see* Oviduct
Tubular exocrine glands, 89
Tubules
  conducting, of male reproductive system, 149-150
  convoluted
    distal, 139, 147
    proximal, 139, 144
  in epididymis, 158
  renal, 138, 139
  seminiferous, 149, 151, 152, 153, 157, 158
  T, 54, 57
    of skeletal muscle, 50
  uriniferous, 138
Tubuli recti, 149, 158
Tunica adventitia, 67, 68, 71, 72
Tunica albuginea, 149, 150, 151, 161
Tunica intima, 67, 68, 71, 72
Tunica media, 67, 68, 71, 72

U

Umbrella cells
  of bladder, 148
  of transitional epithelium, 15
Unicellular exocrine glands, 89
Unmyelinated nerve in connective tissue, 64
Unmyelinated nerve fibers, 60
Ureter, 138, 139, 147
  wall of, 147
Urethra, 138, 139
  penile, 160
Urinary bladder, 138, 139, 148
  transitional epithelium of, 15, 148
Urinary pole of renal corpuscle, 138
Urinary space, 138
Urinary system, 138-148
Urinary tract, 138, 139
Urine, 138
Uriniferous tubules, 138
Uterine cycle, phases of, 169
Uterine tube; *see* Oviduct
Uterus, 162
  endometrium of, 169
  epithelial cells of, 169
  during menstruation, 169

V

Vagina, 162, 170
  epithelium of, 80, 170
Valve, ileocecal, 110
Vas deferens, 149
Vasa rectae, 138
Vasa vasorum, 68
Vascular compartment of bone marrow, 42
Vascular pole of kidney, 138
Veins, 68, 76
  central, of liver, 124, 126, 129
  ovarian, 161
  portal, 127, 128
  pulmonary, 130
  renal, 138
  of spleen, 78
  subclavian, 81
  testicular, 149

Vena cava, 76
Ventricles, 67
  wall of, 70, 71
Venules, 68, 75
  portal, of liver, 124
  postcapillary, 83
    in lymph node, 75
  seminal, 149, 150, 160
Vessels, lymphatic, 78
Vestibular folds, 132
Villus, 116
  intestinal, 110
    epithelium of, 116, 117
VIP, 118
Visceral components of nervous system, 59
Visceral epithelial cells of kidney, 142
Visceral epithelium, of kidney, 138
Vocal cords, 130, 132

W

Waldeyer's ring, 77
Wandering granulocyte, 3
White blood cells; *see* Leukocytes
White matter, 60
White pulp of spleen, 78, 84
  central arteries of, 78
Woven bone, 32

Z

Z lines, of skeletal muscle, 50
Zona fasciculata, 96, 101
Zona glomerulosa, 96, 101
Zona reticularis, 96, 101
Zone
  of calcification of epiphyseal plate, 37
  of hypertrophy of epiphyseal plate, 37
  marginal, of spleen, 78
  of proliferation, of epiphyseal plate, 37
Zonula adherens, 18, 20
  actin filaments from, 14
Zonula occludens, 20, 68, 117
Zonula occludens junction, 18